Health Assets in a Global Context

Antony Morgan · Maggie Davies · Erio Ziglio
Editors

Health Assets in a Global Context

Theory, Methods, Action

Springer

Editors
Antony Morgan
Department of Public Health Sciences
Karolinska Institutet
SE-171 77 Stockholm
Sweden
and
National Institute for Health and Clinical Excellence (NICE)
High Holborn 71
London
UK
Antony.Morgan@nice.org.uk

Erio Ziglio
WHO European Office for Investment for Health and Development, Venice
WHO Regional Office for Europe
Campo S. Stefano
San Marco 2847I-30124
Venice, Italy
ezi@ihd.euro.who.int

Maggie Davies
Health Action Partnership International (HAPI)
Tavistock House (Entrance D)
Tavistock House
London WC1H 9LG
England
maggie.davies@hapi.org.uk

ISBN 978-1-4419-5920-1 e-ISBN 978-1-4419-5921-8
DOI 10.1007/978-1-4419-5921-8
Springer New York Dordrecht Heidelberg London

Library of Congress Control Number: 2010930690

Printed on acid-free paper

Springer is part of Springer Science+Business Media (www.springer.com)

Editorial Board

Acknowledgements

We hope the ideas and concepts in this book will inspire those interested in improving the lives of populations across the world to think positively about what can be done to maximise the chances of individuals, groups and communities to attain and sustain, long happy and fulfilled lives.

The overarching framework for this book - 'the asset model' was developed over a period of time during meetings in London, Venice and Budapest. The editors would like to thank a number of people who have contributed to the process and thinking along the way. They are Enis Baris Anja Baumann, Chris Brown, Harry Burns Concha Colomer, Cristina Comunian, Mariano Giacchi Theadora Koller, Marcia Faria-Westphal, Dominic Harrison, Lowell Levin, Aldo Morrone and Elisa Radisone.

The book is dedicated to two people, Renzo Lira and Joanne Morgan – no longer with us but who demonstrated the spirit of the book each and every day of their lives.

Preface

Very few people argue with the need to address the social determinants of health. The Commission on the Social Determinants of Health (CSDH) affirms that the conditions in which people grow, live work and age have a powerful influence on health. The Commission's holistic view of these determinants calls for sustained action, globally, nationally and locally to overcome the unequal distribution of power, income, goods and services which often lead to unfair access to health care, schools and education and an individual's chance of leading a flourishing life (CDSH 2008).

Asset based approaches offer one means of contributing to these goals by recognizing that traditional epidemiological risk factors approaches to health development such as programmes on smoking cessation, healthy eating and physical activity are insufficient on their own to ensure the health and well-being of populations. In particular, many of the solutions to addressing the social determinants of health rely on the ability of professionals to recognize that individuals, communities and populations have significant potential to be a 'health resource' rather than just a consumer of health care services. The Asset Model described by Morgan and Ziglio (see Chap. 1) provides a framework for establishing fresh insights into how best to collect and collate scientific evidence to demonstrate the benefits of the asset approach for population health and how to harness the sorts of effective practice that strengthen community capacities, promote independence and autonomy. They also have the potential to secure sustainable and cost containment approaches to health and development.

There are two things that should be noted about the asset approach as described in this book. Firstly, it is not in itself a new concept or approach – but aims to add value to other existing concepts and ideas by bringing them together in such away as to promote a more systematic approach to assembling and applying knowledge for health solutions. Secondly, it would be naïve to think that the asset approach could exist in isolation from the more predominant deficit tradition to health promotion. There will always be some situations where individuals, communities or broader populations are exposed to health threats or increased exposure to known health risks and therefore need the immediate attention of health professionals and access to services. However the identification and strengthening of health assets should be a key component of a country's overall development strategy, because they can act as a buffer or resilience factor to disease risk exposure and importantly can produce health as a positive entity with a focus on quality of life and wellbeing. It is possible to identify health promoting/protecting assets from across all the domains of health determinants including our genetic endowments, social circumstances, environmental conditions, behavioural choices and health services. An inventory of health and development assets would, as a minimum, include family and friendship (supportive) networks, intergenerational solidarity, community cohesion, environmental resources necessary for promoting physical, mental and social health, employment security and opportunities for voluntary service, affinity groups (e.g. mutual aid), religious tolerance and harmony, life long learning, safe and pleasant housing, political democracy and participation opportunities, social justice and enhancing equity (Harrison et al. 2004).

The overarching aim of this book is to stimulate researchers, policy makers and practitioners to think differently about how they approach their goal of improving the health of populations particularly to minimise the risks of exacerbating or widening health inequities. It brings together the work of a number of well known authors who have been working in fields that have direct relevance to the asset model. The 18 chapters included in it provide illustrations as how asset based approaches can be brought to fruition. Of course, it presents only a starting point for further work, particularly in research – but hopefully its immediate impact can be to change the mindsets of those in decision making positions to think of the 'glass half full, not half empty' scenario.

We introduce each chapter here, to highlight how they can help us advance the asset approach to ensure it can demonstrate its potential to contribute to the production of health and reduction of health inequities through science and practice.

The Chapters

Chapter 1 provides the overarching framework for the rest of the contributions to the book. It sets out the rationale for asset based approaches and provides a systematic way of thinking about how to build an evidence base which can identifies the most important assets for health; help us understand the potential cumulative effect of a range of different assets; and clarify their relative importance over the more well established determinants of health such as absolute and relative poverty. It also provides insights in to the sorts of practices that are conducive to the approach. The chapter highlights a number of existing concepts which can be helpful in developing this evidence base and together help to bring the asset model to life. Salutogenesis is introduced as a concept which can help us to think outside of the deficit, disease orientated approach to health and health services as by its very definition asks what creates health, what helps us to manage and understand the world we live in. By doing so it immediately highlights some of the key assets necessary for the development of health and wellbeing. Lindstrom and Eriksson explore the potential of this concept in more detail in Chaps. 2 and 18. The very well known concepts of resilience and social capital are also included in the model as ones with potential to identify a set of indicators for monitoring and evaluating the impact of investing in programmes which emphasis the positive rather than negative. Specifically, in this context, the asset model demonstrates how social capital can be applied for health benefit – offsetting some of its criticisms concerning its 'dark-side' (Portes 1996). Chapters by Bartley, Kawachi and Baum (6, 9 and 16, respectively) all elaborate the potential for these concepts to contribute to the model.

Another important idea intrinsic to the model is that of asset mapping – this technique seeks to build capacity within local communities by making the most of the existing competencies of individuals, the resources of organisations and institutions and the collective ability of groups take control of their own health (see Chap. 4 by McKnight). The model also identifies the need to develop new indicators and evaluation techniques that can take account of the asset approach and ultimately demonstrate the benefits of investing in it (see Chaps. 5 and 7).

The concept of lifecourse is also important to the model – as the potential for health assets to be offset by all those risks that individuals and communities inevitably face during the life experience, can be understood if we assess those assets that can be accrued at different life stages. Chapters 8 by Morrow and 17 by Baban illustrate the importance of applying the approach to young people's health and development.

Of course, none of the ideas, concepts or techniques mentioned above can be brought to practical value unless researchers, practitioners and policy makers embrace positive approaches to health and importantly focus on health and wellbeing rather than disease and dying. One of the reasons why politicians at least might favour the latter is on the surface it is easier count death and measure progress against it. The asset model provides an opportunity to make more explicit the concepts of wellbeing and its associated precursors and to demonstrate how they can be measured. The asset model challenges all professionals involved in health development to re-think their strategies for promoting health and to balance their activities between the asset and more familiar needs based approach – more thoughtful investments might then bring the longer term gains required to promote the best health we can and help us manage the limited resources available in our health systems.

Lindstrom and Eriksson (Chap. 2) consider the theoretical and empirical work relating to the salutogenic framework. This framework focuses on positive health, in contrast with the traditional disease-orientated approach.

Salutogenesis centres on two core concepts: Generalised Resistance Resources (GRR) and the Sense of Coherence (SOC). The GRRs are biological, material and psycho social factors that make it easier for people to perceive their lives as consistent and structured. 'The GRRs lead to life experiences that promote a strong sense of coherence – a way of perceiving life and an ability to successfully manage the infinite number of complex stressors encountered in the discourse of life.'

The authors review a range of other concepts and their relationship with salutogensis. These include hardiness, theories on welfare and quality of life, learned resourcefulness, resilience and theories relating to social and cultural contexts. The review indicates that salutogenesis draws a range of other related concepts.

The SOC questionnaire has been used to understand and test the role of SOC in explaining health outcomes. SOC has been shown to be strongly related to health, especially mental health. Lindstrom and Eriksson state that SOC, although not the same as health, 'is an important disposition for people's development and maintenance of their health'.

These findings suggest that the real potential of a salutogenesis approach relates to the adoption of healthy public policies. Historically public health has operated in a risk framework, while salutogenesis makes other solutions available for improving health. Two themes have evolved within salutogenic research-resilience and sense of coherence – that can now guide action that addresses social and mental wellbeing in a post-modern world.

Kelly (Chap. 3) highlights the importance of complexity of understanding how to create the optimum conditions for health by introducing the notion of the lifeworld. This chapter explores the relationships between those assets that help to protect health and those conditions which create vulnerabilities to ill health. It explains how these are located in the lifeworlds of ordinary human experience and the health benefits and disbenefits which accumulate over the life course. Kelly explains that the lifeworld and lifecourse together are the bridge between social structure and individual human biology. Together they constitute the focal point where society and biology intersect and interact. The lifeworld and lifecourse are the mechanisms through which the social determinants of health produce biological outcomes in individuals. Theorising this vital causal link from the social to the biological and from society to individuals, is essential for ensuring the success of the asset approach in practice. Assets and vulnerabilities are the crucial mediating or intervening variables between the wider determinants of health and the human body and it is those intervening variables that produce individual differences in health. Researchers can help us to understand how through the identification of key health assets these differences in health can be minimised.

Asset mapping is introduced in *Chap. 4* as a means of capturing the spirit and energies of communities to assert their ownership on health development. McKnight highlights how policy makers have tended to create hierarchical systems where a small number of people are in charge of the mass production of standardised goods. Clients/consumers in large numbers grow dependent on this cycle of production. Such systems create dependency rather than empowerment. He argues that in creating maps to reflect the way in which these systems work we have tended to neglect the notion of "associated community"; where there is a dependence on consent, choice, care and citizen power. Systems are seen to exploit need in individuals, whilst communities, in contrast nurture existing skills and capacity. Systems identify with "the glass half empty" approach, whilst communities with "the glass half full". The service culture produces "clients", whilst the community culture produces "citizens".

This chapter explores the nature of the relationship between systems, communities and citizens, and looks at the shift, in developed society, from equal relationships between citizens and communities to a relationship where systems are dominant. The authors argue that the move towards an increasingly "consumerist society" has marginalized the role of the citizen. In order to encourage and build healthy communities we must recognise and appreciate the unique capabilities that communities offer in developing, nurturing and caring for their citizens.

Hills and colleagues (Chap. 5) discuss the limitations of current evaluation frameworks and methods for evaluation of an asset based approach. The challenges that need to be addressed for developing the evidence base on effectiveness are highlighted.

The authors assert that a new paradigm is required for evaluation of a health assets based approach. The orthodox approach, based on the epidemiological discipline, has limited utility for evaluating the effectiveness of community assets, capabilities, risks and protective factors; and for the synthesis of evidence across studies.

There are major challenges for the evaluation of complex initiatives and programmes. There is a need for greater theoretical and methodological precision, particularly with respect to definition of health assets and their operationalisation through appropriate indicators. A more integrated approach to process and outcomes evaluation, formative and summative approaches is required. 'Improvements in specific health assets need to be seen as intermediate outcomes in a linked chain of progress towards improving overall health and social outcomes.' Participatory evaluation approaches need to be adopted that provide greater understanding of the processes involved in implementing programmes and their impact on the outcomes of the programme. Evaluators need to have a more direct role in programme development: evaluation becomes 'reflective practice'.

Realist synthesis is applied to determine the effectiveness of a Canadian Community Interventions Project. This provides an example of an alternative methodology that enables the synthesis of evidence from different initiatives and programmes. Programmes are viewed as the interaction between context, mechanism and outcomes. Systematic review is concerned with understanding 'families of mechanisms' across programmes. The 'mechanisms' operating in the Community Interventions Project are illustrated, and relate to elements of collaborative planning, community organisation and action, and transformational change. The authors indicate that evaluation of the assets based approach is possible, but will required development of such innovative methodologies.

Bartley et al. (Chap. 6) examine evidence relating to positive adjustment and resilience as an asset which can promote health even in adverse conditions.

Studies show that individuals and families experiencing difficult conditions are more likely to experience negative health consequences. However the processes by which individuals and communities adapt have received less research attention.

Three models of resilience have been identified based on a review of evidence in this field. These three models (compensatory, protective and challenge) are described.

A link has also been made between the study of resilience and research on the life course processes involved in chronic diseases. This has highlighted the need to examine the accumulation of both risks and resources or assets. Health assets are shaped by the social and physical environment. Resilience is a set of conditions that allow individual adaptation to different forms of adversity. Resilient practices and processes may be viewed as health assets. Such processes need to be identified and promoted by social and economic policies.

The authors discuss issues relating to resilience and freedom. Sen's work indicates that the ability to adapt in the face of adversity can increase an individuals perception of their own freedom to lead a valued life, i.e. resilience increases capability. 'It is important for the individual to have the freedom to pursue health itself, and therefore to understand constraints on that freedom': such as being forced by financial necessity to accept stressful working conditions, and to live in polluted areas.

This means that policy should be concerned with enabling people to make healthy choices while faced with these challenges; different policy responses will be required to address different threats to freedom.

Bartley and colleagues consider a number of cases that show how health resilience can be promoted in communities that are disadvantaged. For example analysis of health inequalities in Europe, has shown that socially disadvantaged populations in Southern European countries, possess a source of resilience in terms of a healthy diet. Although these countries have clear income inequalities, these populations have long life expectancy and less heath inequalities. More research is required to understand diet as a source of health resilience but there are potentially important implications for wider policies.

The authors explore how that process of modernisation may lower the economic capability societies with detrimental health consequences. The role of women in the nurture of children and families has added value in traditional economies. However the changes in this role in modern societies (a shift between home and work) are not fully understood and the authors assert that skills in the conduct of family relationships as a major health asset are being neglected – there is loss of 'free emotional labour' and … 'It is important to increase the capacities of both men and women to choose a way of life they can sustain themselves in terms of both physical and emotional self care'.

Bartley and colleagues argue that there are many aspects of human relationship that function as health assets for individuals and communities. However they are only acknowledged when they are lost. The assets based approach provides the potential for recognising and understanding the processes necessary to development of these capabilities in the modern context.

Wille and Ravens-Sieberer (Chap. 7) consider approaches to the measurement of resilience. Research in resilience does not address pathological responses of individuals to stress but investigates health protecting mechanisms, i.e. the ability of individuals to maintain good health despite considerable stressors.

Resilience research has aimed to identify protective factors or developmental assets that can modify a child's response to adversity. This understanding provides the basis for designing prevention programmes that promote factors that buffer effects of adversity.

Conceptually resilience is characterised by good outcomes despite of serious threats to adaptation or development. Two conditions pertain: the presence of demonstrable risk and competence in response. There is an interactive process involving a person's constitution as well as functional qualities of its environment.

There are certain conceptual challenges. For example there is some inconsistency in how the term 'protective' is used. Certain authors only use 'protective' to factors that operate in the presence of adversity-buffering the effect of risks, but it is also applied more broadly.

From a salutogenic perspective there is a case for a population based approach for supporting resilience among children and adolescents through direct amelioration as well as buffering of protective factors. Large population based studies that assess a variety of risks and resources can support the design of effective public health interventions. Such studies are rare; however the BELLA study provides an important example of a study that is focusing on mental health problems in children and adolescents and associated risks and resources. The range of measures used to assess risk factors and protective factors are described. The chapter demonstrates the need for researchers to pay attention to better measurement so that their work can be more easily applied to policy action.

Morrow and Mayall (Chap. 8) explore the concept of children's well-being, how it is measured and how it is being researched. The authors indicate that the concept of well-being is not well defined, yet it has become part of public, political and policy discourse particularly in the UK. Given the emphasis of wellbeing in the asset model, this chapter provides important reflections on the issues involved in assessing how best it should be conceptualized and measured.

A number of important questions are raised, including whether other European countries would simply refer to 'children's welfare'; and whether the focus on well-being is 'inherently individualistic', and detracts from a concern for welfare and responsibilities of governments towards children.

The authors conclude with a number of suggestions. Care needs to be taken with conceptualisation of complex concepts such as 'well-being'. There remains a 'danger that a focus on well-being is ultimately an individualistic, subjective approach that risks depoliticising children's lives'. Caution is required when reporting research relating to children, as there is a risk of over-simplification through international comparisons. Both qualitative and quantitative approaches should be used. Children and young people should be involved in the conceptualisation of well-being. There should be greater understanding of UN Convention on the Rights of the Child in moving towards a 'genuinely rights-based approach to monitoring children's everyday lives' that confronts the low social status of children in western societies.

Kawachi (Chap. 9) summaries the nature of the knowledge base concerning social cohesion as a community level asset and determinant of health – covering theories of causation, measurement approaches, empirical evidence and also the potential of social capital as a public health intervention.

Social cohesion is clearly related to an assets based model of health – enhancing the capacity of communities to preserve and maintain. Residents of cohesive communities can access and mobilise to protect their health consist of norms, trust, and the exercise of sanctions. These assets are translated into improved health status through a number of social processes – socialisation, informal social control, and collective efficacy.

Recent reviews of the empirical evidence link community cohesion to health outcomes. Studies indicate a link between community cohesion and physical health outcomes (including self rated health) and health related behaviours. The evidence on mental health is more sparse and mixed. The majority of studies have been conducted in developed countries. Community cohesion (as a health asset) appears to be more salient in societies characterised by the deficient provision of material infrastructure.

There is debate about the value of investing in social cohesion as a public health improvement strategy. Social cohesion is not a panacea for population and can sometimes have negative consequences. For example strong social networks may demand conformity and restrict individual freedoms. Kawachi identifies a number of principles that should guide investment in building social capital. Broader structural interventions (such as job creation and improved working conditions) aimed at boosting the capacity of individuals and communities to organisation should be considered along side building social capital locally. Attention needs to be given to the type of social capital; building bridging social capital rather than bonding social capital. For example the linking of unemployed youth to employed adults can provide access to role models and mentoring. The distribution of costs and benefits should be assessed to avoid unintended consequences. For example women may disproportionately be expected to provide support. There is also a need for governments to be actively involved in building social capital, voluntary efforts are insufficient.

Popay (Chap. 10) focuses on activities concerned with enabling communities to have greater control over decisions that affect their lives with the aim to improve population health and or reduce health inequalities.

The author provides definitions of community development, community empowerment and community engagement and involvement. A theoretical framework is presented that defines a number of interlinked pathways between activities aimed at increasing community engagement and/or empowerment and health outcomes including both improved population health and reduced health inequalities. In theory different pathways to health outcomes will be operating at different levels of empowerment and/or engagement. Activities involved in giving communities more power and control over decisions that affect their lives are more likely to have positive impacts on service quality, social capital, socio economic circumstances, community empowerment and ultimately on population health and health inequalities.

Popay states that community engagement and development have a long history both in the UK and internationally. Current UK policy across many different areas view engagement and empowerment as the means to finding local solutions and a pre requisite for success and sustainability. However evidence highlights that there are a range of barriers to effective community development which relate to a lack of both community and organisational capacity.

Popay discusses the challenges and limitations relating to the evidence base and provides a comprehensive set of issues that need to be addressed in conducting evaluations. Given the diversity of the evidence base, there is a strong case for constructing a review of evidence that tests theoretical models of the pathways between different approaches to community empowerment and engagement (and specific methods) and different intermediary and longer term outcomes.

Rutten (Chap. 11), Mukhopadhyay (Chap. 12), Franceschini (Chap. 13) and Houeto (Chap. 14) all provide examples of the issues involved in the development, implementation and evaluation of asset approaches to community health in different country contexts. The experiences from Germany, India, Latin America and the Caribbean and West Africa, demonstrate the commonalities and differences of applying the model in different circumstances.

Rutten et al., (Chap. 11) uses the concept of asset mapping to improve opportunities for women living in difficult life situations in Germany to engage in physical activity or 'movement' as they define it. It demonstrates how the model can be used to challenge power structures within communities to overcome how professionals in positions of power can work with representatives from the community to achieve their health goals. Importantly they describe a process that could be replicated in different country contexts to help overcome some of the barriers that local communities face in try to have their voices heard by professionals in positions of power. They also highlight how the processes important to the success of community focused initiatives can be captured by mixed method approaches to evaluation and use of indicators that represent the assets necessary for improving the opportunities for health and access to facilities and services.

Chapter 12 focuses on sustainable community based health and development programmes in rural India. It introduces the Khoj project, a community based development programme which exemplifies the power of the asset approach to change the life circumstances of people living in poorer circumstances. Mukhopadhyay and Gupta describe their experience of strengthening the capacities of local communities in remote rural parts of India. The project is set within the broader context of Indian state's commitment to achieve "health for all". The overall vision of Khoj is to create an enabling climate for the sociopolitical development of communities living in difficult terrains of the country. The chapter highlights the successes of a non government group through implementation of a range of cross cutting interventions aiming to bring about a holistic change in the lives of the communities by uplifting their socioeconomic and health status. The Khoj projects emphasizes that there is no concept of recipients, as the community is involved in managing the development of the project including efforts access and obtain the resources needed. The chapter outlines the broader context within in which the project takes place with a brief description of the health sector in India and highlights the features of the community centric sustainable strategies of Khoj that brought about improvements in the overall well being of the population.

Chapter 13 by Franceschini and colleagues use the settings approach to highlight what can be achieved in Latin American countries (LAC) where policies and interventions to tackle poverty and inequalities in health have tended to focus on disease prevention and treatment. The authors argue that to create sustainable strategies it is more beneficial to follow a "settings approach", based on the belief that determinants of poverty and equity, and their influence on health, can be tackled through activities, which embrace and work with existing community networks and infrastructures. This may include the creation of appropriate public policies and laws and places particular emphasis on the importance of working with regional and local governments.

This chapter looks at the Healthy Municipalities and Communities movement, developed in the 1990s, whose aim was to look at underlying living conditions and build on existing assets. The focus is deliberately shifted from a focus on illness and disease to tackling the determinants of health. The chapter concludes by highlighting the constraints of traditional evaluation methods in their ability to record and assess the significance and impact of "asset building" in projects. Participatory evaluation techniques, it is proposed, may be an effective methodology to engage people in a joint reflection and learning process.

Houeto and Deccache (Chap. 14) provide an example from Benin, West Africa of how parental and community assets can help to control under five child malaria. This chapter reviews the issues around the burden of malaria in the region and details the successful facets of a community-led, assets based, anti-malarial project.

Chapters 15–18 (Makara, Baum, Baban and Eriksson, respectively) consider the asset model through the policy lens and the range of issues that need be addressed by those in positions of power to ensure that appropriate attention is given to the approach.

Chapter 15 (Makara et al.) reflects on the Hungarian experience of adopting assets based approaches and the timeliness of adopting the asset approach as the country faces the challenges of the social and health impact of the economic and financial crisis. A greater focus on assets based approaches could help unlock some of the existing barriers to effective action on health inequities. The chapter highlights that Hungary has a history of asset based approaches in local communities. However, if an asset approach is to be realised, a number of things need to be in place to ensure that the aims and objectives of the New Hungary Development Plan (NHDP) can be reached. This chapter sets out the lessons learnt from the past and highlights the critical conditions for policy to assure they take account of the country's assets at the national, regional and local level.

In *Chap. 16, Baum* examines the role of social capital in bringing about equity based policies that are central to achieving healthy populations. This involves a review of theories and evidence on the relationship between different forms of social capital (bonding, bridging and linking), equity and health outcomes.

Baum explores in detail how health inequities are created through social and economic structures, opportunities and networks, and psychosocial and behavioural mechanisms, and how social capital can play a role in making the outcomes more equitable. 'A high social capital society has high social and civic participation with bonded, bridging and linking networks which produce co-operation and trust among the citizens and a desire to provide a fair go, for all members of the community'.

But there is an issue of direction of causality. Wilkinson's work indicates that equity of income distribution in a population leads to a society with these high social capital attributes However Baum points out that it is possible to assume that high social capital society will result in more equitable health outcomes and that social capital is easier to generate in more equitable societies. A virtuous cycle can be established.

The role of governments in creating and supporting social capital, and how social capital can effect political processes, is also examined. Linking social capital implies can be particularly important in bringing about redistributive and progressive policies. A number of historical and contemporary examples are cited that demonstrate how movements of solidarity and democratization can impact on equity that there is a sense of obligation from powerful institutions in society towards the less powerful.

Thus a crucial public policy question is what are the conditions under which a society demonstrates higher degrees of linking social capital and solidarity? How can these attributes be fostered especially in an age in which economic globalisation stresses the value of individual autonomy.

Baum concludes that further research on social capital and its relationship to health equity that is more strongly informed by political economy theory will be important for better understanding of its role as a health asset.

Chapter 17 by Baban and Craciun focuses on the assets required for the health and wellbeing of adolescents living in Romania. They use data from the Romanian Health Behaviour in School Aged Children survey to examine how 'internal and external assets' relate to the mental health and health behaviour of this group of young people. In particular they investigate the relationship between school social capital and mental health and consider the implications for health promoting school based policies. The authors argue that the assets based model for health provides a useful framework, demonstrating how school health promotion should focus on building internal and external resources, helping young people to become active agents in the promotion of their own mental well being and health behaviour. Results demonstrate that changes in family structure, parenting patterns and the easy availability of unhealthy lifestyle options means that the contemporary role played by school in the health education of teenagers has assumed greater importance than in the past. Gender differences also emerged from the study, with boys demonstrating more internal and external resources than girls. Data such as this can be useful in developing national school policy, promoting student centred methods that help increase self efficacy and self esteem.

Eriksson and Lindstrom in the final Chap. 18 assess the potential of the salutogenic approach as the basis for tackling public health challenges. The salutogenic approach focuses on assets for health and the processes that can promote health.

Salutogenic theory is conceptually and empirically sound. The application of the sense of coherence scale (SOC) demonstrates the evidence potential as for research and practice.

Potentially the salutogenic approach embraces a number of concepts that are concerned with assets for promoting health. The *sense of coherence* has similarities, as well as differences with a range of other concepts including resilience, hardiness, self efficacy, empowerment and habitus and cultural capital.

There is potential to integrate the sense of coherence as an indicator within the health indicator system. It is important that SOC as a health indicator is assessed on a population level, and the authors propose introducing a new concept RALY – Resource Adjusted Life Year as a measure to include in vital statistics – applied on a general population level. The inclusion of SOC as a health indicator is important for the deeper integration of the salutogenic perspective on healthy public policy – a policy development approach that 'gives people the possibility to live the life they want to live'. The salutogenic model can also provide a comprehensive cross sectoral framework and coherence for policy making.

The salutogenic framework is also important for public health and health promotion research. The authors introduce a model that draws on a number of theories and brings together 'research on risk factors for vulnerability and adversities, protective factors for survival and good health outcomes with salutary factors promoting health and Quality of life'.

Together the chapters demonstrate what we already know about positive approaches to population health. In doing so, they raise the issues that need to be addressed if we are to move towards a robust and systematic evidence base that highlights the benefits of investing in the assets of individuals, communities and populations for long term sustainable health and development.

London, UK — Antony Morgan
London, UK — Amanda Killoran
London, UK — Maggie Davies
Venice, Italy — Erio Ziglio

References

Commission on the Social Determinants of Health (CSDH). (2008). *Closing the gap in a generation – health equity through action on the social determinants of health. Final report of the Commission on the Social Determinants of Health*. Geneva: World Health Organisation

Harrison, D., Ziglio, E., Levin, L., & Morgan, A. (2004). *Assets for health and development: developing a conceptual framework*. European Office for Investment for Health and Development, Venice: World Health Organization

Portes, A. & Landolt, P. (1996). The downside of social capital. *The American Prospect* **26** 18–21

Disclaimer

The views expressed herein are solely those of the authors and do not claim to represent those of the author's affiliations

The Commission on Social Determinants of Health has defined health equity as: 'the absence of unfair and avoidable or remediable differences in health among social groups' (Solar & Irwin, 2007), adapted from Margaret Whitehead's definition of health equity (Whitehead, 2006). Health inequity is therefore defined as unfair and avoidable or remediable differences. However, the terms, health inequity and health inequalities are often used interchangeably. In the context of this book, each author has used their preferred term but the meaning is the same.

Solar O, Irwin A. (2007) A Conceptual Framework for Action on the Social Determinants of Health. Discussion Paper for the Commission on Social Determinants of Health. Commission on Social Determinants of Health, World Health Organization, Geneva, Draft April 2007. Available at http://www.who.int/social_determinants/resources/csdh_framework_action_05_07.pdf .

Whitehead M, Dahlgren G. (2006) Levelling up (part 1): a discussion paper on concepts and principles for tackling social inequities in health. Studies on social and economic determinants of population health, No.2, WHO Regional Office for Europe.

Contents

Editors

Antony Morgan is an Epidemiologist and is currently an Associate Director at the Centre for Public Health Excellence, National Institute for Health and Clinical Excellence (NICE), England. Originally an applied chemist, Antony later trained in information science and epidemiology and has worked in Public Health in the English NHS for the last 25 years, at district, regional and national level. Antony is a Fellow of the UK Faculty of Public Health and has Honorary Research Appointments at the Universities of Hertfordshire and Edinburgh. At NICE he is currently responsible for producing public health guidance across a range of public health topic areas, including inequalities, community engagement, mental well being and children, and sexual health. Special areas of research interest and expertise include social action for health (using the concept of social capital); assets approaches to health and development (particularly in relation to adolescent health) and new methodologies for building an evidence base on the social determinants of health. Antony is currently the Principal Investigator for England on the World Health Organization (WHO) Health Behaviour in School Aged Children Study.

Maggie Davies is the Principal Advisor on International Health Improvement at the Department of Health, England. She is on secondment from the National Institute of Health and Clinical Excellence (NICE) where she is Associate Director of Development. Maggie is also the lead tutor on the Distance Learning MSc in Health Promotion for the London School of Hygiene and Tropical Medicine. Maggie is President of the Pan-European network Eurohealthnet, which deals with equity and health issues, and is Global Vice President for Conferences for the International Union of Health Promotion and Education.

Previously a lecturer in semiotics, Maggie has over 20 years experience of work in the field of public health which has ranged from managing local services to large-scale international projects. This includes work for organisations such as World Health Organization (WHO) and the World Bank.

Maggie has also been a volunteer for non-government agencies and has been a Director of the Terrence Higgins Trust and Rape Crisis, Croydon.

Maggie has a record of publication in the field and most recently has edited two books for the Oxford University Press on Health Promotion Theory and Practice.

Maggie has post graduate qualifications in health management and is a fellow of the Faculty of Public Health.

Erio Ziglio is currently Head of the World Health Organization (WHO) European Office for Investment for Health and Development in Venice. He has worked for over 15 years in the academic world both in Europe and in North America. Between 1978 and 1990, he lectured for the Department of Social Policy at the University of Edinburgh and carried out research at the University's Research Unit in Health and Behavioural Change. In 1985, he was awarded his PhD at the University of Edinburgh.

In North America he was Visiting Professor at the University of Toronto, Department of Community Medicine (1983) and at Carlton University, Department of Social Studies, Ottawa, (1986). Dr Ziglio was also a member of the International Faculty of the School of Public Health at Yale University from 1996 to 2003.

Dr Ziglio has lectured internationally and published widely on subjects such as: health promotion; health policy and planning; social determinants of health; health inequities and health and development issues. He held an Honorary Professorship from the University of York, and has been an Honorary Research Fellow at the University of Edinburgh.

In the late 1980s he worked for 3 years as a Public Health Consultant for the European Commission in the early 1990s, joined the WHO Regional Office for Europe in Copenhagen taking on responsibility for Health Promotion and the Investment for Health Programme. Since 2002, Dr Ziglio has headed the WHO European Office for Investment for Health and Development in Venice.

During his professional career he has had the opportunity to conduct extensive field work in many countries, including the United Kingdom, USA, Canada, Finland, Slovenia, Hungary, Romania, Czech Republic, Malta, Spain, Portugal, Italy and Brazil. Dr Ziglio's work has been published and translated into several languages including English, German and Italian.

Authors

Karim Abu-Omar, PhD works as a researcher at the Institute of Sports Science and Sport of the Friedrich-Alexander-University Erlangen-Nuremberg. He has a MA degree in Sociology and did his PhD in Medical Sociology at the University of Alabama at Birmingham (UAB), United States. His research interests include health promotion policy development and implementation, and physical activity surveillance.

Adriana Baban is a professor of health psychology at Babes-Bolyai University, Cluj, Romania. She has extensive international experience in research and programs on women health, violence against women and girls, children trafficking, working in collaboration with the United Nations agencies, including their Children's Fund (UNICEF). Currently, Dr. Baban is interested in studying both individual and social determinants of adolescents' well-being and positive health. She is author of six books, and more than 50 chapters and articles.

Mel Bartley is Professor of Medical Sociology in the Department of Epidemiology and Public Health, University College London, and director of the Economic and Social Research Council (ESRC) International Centre for Life Course Studies in Society and Health. Her background is in philosophy, medical sociology and social policy. While writing this chapter she was Research Co-ordinator of the ESRC Research Priority Network on Human Capability and Resilience. Her research interests also include health inequality, gender differences in health, and the relationship between unemployment and health in different welfare regimes.

Fran Baum is an Australian Research Council Federation Fellow and Professor of Public Health sat Flinders University, Adelaide, Australia. She is also Foundation Director of the Southgate Institute for Health, Society and Equity & the South Australian Community Health Research Unit. She has been an active member of the People's Health Movement – a global network of health activist (www. phmovement.org) – since its formation in 2000 and currently serves as the Co-Chair of its Global Steering Council. She also served as a Commissioner on the Commission on the Social Determinants of Health from 2005 to 2008. She is a Fellow of the Australian Academy of Social Science and of the Australian Health Promotion Association and is also a past National President and Life Member of the Public

Health Association of Australia. Her research focuses on the social and economic determinants of health and community based health promotion.

David Blane is Professor of Medical Sociology in the Department of Primary Care and Social Medicine at Imperial College London Medical School. He is deputy director of the Economic and Social Research Council (ESRC) International Centre for Life Course Studies in Society and Health. His background is in medicine, sociology and public health, and his work has included the development of the 'life grid' method and the CASP measure of quality of life in older age, now used on all major studies of ageing.

Simon Carroll has had a long interest in the health research field, completing his doctoral work on alternative approaches to assessing the effectiveness of complex health interventions at the University of Victoria. More recently he has worked closely with both the Pubic Health Agency of Canada's Effectiveness of Community Interventions Project, the North American Region of the International Union for Health Promotion and Education's effectiveness project, and the Pan-American Health Organization's Health Promotion Effectiveness Working Group. He was the Associate Director of the Community Health Promotion Research Centre at the University of Victoria, British Columbia (2007–2009).

Dr. Carroll is currently developing a variety of social theory approaches to assessing the effectiveness of complex health interventions, particularly in relation to the integration of the contextual dimension into effectiveness analysis. He has a special interest in the application of critical realism in this area, along with methodological reflections on context inspired by ethnomethodology.

Catrinel Craciun is a teaching assistant in the field of health psychology at the Babes-Bolyai University, Cluj, Romania. She is also a PhD candidate at the Freie Universität Berlin where she is working on evidence-based behavior change interventions in skin cancer prevention. As part of the research team of the Romanian Health Psychology Association she is currently interested in designing health programs that focus on promoting assets in adolescents and children.

Alain Deccache is a professor of Health Promotion and Health Education at the School of Public Health, Catholic University of Louvain, Brussels, Belgium. Former Director of the School of Public Health, he is the Director of Health Promotion and Health Education Unit which is a World Health Organization (WHO) collaborative centre for Health Promotion documentation since 1989. His main research interests include individual empowerment in chronic disease care and community intervention.

Sylvie Desjardins is the Scientific Director of the World Health Organization (WHO) Collaborating Center on Chronic Disease Policy, and lead the multi-disciplinary team. Sylvie is a PhD candidate in Public Health at the University of Montreal, a Masters Degree in Economics and Health Administration, and Bachelor degree in Economics. As an applied micro-economist, Sylvie has 10 years experience in public health sector analysis in which she has conducted a wide range of economic investigations on the return of investment of policy and community intervention, the direct and indirect costs of illness, the cost-effectiveness and outcomes of treatment, and health care payment and reimbursement practices. She has leveraged this knowledge of large-scale public and private databases to conduct causation and impact assessments on policy decision. As a teacher, researcher and senior health economist, Sylvie brings a unique and practical lens to population health discussions on the effectiveness of interventions and evidence-based policy making. Her expertise lies in researching the linkages between investments in health promotion and the reduction of economic burden of chronic diseases.

Monica Eriksson, PhD, PM, PL, is a Senior Researcher presently running several projects and a research synthesis on salutogenesis at Folkhälsan in Helsinki. Monika completed her dissertation on Salutogenesis in 2007, and studies in public health and health promotion at the Nordic School of Public Health, Sweden. Monika has many years occupational experience as social worker, especially with disabled people. She was also a former investigator at a Nordic Institution of the Nordic Council of Ministers, Project Leader of the Salutogenic Project, Nordic School of Public Health (NHV), and Sweden and Public Health Investigator, Government of Åland.

Maria Cristina Franceschini is a Technical Officer with the Sustainable Development and Environmental Health Unit of the Pan American Health Organization (PAHO) working with issues related to health promotion and health determinants. Ms. Franceschini has been working with PAHO for the past 6 years. She holds a degree in anthropology and a masters degree in international health.

Cristina Raquel Caballero Gracia is a PhD student at the National Institute of Public Health of Mexico with primary interest in health systems, health promotion, dental health services and quality of life research, and health and social disparities. She is an Assistant Professor with the National University of Asunción, School of Dentistry, Paraguay. She holds a degree in dentistry, a specialty certification in restorative dentistry and a masters degree in public health administration.

Anjali Gupta is MPhil in Community Health and Social Medicine from the Jawaharlal Nehru University, India. Currently she is working as Senior Programme Officer with Voluntary Health Association of India (VHAI). She is also the Associate Editor for Health For the Millions public health journal.

Marcia Hills, RN, PhD is a professor in the School of Nursing at the University of Victoria. She is the former Director of the Canadian Consortium for Health Promotion Research (CCHPR) and the founding Director of the Centre for Community Health Promotion Research (cchpr) at the University of Victoria. She is a globally elected member of the International Union for Health Promotion and Education (IUHPE) Board of Trustees and the President of the Canadian Association of Teachers of Community Health (CATCH). She has worked with IUHPE, the Pan American Health Organization (PAHO) and the Public Health Agency of Canada (PHAC) to develop participatory evaluation and new methodologies for synthesizing the effectiveness of complex health promotion interventions. She has been a visiting scholar in England, Australia and Brazil.

David Houéto, MD (University of Abomey-Calavi, Benin), holds a Masters degree in Public Nutrition and Health System Organization (Senghor International University of Alexandria, Egypt) and a PhD in Health Promotion (Catholic University of Louvain, Brussels, Belgium). He is the Regional Advisor in Health Promotion for Africa of the Preventive Medicine Agency (AMP, www.aamp.org) and the President of the Francophone Network for Health Promotion (REFIPS, www.refips.org). His main research interests include community development and health system strengthening with health promotion approach.

Ichiro Kawachi is Professor of Social Epidemiology, and Chair of the Department of Society, Human Development and Health at the Harvard School of Public Health. Kawachi received both his medical degree and PhD (in epidemiology) from the University of Otago, New Zealand. He has taught at the Harvard School of Public Health since 1992. Kawachi has published widely on the social determinants of population health. He was the co-editor (with Lisa Berkman) of the first textbook on Social Epidemiology, published by Oxford University Press in 2000. His books include The Health of Nations (The New Press 2002) and Social Capital and Health (Springer 2008). Kawachi currently serves as the Senior Editor (Social Epidemiology) of the international journal Social Science & Medicine, as well as an Editor of the American Journal of Epidemiology.

Michael P. Kelly is Director of the Centre of Public Health Excellence at the National Institute for Health and Clinical Excellence (NICE). He originally graduated in Social Science from the University of York, holds a Masters degree in Sociology from the University of Leicester, and undertook his PhD in the Department of Psychiatry in the University of Dundee. Before joining NICE he was Director of Evidence and Guidance at the Health Development Agency. He has held posts at the Universities of Leicester, Dundee, Glasgow, Greenwich and Abertay. He now has an honorary chair in the Department of Public Health and Policy at the London School of Hygiene and Tropical Medicine, University of London and is a Fellow of the Faculty of Public Health.

Professor Kelly is a medical sociologist with research interests in evidence based approaches to health improvement, methodological problems in public health research, evidence synthesis, coronary heart disease prevention, chronic illness, disability, physical activity, health inequalities, social identity and community involvement in health promotion.

Bengt Lindström, PhD, drPH, MD, Paediatrics, is Professor of Health Promotion and Director of Research. Bengt has been involved in Public Health and Health Promotion at the Nordic School of Public Health since 1984. His dissertation was on the Quality of Life of Children. Bengt met Aaron Antonovsky in the 1980s and 1990s and discovered that the combination of salutogenesis and quality of life gives efficient instruments for health promotion. At present Bengt is running the

International Union for Health Promotion and Education (IUHPE) Global Working Group on Salutogenesis from Helsinki.

John McKnight has partnered with Jody Kretzmann for nearly 3 decades on research on community organizations and neighborhood policy. Additionally, Professor McKnight has conducted his own research on social service delivery systems, health policy, the inclusion of marginalized people, and institutional racism. He currently contributes to the Asset-Based Community Development Institute efforts and continues his own research and community work.

Péter Makara has a PhD in Sociology. He is author of several publications in the field of health promotion, disease prevention and health policy analysis. He is an associate professor in the Master School of Health Policy, University of Debrecen.

Sabine Mayer is a lecturer at the Institute of Sport Science and Sport of the Friedrich-Alexander-University Erlangen-Nuremberg. She has a degree in Sport Science and has been working in a number of fields of research, including sport sociology and rehabilitation science. She has been involved in the planning and implementation phase of the BIG project, contributing mainly to the design and analysis of the physical activity interventions. For her doctoral thesis, she was involved in the SEFIP (Senior Fitness and Prevention) Study, which investigated the effects of a general rehabilitation sports program on multiple impairments and diseases among older women.

Berry Mayall is Professor of Childhood Studies at the Institute of Education, University of London. She has worked for many years on research projects focusing on children's and parents' experiences and understandings of childhood. Currently she teaches the sociology of childhood on an MA in the Sociology of Childhood and Children's Rights. Among her many publications are: Conceptualising Child–Adult Relations (2001, edited with Leena Alanen); Towards a Sociology for Childhood (2002); Childhood in Generational Perspective (2003, edited with Helga Zeiher). Currently she is working with Virginia Morrow on a book exploring English children's contributions to the war effort (1939–1945).

Richard Mitchell is Professor of Health and Environment at the Faculty of Medicine, University of Glasgow. His research focuses on the interactions between, and impacts of, social and physical environments in determining health inequalities. He is currently particularly interested in the capacity that certain social and physical environments may have to foster or protect population health; the 'salutogenic' aspects of environment, rather than the 'pathogenic'. He combines methods from epidemiology and geography in this research.

Antony Morgan

See Editors

Virginia Morrow is Reader of Childhood Studies at the Institute of Education, University of London, where she is Programme Leader of the MA Sociology of

Childhood and Children's Rights. Children and young people have been the focus of her research activities since 1988. Her main research interests are the history and sociology of child labour and children's work; methods and ethics of social research with children; sociology of childhood and children' rights; social capital in relation to children and young people; children' understandings of family and other social environments. She is also the author of numerous papers and reports, and is currently working as advisor to Young Lives, a longitudinal study of child poverty (www.younglives.org.uk). She is co-editor of Childhood: a global journal of child research.

Jennie Popay is a sociologist working in the fields of social policy and public health. She has held posts in academia, the voluntary sector and the NHS. Her research interests include the social determinants of health and health equity, lay expertise about health, illness and health inequalities, community engagement/empowerment and methods for the synthesis of evidence for public health action. She chaired a global knowledge network supporting the World Health Organization (WHO) Commission on the Social Determinants of Health by collating international evidence on action to promote health equity by addressing social exclusion and has held public appointments as a member of the UK Commission for Health Improvement and the English Commission for Patient and Public Involvement in Health.

Alok Mukhopadhyay is the Chief Executive of Voluntary Health Association of India(VHAI). VHAI is a Federation of 27 State Voluntary Health Associations and 4,500 member organisations, working in the field of health promotion and health care throughout the country. He is a member of the National Commission on Macroeconomics & Health; National AIDS Control Board; Empowered Action Group, Government of India. He has been an Advisor to the World Health Organization (WHO), The World Bank as well as to the Asian Development Bank. His contribution in developing community based health and development programmes in India is well recognized. He has conceptualized, produced and directed popular films on social issues for national TV channels.

Zsófia Németh studied psychology and public health and is working on her PhD at the ELTE University. She is employed by the Hungarian National Institute for Health Development.

Ulrike Ravens-Sieberer, Professor for Child Public Health, University Clinic Hamburg-Eppendorf, Germany. As a psychologist with postgradual training in public health Ulrike has been involved in Health related Quality of Life (HRQoL) research since 1990. This work also includes developing methods for assessing HRQoL and mental well-being in the pediatric population in order to promote cross-cultural quality of life research and assessment as well as the application of quality of life measures in health reporting and health surveys. Ulrike served as head of the research group 'Child and Adolescent Health' at the Robert Koch Institute in Berlin, the federal public health research institution in Germany. She then became a full professor for Public Health and Health Psychology at the

University of Bielefeld, School of Public Health, Germany, and director of the World Health Organization Collaborating Centre for Child and Adolescent Health Promotion. Ulrike has been a full professor and Head of the research section 'Child Public Health' since 2008. In this position she is responsible for coordinating and conducting German and European health surveys on health behaviour, HRQoL, and mental health in children and adolescents. This includes the implementation and analysis of the international study 'Health Behaviour in School Aged Children' for Germany.

Marilyn Rice is the Senior Advisor in Health Promotion for the Pan American Health Organization (PAHO), the Regional Office for the Americas of the World Health Organization (WHO). She has worked for PAHO for 15 years and the Global Office of WHO for 7 years. Ms. Rice is also the Vice President for the North American Regional Office of the International Union for Health Promotion and Education (IUHPE). She holds a degree in sociology and masters training in public health and health education.

Alfred Rütten is the head of the Institute of Sports Science and Sport of the Friedrich-Alexander-University Erlangen-Nuremberg. He was visiting research Professor at the Departments of Sociology and Medicine of the University of Alabama at Birmingham (USA), and visiting Professor of Public Health at the Department of Epidemiology and Public Health at Yale University, New Haven (USA).

Prof. Rütten is the principal investigator of the BIG project. He is currently leading the EU funded projects 'Improving Infrastructures for Leisure-Time Physical Activity in the Local Arena – Good Practice in Europe (IMPALA)' and 'Building Policy Capacities for Health Promotion through Physical Activity among Sedentary Older People (PASEO)'.

Ingrid Schoon is a developmental social psychologist with expertise in the study of risk and resilience, i.e. the factors and processes shaping human development in the face of adversity. Her research interests lie with the study of life course development in context, focusing in particular on the realization of individual potential, social equalities in attainment and health, and the intergenerational transmission of (dis)advantage. Her current research addresses issues related to the wellbeing of children and productive youth development. She is the author of more than 100 scholarly articles, book chapters, and reports. Her recent publications include a monograph on 'risk and resilience' and an edited volume on 'transitions from school to work', both published by Cambridge University Press.

Sabine Seidenstücker works for the City of Mannheim in the Department of Health. She has been a researcher at the University of Koblenz-Landau and the Friedrich-Alexander-University Erlangen-Nuremberg. Sabine has been involved in the planning and implementation phase of the BIG project.

Ágnes Taller studies social policy. She is a technical officer in the National Institute for Health Development.

Nora Wille works at the 'Child Public Health' Research Section, University Clinic Hamburg-Eppendorf, Germany. As a psychologist with postgradual studies in public health and epidemiology, Nora's main research interests are in psychiatric epidemiology and quality of life research. Her involvement in this field started in 2005 within the framework of the international KIDSCREEN project on health-related quality of life (HRQoL) in children and adolescents. In 2006, as a researcher at the Robert Koch Institute in Berlin, Nora took responsibility for conducting the BELLA study, the mental health module of the German Health Interview and Examination Survey for Children and Adolescents (KiGGS). This longitudinal study collects comprehensive data on mental health and HRQoL as well as relevant predictors in a large and representative sample of families in Germany. Nora continued the project management of the BELLA study at the World Health Organization (WHO) Collaborating Centre for Child and Adolescent Health Promotion, University of Bielefeld, Germany. She currently works at the University Clinic Hamburg-Eppendorf, where she continues to coordinate the BELLA study and analyses the role of risks and resources for young people's mental health. Beyond this, Nora is involved in further studies, such as intervention studies in overweight youth or the development and pilot testing of the EQ-5D-Y.

Erio Ziglio

See Editors

Abbreviations List

Chapter 1

ESRC	Economic and Social Research Council
WHO	World Health Organization

Chapter 2

GNP	Gross National Product
GRR	Generalised Resistance Resources
OECD	Organisation for Economic Co-operation and Development
SOC	Sense of Coherence
UN	United Nations
UNESCO	United Nations Educational Scientific and Cultural Organization
UNICEF	United Nations Children's Fund
WHO	World Health Organization

Chapter 3

CSDH	Commission on the Social Determinants of Health
EU	European Union

Chapter 4

There are no abbreviations used in this chapter.

Chapter 5

ECIP	Effectiveness of Community Interventions Project
HC	Health Canada
IFH	Investment for Health
PHAC	Public Health Agency of Canada

Chapter 6

ESRC	Economic and Social Research Council

Chapter 7

ER89	Ego Resilience scale

Chapter 8

HBSC	Health Behaviour in School-Aged Children
OECD	Organisation for Economic Co-operation and Development
UN	United Nations
UNCRC	UN Convention on the Rights of the Child
UNICEF	United Nations Children's Fund

Chapter 9

ICC	Intra-Class Correlations

Chapter 10

CDP	Community Development Project
WHO	World Health Organization

Chapter 11

HEPA	Health-Enhancing Physical Activity
WHO	World Health Organization

Chapter 12

ANC	Antenatal Care
ARI	Acute Respiratory Infection
GARVIS	Gramin Vikas Vigyan Samity
GDI	Gender Related Development Index
GNP	Gross National Product
GOI	Government of India
IEC	Information Education and Communication
IGP	Income Generation Programme
IMR	Infant Mortality Rate
MM	Mahila Mandal
NFHS	National Family Health Survey
NGO	Non Government Groups
OPD	Out Patient Department
SHG	Self Help Groups
TBA	Traditional Birth Attendant
TB	Tuberculosis
TT	Tetanus
VDC	Village Development Committee
VEC	Village Education Committee
VHAI	Voluntary Health Association of India
VHW	Village Health Worker
VOPAs	Village Old People's Associations

Chapter 13

HMC	Healthy Municipalities, Cities and Communities
LAC	Latin America and the Caribbean
PAHO	Pan American Health Organization
PHC	Primary Health Care
SDH	Social Determinants of Health
WHO	World Health Organization

Chapter 14

ACT	Artemisinin Combined Therapy
CMW	Community Health Worker
HMM	Home Malaria Management
IEC	Information, Education and Communication
IITA	International Institute of Tropical Agriculture

IMCI	Integrated Management of Childhood Illness
IMN	Impregnated Mosquito Nets
MDG	Millennium Development Goals
SSA	Sub-Saharan Africa

Chapter 15

EU	European Union
GDP	Gross Domestic Product
MoH	Ministry of Health
NHDP	New Hungary Development Plan
WHO	World Health Organization

Chapter 16

NHS	National Health Service

Chapter 17

EU	European Union
HBSC	Health Behaviour in School-Aged Children
HPS	Health Promoting School
MoER	Ministry of Education and Research
MoPH	the Ministry of Public Health
NGOs	non government groups
SOC	Sense of Coherence
SSC	School Social Capital
UNDP	United Nations Development Programme
UNICEF	United Nations Children's Fund
USAID	United States Agency for International Development
WHO	World Health Organization

Chapter 18

DALY	Disability Adjusted Life Years
GRR	General Resistance Resources
HMP	Health Monitoring Programme
ICF	International Classification of Functioning
IUHPE	International Union for Health Promotion and Education
RALY	Resource Adjusted Life Years
SOC	Sense of Coherence
WHO	World Health Organization

Part I
Conceptualising the Notion of Health Assets

Chapter 1
Revitalising the Public Health Evidence Base: An Asset Model

Antony Morgan and Erio Ziglio

Keywords Asset mapping • Evaluation • Health assets • Inequities • Salutogenesis

1.1 Introduction

In an increasing number of countries, politicians, policy makers and practitioners are now convinced about the need to tackle health inequities both between and within countries to ensure that these heath inequities are increasingly recognised as a global problem. In 2000, the 189 states of the United Nations reaffirmed their commitment to work towards a world in which eliminating poverty and sustaining development would have the highest priority (WHO 2003). Nonetheless, whilst there are many examples of national governments developing comprehensive strategies, programmes and initiatives to tackle inequities (DH 2003; MHSA 2003; King 2000), countries vary in their awareness and commitment to take action (Judge et al. 2006).

Despite the growing number of policy commitments to tackle inequities, overall improvements in health since the 1950s are coupled with persistent differences in health between different social groups. Evidence demonstrates that even in Europe today, there are many examples of systematic differences in health between different social groups and in all European countries most disadvantaged groups have worse health and higher mortality (Whitehead and Dahlgren 2006). This suggests that some of the policies and interventions put in place to alleviate these differences are failing some sections of our societies. Moreover in some instances, some of these well-intentioned policies may in fact be having some negative unintended consequences. Despite calls for all health policies to be "equity proofed" (Acheson 1998; Stahl et al. 2006) many cross-government policies are implemented without adequate attention to their impact on health inequities.

A. Morgan (✉)
Centre for Public Health Excellence, National Institute for Health and Clinical Excellence (NICE), 71 High Holborn, London WC1V 6NA, UK; Karolinska Institute, Stockholm, Sweden
e-mail: antony.morgan@nice.org.uk

A. Morgan et al. (eds.), *Health Assets in a Global Context: Theory, Methods, Action*,
DOI 10.1007/978-1-4419-5921-8_1, © Springer Science+Business Media, LLC 2010

Why should this be? Firstly, it is well recognised that the multifaceted causes and solutions required to address the underlying determinants of inequities pose particular problems for policy makers, in that policies need to be long term, require intersectoral collaboration (Exworthy et al. 2003) and continued resources if goals of sustainability are to be reached.

Secondly, whilst there is a wealth of data (Marmot et al. 1991; Wilkinson 1996) documenting the amount and type of inequities that exist in populations, there is little empirical evidence about the effectiveness of strategies for reducing them (Mackenbach and Bakker 2002; Whitehead and Dahlgren 2006). Moreover, the evidence that does exist tends to be of a higher general order, describing the types of actions that are required but stopping short of how these actions might work for different population groups in different contexts. In addition, the mechanisms giving rise to inequities are still imperfectly understood and evidence remains to be gathered on the effectiveness of interventions to reduce such inequities (Woodward and Kawachi 2000; WHO 2005).

Thirdly, a lack of attention to follow through well-intentioned policies and programmes with sophisticated action plans for implementation, often leads expectations by Government, professionals and the general public to be undermined. Action plans which don't pay attention to the need for adequate performance management, insufficient integration between policy sectors, and contradictions between health inequities and other policy imperatives may fail (Exworthy et al. 2002).

Fourthly, in the context of this paper we argue that in its quest to improve health and combat disease, public health has focused on gathering evidence about "what works" from a deficit point of view. That is, there is a tendency to focus on identifying problems and needs of populations that require professional resources and high levels of dependence on hospital and welfare services (Morgan and Ziglio 2006; Ziglio et al. 2000). This leads to policy development which focuses on the failure of individuals and local communities to avoid disease rather than their potential to create and sustain health and continued development.

Whilst deficit models are important and necessary to identify levels of needs and priorities, they have some drawbacks and need to be complemented by asset perspectives. The asset model presented here aims to redress the balance between evidence derived from the identification of problems to one which accentuates positive capability to jointly identify problems and activate solutions, which promotes the self-esteem of individuals and communities leading to less dependency on professional services. This can lead to an increase in the amount and distribution of protective/promoting factors that are assets for individual and community level health. Redressing the balance, however, does not mean that one approach is better than the other. But in evidence terms at least, the asset model may help to further explain the persistence of inequities despite the increased efforts by governments internationally to do something about them.

The asset model described here draws on a number of perspectives to help us more systematically understand the causes and mechanisms of inequities in health and what to do about them by:

- Drawing on the theory of salutogenesis to investigate the "key factors" or "health assets", which support the creation of health rather than the prevention of disease.

- Applying the concept of asset mapping to help create more effective solutions to implementation working with the existing capabilities and capacities of individuals and communities and building on them.
- Employing the use of a new set of asset indicators with multi-method evaluations to assess the effectiveness of community based approaches to tackling health inequities.

1.2 What Are Health Assets?

The World Health Organization (WHO) European Office for Investment for Health Development based in Venice, Italy, is using the term "health assets" to mean the resources that individuals and communities have at their disposal, which protect against negative health outcomes and/or promote health status. These assets can be social, financial, physical, environmental or human resources (e.g. education, employment skills, supportive social networks, natural resources, etc.) (Harrison et al. 2004).

As such, a "health asset" can be defined as any factor (or resource), which enhances the ability of individuals, groups, communities, populations, social systems and/or institutions to maintain and sustain health and well-being and to help to reduce health inequities. These assets can operate at the level of the individual, group, community, and/or population as protective (or promoting) factors to buffer against life's stresses.

It is possible to identify health promoting/protecting assets from across all the domains of health determinants including our genetic endowments, social circumstances, environmental conditions, behavioural choices and health services. An inventory of health and development assets would, as a minimum, include:

- At the *individual* level: social competence, resistance skills, commitment to learning, positive values, self-esteem and a sense of purpose. For example, with respect to young people an asset approach to health and development could involve prevention activities which focus on protective factors which build resilience to inhibit high-risk behaviours such as substance abuse, violence, and dropping out of school.
- At the *community* level: family and friendship (supportive) networks, intergenerational solidarity, community cohesion, affinity groups (e.g. mutual aid), religious tolerance and harmony. For example, the cohesiveness of a community measured by a set of strong and positive interlocking networks may be seen as a health asset. In this instance, the asset has the potential to be health promoting irrespective of the levels of disadvantage in that community.
- At the *organisational or institutional* level: environmental resources necessary for promoting physical, mental and social health, employment security and opportunities for voluntary service, safe and pleasant housing, political democracy and participation opportunities, social justice and enhancing equity. For example, health systems across Europe are under utilised instruments for social and economic development. In an asset model, planners would ask how health services can make

best use of their resources (and maximise their assets) to help reduce health inequities by impacting on the wider determinants of health, to build stronger local economies, safeguard the environment and to develop more cohesive communities.

1.3 Developing the Asset Model

Working together, assets based approaches add value to the deficit model by:

- Identifying the range of protective and health promoting factors that act together to support health and well being and the policy options required to build and sustain these factors.
- Promoting the population as a co-producer of health rather than simply a consumer of health care services, thus reducing the demand on scarce resources.
- Strengthening the capacity of individuals and communities to realise their potential for contributing to health development.
- Contributing to more equitable and sustainable social and economic development and hence the goals of other sectors.

In reality, both models are important, however, more work needs to be done to redress the balance between the more dominant deficit model and the less well-known (and understood) asset model. The asset model presented here promotes a more systematic approach to understanding the science and practice of an asset approach to health and development. In doing so, it has the potential to create a more robust evidence base that demonstrates why investing in the assets of individuals, communities and organisations can help to reduce the health gap between those most disadvantaged in society and those who achieve best health.

The asset model draws on a number of current and resurgent ideas found in the literature. The first of these is the concept of salutogenesis, coined by Aaron Antonovsky (1987, 1996) to focus attention on the generation of health as compared to the pathogenesis focus on disease generation. Salutogenesis asks, *"what causes some people to prosper and others to fail or become ill in similar situations?"* It emphasizes the success and not the failure of the individual and it searches for the foundations of positive patterns of health rather the foundation of negative outcomes.

The asset model also incorporates the idea of asset mapping as a way of promoting effective implementation of equity focused policies by taking a positive approach to measuring and diagnosing community capacity to engage in health development activities. Kretzmann and McKnight (1993) describe asset mapping as a process of building an inventory of the strengths and gifts of the people who make up a community prior to intervening. Asset mapping reveals the assets of the entire community and highlights the interconnections among them, which in turn reveals how to access those assets. McKnight (1995) claims that asset mapping is necessary if local people are to find the way toward empowerment and renewal.

The asset model also promotes a multidisciplinary approach to the evaluation of complex interventions, deriving a new set of "salutogenic" indicators useful for measuring the effectiveness of these interventions in different contexts.

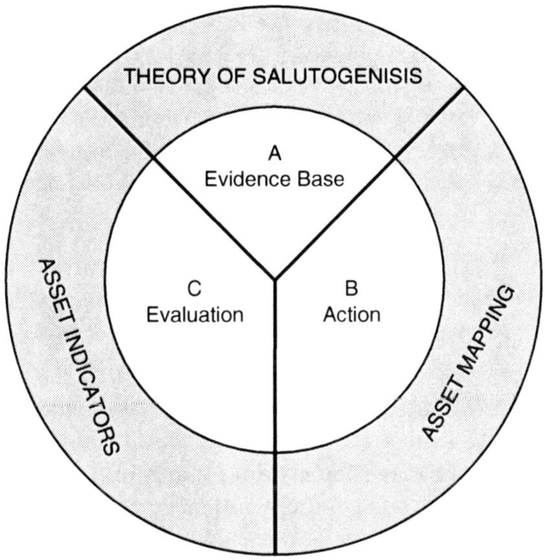

Fig. 1.1 An asset model for public health

Figure 1.1 highlights how the asset model can be utilised to:

- Generate a "salutogenic" evidence base that identifies the most important health promoting and/or protective factors for health and the actions that need to be taken to create the necessary conditions for health.
- Assess how most effectively to implement the actions required to create these conditions for health.
- Develop the most appropriate measures and evaluation frameworks to assess the effectiveness of these actions.

1.4 Using Salutogenesis to Build an Evidence Base for Health

Evidence-based public health is now well established and forms an integral part of the decision making process for health development. Much work has already been done to create the scientific base for action (IUHPE 2000), and a range of methodologies developed to evaluate these actions. The asset model seeks to complement these achievements by building a more systematic approach to collecting and synthesising evidence based on the theory of salutogenesis.

The "salutogenic" perspective or "the origin of health" allows us to identify those factors which keep individuals from moving toward the disease end of the health and illness spectrum (Lindström and Eriksson 2006). It can help us to identify the combination of "health assets" that are most likely to lead to higher levels of overall health, well-being and achievement. Specifically, the concept embraces the need to focus on people's resources and capacity to create health. It argues that the more that individuals understand the world they live in, which is manageable and has meaning, the more they can utilise the resources they have themselves and around them to maintain their own health. Lindström and Eriksson (2005) argue that the concept can be applied at an individual, group and societal level.

A "salutogenic" approach to building an evidence base for public health would include the need to identify those health promoting or protective factors (assets) that are most important in creating health and to understand the implications for action.

At its core, salutogenesis asks:

- What external factors contribute to health and development?
- What factors make us more resilient (more able to cope in times of stress)?
- What opens us to more fully experience life?
- What produces overall levels of well being?

Applying this concept to the search for evidence on the determinants of health and the evidence of the most effective actions has the potential to explain further what is required to tackle inequities in health. It also encourages the discipline of modern epidemiology to move towards finding answers to what creates health, rather than its traditional focus of generating evidence about the causes and distribution of disease and early death. The asset model therefore calls for a rethinking of the theoretical basis on which the public health evidence base is built.

The key questions for an epidemiology of health would include:

- What are key assets for health and development at each of the key life stages?
- What are the links between these assets and a range of health outcomes?
- How do these assets work in combination to bring about the best health and well being outcomes?
- How may these factors be used to contribute to reductions in health inequities?

Of course, there are many examples where this approach to research is already being taken. The asset model aims to encourage a more systematic way of collecting and synthesising this research to ensure that it features in the ongoing practice of evidence-based public health which is still dominated by a positivist biomedical approach to understanding "what works."

Notable examples include the work of the Economic and Social Research Council (ESRC) Priority Network (http://www.ucl.ac.uk/capabilityandresilience/) and the Search Institute (http://www.search-institute.org/).

The ESRC Priority Network (Bartley 2006) has compiled the most recent evidence on the best ways to promote "capability and resilience" two concepts used to refer to the ability to react and adapt positively when things go wrong. This research recognizes resilience as an asset because it allows individuals to rise above poor circumstances and succeed either to avoid high risk taking behaviour or to thrive in the face of these circumstances.

The concept of resilience has been identified as an example of an important health asset to support the healthy development of young people particularly those who are growing up in difficult circumstances. Resilient young people possess problem solving skills, social competence and a sense of purpose, which can be utilised as an asset that can help them rebound from setbacks, thrive in the face of poor circumstances, avoid risk-taking behaviour and generally continue on to a productive life.

The Search Institute has developed 40 essential developmental assets for young people, particularly during adolescent years, which foster resilience capabilities and support growing up as healthy, caring and responsible people. Many of the factors associated with resilience in young people relate to the social context within which they live.

1.5 Assets in Action

The Acheson Report on Inequalities in Health (Acheson 1998) recognized that the solutions to major public health problems such as heart disease, cancers, mental health and accidents are complex. These problems require interventions, which cut across sectors to take account of the broader social, cultural, economic, political and physical environments which shape people's experiences of health and well-being.

Some evidence exists to demonstrate that communities which are more cohesive, characterized by strong social bonds and ties are more likely to maintain and sustain health even in the face of disadvantage (Putnam 1995; Kawachi et al. 1997).

The cohesiveness of a community measured by a set of strong and positive interlocking networks and their positive impact on well-being may be seen as a health asset. In this instance, the asset has the potential to be health promoting irrespective of the levels of disadvantage in that community.

Supporting the development of strong cohesive communities is now commonplace in many government strategies to tackle health inequities and most people working with local populations realise that good community capacity is a necessary condition for the development, implementation and maintenance of effective interventions (Morgan and Popay 2007). However, Jordan et al. (1998) argues that whilst the nature and extent of public involvement in determining the most appropriate ways of developing health has increased, the quality of consultation remains questionable. One reason for this is that policy makers under heavy pressure to achieve very specific national policy targets may feel that the involvement of the community is time consuming and that they can suffer a loss of control. This can lead to community involvement activities becoming tokenistic and separated from the main decision making processes of professionals.

Another problem associated with poor community involvement is that professionals tend to define communities by their deficiencies and needs. These needs are often translated into deficiency-orientated policies and programmes which rightly identify the problems and try to address them. A possible downside to this approach is highlighted by Kretzmann and McKnight (1993), who claim, from their work with communities, that many low-income urban neighbourhoods have become environments of service where behaviours are affected because residents come to believe that their well-being depends upon being a client. They therefore suggest that rather than focus on deficits an alternative approach would be to develop policies and activities based on the assets, capabilities and the skills of people and their neighbourhoods.

Learning how to ask what communities have to offer begins a process of building and developing local capacities for creating health. It brings knowledge, skills, and capacities out into the open, where they can work together to everyone's benefit. As the web of assets grows, so does the potential for the community to work with professionals as co-producers of health, which can also contribute to a sense of belonging and more cohesive communities.

Community asset mapping processes, as outlined by Kretzmann and McKnight, help to initiate a process that fully mobilizes communities to use their assets around a vision and a plan to solve their own problems. They illustrate the differences between the traditional approach to assessing need and the asset approach, which identifies the following distinct categorisations for asset identification:

- *Primary building blocks*: assets and capacities located inside the neighbourhood and largely under neighbourhood control (e.g. skills, talents and experience of residents, citizen associations etc).
- *Secondary building blocks*: assets located within the community but largely controlled by outsiders (physical resources such as vacant land, energy and waste resources; public institutions and services).
- *Potential building blocks*: resources originating outside the neighbourhood outside the neighbourhood controlled by outsiders (e.g. public capital improvement expenditures).

Guy et al. (2002) promote asset mapping as a positive, realistic (starting with what the community has) and inclusive approach to building the strengths of local communities towards health improvements for all. Asset maps provide a starting point for taking action in a way which builds trust between professionals and local communities.

Asset mapping is therefore a key step in the process of implementing well-intentioned policies aiming to tackle health inequities. Good health needs assessment should provide a means of identifying the health assets and needs of a given population to inform decisions about service delivery. Combined with more traditional ways of measuring need, asset mapping can provide health promoters with an understanding of how best to create the conditions required to maximise the potential for health.

Asset mapping also helps us to conceptualise what is "salutogenic" – health enhancing in the contexts of people's physical, emotional, economic and cultural environments. In doing so, it begins the process of identifying the most appropriate "asset indicators" to be used in the evaluation of strategies aiming to create the conditions for health.

1.6 Assets and Evaluation

The asset model encourages the use of a new set of indicators to evaluate those programmes and initiatives that are developed to promote health and the reduction of health inequities, as defined in this article. Work is already under way to classify a set of "salutogenic" indicators that can be used for this purpose (Bauer et al. 2006). The development of these indicators is the first step in producing a revitalised evidence base developed through an asset approach to health and development.

The next, perhaps more challenging, step is to find appropriate methods and means of evaluating these programmes to help demonstrate the value in investing in the asset based approach. Some of this evidence already exists, however, as Hunter and Killoran (2004) note, much of the relevant evidence base available to provide answers on the best way of tackling inequities does not match the traditional requirements in evidence based medicine. Evidence arising from a "salutogenic" approach to health and development probably lies in this domain.

Savedoff et al. (2006) argue that this evaluation gap has arisen because governments and official donors do not demand or produce enough impact evaluations which aim to tell us the types of social interventions that succeed, and those which are commissioned are often methodologically flawed.

In addition, whilst there is much rhetoric in policy and research about the need to employ a multidisciplinary approach to finding evidence about the social determinants of health, the positivist model of synthesising evidence on the whole remains in the biomedical tradition.

The asset model uses an evaluation framework that follows the general shifts in policy thinking over the last few years which have refocused interventions (Hills 2004):

- From a disease prevention model targeting morbidity and mortality to a more positive approach targeting general health and well-being.
- From a model of single disease causality to a multiple dynamic model of health and its determinants.
- From individual style interventions to more community based and system level interventions.
- From the notion of passive recipients of health programmes to a more active public participation movement in health.

The asset model approach to evaluation endorses the framework put forward by Wimbush and Watson (2000) which demonstrates that there are many stages and forms of evaluation which contribute to the development of effective interventions. They call for a more explicit expression of the types of questions that need answering, for whom and for what purpose. Focusing evaluations on outcomes and effectiveness may meet the information needs of strategic planners but often fall short of answering questions for stakeholders involved in other parts of the implementation chain. In addition, as Koelen et al. (2001) argue, "methods of research have to be determined, among others, by the purpose of the study the context and the setting, the theoretical perspectives, the applicability of the measurement tools and the input of community participants."

More emphasis on evaluation that helps us to understand the mechanisms of change and the underpinning theories upon which programmes are based may help us to overcome the evaluation gap on how best to tackle health inequities. Pawson and Tilley's (1997) notion of realistic evaluation is helpful as it promotes theory-driven evaluations which help to capture the linkages between the context (the necessary conditions for an intervention to trigger mechanisms), mechanisms (what is it about a particular intervention that leads to a particular outcome in a given context) and outcomes (the practical effects produced by causal mechanisms being triggered in a given context).

The values of the asset model fit comfortably with these approaches to evaluation. Its framework for evaluation incorporates an analysis of different stakeholder perspectives, in particular, the voices of local communities in the evaluation process, and addresses the need to ask questions not only about what works, but for whom and in what circumstances. In doing so, it draws on a range of approaches and methods to produce a single coherent model for assessing the effectiveness of "salutogenic" approaches to health and development.

The asset model evaluation framework also answers the call by Hunter and Killoran (2004) for interventions to reflect theoretical approaches to understanding social and environmental sources of structural inequities. As many of the important assets for health and development lie within these domains, it promotes the need to answer questions of how these factors interrelate, how they are mediated and how they are constructed over an individual life history.

The asset model encourages the art of systematic reviewing to pay more attention to how different kinds of evidence can be brought together to help with the task of piecing together an "evidence jigsaw" (Whitehead et al. 2004). Such a "jigsaw" would encompass different types of evidence – for example, evidence about the potential effectiveness of policies (from experimental, quasi-experimental, and observational studies); evidence on the diagnosis and/or causes of problems that could contribute to the development of appropriate interventions/programmes; and evidence on costs and cost-effectiveness.

Therefore, it may not be a lack of evidence that is necessarily the problem, but the ways in which we conceptualise issues and where we look to find the evidence. Judd et al. (2001) advocates a shift away from a pathogenic risk factor and outcomes-orientated perspective of evaluation towards a more balanced menu of possible targets for change and accompanying standards for defining success. They argue that this is not at odds with standards that are systematic and supportive of accountability. A more "salutogenic" approach to evaluation will allow the process and outcomes of community based evaluations to be relevant to community stakeholders, policy makers and funders.

The asset model has the possibility to help to reconstruct better evaluation frameworks because:

- It seeks to understand the combination of factors required to effect population heath.

- It majors on the need to employ community-based approaches to health development and in so doing recognises that evaluations should articulate process, impact and experience.

1.7 Conclusions

The values and principles of the asset model reflect those originally articulated in the Ottawa Charter (WHO 1986). In particular, it emphasises the need to strengthen local communities – the model, through asset mapping, promotes the process of community empowerment to encourage *"their ownership and control of their own endeavours and destinies"* (McKnight 1995). It also supports the development of personal skills through its "salutogenic" approach to health development. It creates supportive environments by helping to identify the key assets which generate living and working conditions that are safe, stimulating, satisfying and enjoyable.

Many of the key assets required for creating the conditions for health lie within the social context of people's lives and therefore it has the potential to contribute to reducing health inequities.

It has the potential to revitalise the evidence-base for public health by helping politicians, policy makers, researchers and practitioners rethink how to conceptualise the concept of health to:

- Raise the self-esteem and resourcefulness of individuals to improve and sustain their own health.
- Provide mechanisms to ensure that all policies and programmes aimed at tackling health inequities take account of the positive attributes already existing in individuals and communities.
- Improve the efficiency of organisations to contribute to the overall well-being of the communities they serve.

The asset model presented here aims to revitalise how policy makers, researchers and practitioners think and act to promote a more resourceful approach to tackling health inequities. The model outlines a systematic approach to asset based public health which can provide scientific evidence and best practice on how to maximise the stock of key assets necessary for promoting health.

In research terms, this evidence-base needs to articulate what the most important assets are for health and development and how policy and practice can support individuals, communities and organisations to utilise them for health and development. Research is also required to convince policy makers of the economic benefits of investing in the positive-centred asset approach. The evidence-base also needs to be drawn from the practical experiences of the people working most closely with communities to understand how these assets can be released in real life settings. If it does this, it has the potential to strengthen the evidence-base for public health, which, to date, has been dominated by deficit models of health.

Redressing the balance between the asset and deficit models for evidence-based public health could help us to unlock some of the existing barriers to effective action on health inequities. This re-balancing would help to better understand the factors that influence health and what can be done about them. It therefore promotes a positive and inclusive approach to action.

Given the increasing global context for health, the asset model also provides an opportunity for innovation and collaboration at an international level so that we can galvanise efforts to revisit existing evidence with an assets frame of reference, and to collect new data that tells us how to maximise the stock of health and development assets, both within and across countries, to help to sustain health for all now and in the future.

Previously published as: Morgan, A. & Ziglio, E. (2007). Revitalising the evidence base for public health: an assets model. Promotion & Education, Supplement 2, 17–22.

References

Acheson, D. (1998). *Independent inquiry into inequalities in health report.* London: The Stationery Office.

Antonovsky, A. (1987). *Unraveling the mystery of health. How people manage stress and stay well.* San Francisco: Jossey-Bass.

Antonovsky, A. (1996). The salutogenic model as a theory to guide health promotion. *Health Promotion International* vol 11, no 1, 11–18.

Bartley, M., (Ed.) (2006). *Capability and resilience: beating the odds.* UCL., London: University College London. http://www.ucl.ac.uk/capabilityandresilience/beatingtheoddsbook.pdf cited May 2009.

Bauer, G., Davies, J. K., & Pelakin, J. (2006). The EUHPID health development model for the classification of public health indicators. *Health Promotion International,* vol 21, no 2, 153–159.

Department of Health. (2003). *Tackling health inequalities: a programme for action.* London: Department of Health.

Exworthy, M., Berney, L., & Powell, M. (2002). How great expectations in Westminster may be dashed locally': the local implementation of national policy on health inequalities. *Policy and Politics,* vol 30, no 1, 79–96.

Exworthy, M., Blane, D., & Marmot, M. (2003). Tackling health inequalities in the United Kingdom: the progress and pitfalls of policy. *Health Services Research,* vol 38, 1905–1922.

Guy, T., Fuller, D., & Pletsch, C. (2002). *Asset mapping: A handbook.* Ottawa, Ontario: Canadian Rural Partnership.

Harrison, D., Ziglio, E., Levin, L., & Morgan, A. (2004). *Assets for health and development: developing a conceptual framework.* European Office for Investment for Health and Development, London: World Health Organization.

Hills, D. (2004). *Evaluation of community levels interventions for health improvement: a review of experience in the UK.* Venice: Health Development Agency.

Hunter, D., & Killoran, A. (2004). *Tackling health inequalities: turning policy into practice.* London: Health Development Agency.

IUHPE. (2000). *The evidence of health promotion effectiveness: Shaping public health in a new Europe.* A report for the European Commission ECSC-EC –EXEC, Brussels. Paris: Jouve Composition & Impression.

Jordan, C., Dowswell, T., Harrison, S., Lilford, R., & Mort, M. (1998). Whose priorities? Listening to users and the public. *British Medical Journal,* vol 316, 1668–1670.

Judd, J., Frankish, J., & Moulton, G. (2001). Setting standards in the evaluation of community based health promotion programmes – a unifying approach. *Health Promotion International*, vol 16, no 4, 367–379.

Judge, K., Platt, S., Costongs, C., and Jurczak, K. (2006). *Health inequalities: a challenge for Europe.* An independent expert report commissioned by the UK Presidency of the EU. http://ec.europa.eu/health/ph_determinants/socio_economics/documents/ev_060302_rd05_en.pdf cited May 2009.

Kawachi, I., Kennedy, B. P., Lochner, K., & Prothrow-Stith, D. (1997). Social capital, income and inequality. *American Journal of Public Health*, vol 87, 1491–1498.

King, A. (2000). *The New Zealand health strategy.* Wellington: Ministry of Health.

Koelen, M., Vaandrager, L., & Colomér, C. (2001). Health promotion research: dilemmas and challenges. *Journal of Epidemiology and Community Health,* vol 55, 257–262.

Kretzmann, J. P., & McKnight, J. (1993). *Building communities from the inside out: a path towards building and mobilising a community's assets.* Evanston, IL: Institute for Policy Research.

Lindström, B., & Eriksson, M. (2005). Salutogenesis – a glossary. *Journal of Epidemiology and Community Health,* vol 59, 440–442.

Lindström, B., & Eriksson, M. (2006). Contextualising salutogenesis and Antonovsky in public health development. *Health Promotion International,* vol 212, no 3, 238–244.

Marmot, M. G., Davey Smith, G., Stansfield, S., Patel, C., North, F., Head, J., White, I., Brunner, E., & Feeney, A. (1991). Health inequalities among British civil servants; the Whitehall II study. *Lancet,* vol 337, 1387–1393.

Mackenbach, J. P., & Bakker, M. J. (2002). *Reducing inequalities in health: the European perspective.* London: Routledge.

McKnight, J. (1995). *The careless society: community and its counterfeits.* New York: Basic Books.

Ministry of Health and Social Affairs. (2003). *National public health strategy for Sweden.* Stockholm: Swedish National Institute of Public Health.

Morgan, A., & Ziglio, E. (2006). Foreword. In *Capability and resilience: beating the odds.* Department of Epidemiology and Public Health, UCL, London: University College London.

Morgan, A., & Popay, J. (2007). Community participation for health. Reducing health inequalities and building social capital. In Scriven, A., & Garman, S., *Public health: social context and action.* London: Open University Press.

Pawson, R., & Tilley, N. (1997). *Realistic Evaluation.* London: Sage.

Putnam, R. (1995). *Making democracy work. Civic traditions in modern Italy.* New Jersey: Princeton University Press.

Savedoff, W., Levine, R., & Birdsall, N. (2006). *When will we ever learn? Improving lives through impact evaluation* Report of the Evaluation Gap Working Group. Washington, DC: Centre for Global Development.

Stahl, T., Wismar, W., Ollila, E., Lahtinen, E., & Leppo, K. (Eds.) (2006). *Health in all policies: prospects and potentials.* Helsinki: Ministry of Social Affairs and Health. http://www.euro.who.int/observatory/Publications/20060915_2 cited May 2009.

Whitehead, M., Petticrew, M., Graham, H., Macintyre, S., Bambra, C., & Egan, M. (2004). Evidence for public health policy on inequalities: 2: Assembling the evidence jigsaw. *Journal of Epidemiology and Community Health,* vol 58, 817–821.

Whitehead, M., & Dahlgren, G. (2006). *Levelling up (part 1): a discussion paper on concepts and principles for tackling social inequalities in health.* Copenhagen: World Health Organization.

Wilkinson, R. G. (1996). *Unhealthy societies: The afflictions of inequality.* London: Routledge.

Wimbush, E., & Watson, J. (2000). An evaluation framework for health promotion: theory, quality and effectiveness. *Evaluation*, vol 6, no 3, 301–321.

Woodward, A., & Kawachi, I. (2000). Why reduce health inequalities? *Journal of Epidemiology and Community Health,* vol 54, 923–929.

WHO. (1986). Ottawa Charter for Health Promotion. *The Move Toward A New Public Health, Ottawa 17–21 November 1986.* World Health Organization.
WHO. (2003). *Millennium development goals. WHO's contribution to tracing progress and measuring achievements.* Geneva: World Health Organization.
WHO. (2005). *Towards a conceptual framework for analysis and action on the social determinants of health.* Geneva: World Health Organization.
Ziglio, E., Hagard, S., & Griffiths, J. (2000). Health promotion development in Europe: achievements and challenges. *Health Promotion International*, vol 15, no 2, 143–154.

Chapter 2
A Salutogenic Approach to Tackling Health Inequalities

Bengt Lindström and Monica Eriksson

Keywords African tribes • Post-modern (society) • Ottawa charter • WHO healthy city project • Learning • Sense of coherence • Quality of Life

2.1 Introduction

In the 1960s the anthropologist Colin M. Turnbull wrote two books that raised much debate – "The Forest People" and "The Mountain People" (Turnbull 1961; Turnbull 1972). The books were about two African tribes, the first living in its original habitat in the forest, thriving and deeply rooted in its culture, rituals and mastery of life in spite of the hard living conditions of the jungle. The other tribe had been driven from its original habitat by "the modern development", to face hunger, disease, and a struggle for survival. The mountain people finally lost their pride and culture, this first created internal conflicts and manslaughter, at the end, a state of mental collapse and total apathy. The debate in the 1960s was about the right to write about the death of a culture in such a depressing way. This still was a time of hope and dreams of a prosperous, independent future in Africa and the ending of colonisation.

Looking back 40 years later at Africa, with the endless series of civil wars, the exploitation and misuse of resources and on top of it the HIV/AIDS catastrophe, one could argue that the picture Turnbull painted was closer to real life than he had ever expected. As an anthropologist he used his stories to draw painful parallels from the developing world and phenomena within Western cultures to highlight universal trends. The state of the mountain people is similar to what has been called the "concentration camp disease" where people just give up because they have lost their meaning in life. On the other hand, we have the stories of people who in spite of these hardships never lose their motivation and out of this hopeless situation create a meaning. This meaning enables them, not only to survive, but to carry on with

B. Lindström (✉)
Folkhälsan Research Centre, Helsinki, Finland and Nordic School of Public Health, Gothenburg, Sweden
e-mail: bengt.lindstrom@folkhalsan.fi

A. Morgan et al. (eds.), *Health Assets in a Global Context: Theory, Methods, Action*, DOI 10.1007/978-1-4419-5921-8_2, © Springer Science+Business Media, LLC 2010

life in full mental and spiritual well-being. This phenomenon came under scientific study about 25 years ago and created the framework for salutogenic research (Antonovsky 1979, 1987). We have just completed a systematic study of salutogenesis and found that there is a strong correlation to mental well-being and quality of life in populations and individuals who have developed a strong sense of coherence – the key mechanism in the salutogenic model. The model has been tested in at least 32 different countries in 33 languages and it was found that the model works in all these diverse cultures (Eriksson and Lindström 2005, 2006).

2.2 Background

The focus of this book is the concepts and models conducive to positive health. One would wish there were universal features and models within health promotion that could be helpful on a global scale and support the general development of mankind. Besides the description of so called "positive concepts" of health our aim here is to look for universal concepts and solutions. At the same time postulating that many of the post-modern trends that upset mental stability are global features that either directly or indirectly influence all countries of the world. It is also clear that Western cultures have a strong focus on the individual and the protection of the rights of the individual as stated in the United Nations (UN) Declaration of Human Rights, as compared to cultures where the collective efforts are considered more important than the individual. From the perspective of health promotion this can make a huge difference, as the emphasis on either the collective or the individual creates different prerequisites for health, including mental health.

2.3 The Present: From Modernity to Post-Modernity

The literature of post-modern or late-modern society is today abundant but diverse (Bauman 1989; Giddens 1990, 1991). While ancient society was based on mythical and religious beliefs, the Modernity from the Enlightenment period until present day holds the rational and logical perspective of science as the ultimate tool for the explanation of reality, in its smallest detail. While public health develops as a construct of modernity. Post-modernity again deals with the deconstruction of society in all respects; everything from the society's central institutions to central values. The world is seen as ahistorical and deinstitutionalised, driven by the subjective ethics of the individual. More moderate theories say that we are in a transition period called the late-modern period (Giddens 1990, 1991). Post-modernists claim man is living in a vacuum without any view of where he is coming from or going to (Bauman 1989). The rationality and logic of science is questioned because it has proved to be unable to explain all aspects of reality. As a consequence, man turns to other models or explanations and forces (like the market or new age ideology) which compete for command of the mind. The post-modern person is alienated from the local community. Instead abstract systems, symbolic values (such as market and media) disturb this relationship and expert systems have become the power to turn to when religion lost its footing (Giddens 1990, 1991). This means that a person, instead of trusting their own judgement or their support network of family and friends, turns to expert advice which takes command of issues that ordinarily could be solved by the person himself. Thus post-modern man can be described as a vulnerable, rather confused, disillusioned person that tries to find his own way in a chaotic and fragmented existence without coherence. At the same time, Western societies carry the ideal of the individual at centre, his freedom of choice and autonomy stands above the needs of the collective (Bourdieu 1993). More activities are available per time unit than ever before, helping to create a ever complicated set of circumstances under which people are expected to build their competence for health and life.

2.4 The Issue of Health Once Again

Much of the critique around various descriptions of health has been that the concepts stem from the orientation of disease where health and disease are placed on the same axis but are diametrically opposed to each other. This would indicate that the same mechanisms would operate in the creation of disease as in the creation of health but in different directions. This is partly true but there are also other options. If one considers in more detail the elimination of a pathogenic condition (a disease) in an organism often means that the specific condition is taken out of the system with little or no consideration of the effect on the health equilibrium. The traditional World Health Organization (WHO) declaration of health from 1948 suffers from the same deficit where "health" is seen as an absolute level which is only achieved when disease is taken out of the system (WHO 1946). Health is therefore defined by the absence of disease. If we instead create a model where there are three different dimensions: disease and its opposite "contra-disease", health and its opposite "contra-health" and quality of life and its opposite "contra-quality of life", one may assume that the state of health, contra-disease and quality of life are situated in the same pole. However, one can combine the positions in any way (partly depending on the definitions of health, disease and quality of life). For example, a person with a high quality of life may have a low degree of health and a high degree of disease, or a person who perceives she has a high degree of well-being in spite of suffering from a disease and limitations of functions. In the same way there are people with a low quality of life who can have a high degree of health and no disease. In fact, one can imagine any combination of the three dimensions.

The WHO only included a fourth dimension, spiritual well-being, to the physical, social and mental dimensions in the 1980s (Mahler 1987). Today, health is seen as an asset for everyday life and not an end product. This is stated in the Ottawa Charter (WHO 1986) on health promotion where health is seen as the process that can lead to the fulfilment of people's life goals. "*Health promotion is the process which enables people to gain control over their health determinants in order to improve their health and thereby be able to live an active and productive life*" (WHO 1986).

One can see this process as three phases, the first recognises the background (the determinants), while the second sets an objective (to lead an active productive life). The third phase is the activity (the enabling process) where the determinants are used to reach the objective in a dialectic relationship between people, the setting and the enablers. While at the heart there is the active, participating human being.

In general there is much more knowledge and information on what causes disease and the treatment of these conditions (the pathogenic orientation) than on what causes and then maintains and develops good health (the salutogenic orientation). Only recently there has been concrete theoretical and empirical constructions oriented towards the salutogenic framework, the most well known is Antonovsky's framework (Antonovsky 1979, 1987).

2.5 An Interdisciplinary Framework to Health?

It is possible that the concept of mental health needs to be examined from other, and joint perspectives, rather than simply as a health science in order to be fully understood (Klein 1990). One approach may be the theory and practice of interdisciplinarity which has evolved as a theoretical framework over the last century.

Klein describes interdisciplinary work as being a way of:

- Answering complex questions
- Addressing broad issues
- Exploring disciplinary and professional relations
- Solving problems that are beyond one discipline
- Achieving unity of knowledge on a limited or grand scale

The understanding of any societal mental health discourse is a complex question involving history, macro-politics, socio-economic development culture and traditions of both individual nations and continents as a whole. Interdisciplinary research has a history over the past century involving most social sciences and especially educational sciences supported by many scientists, intellectuals and organisations (such as the Organisation for Economic Co-operation and Development (OECD), and United Nations Educational, Scientific and Cultural Organization (UNESCO)). It has been particularly apparent in the critical movements such as structuralism and deconstruction (Lévi-Strauss, Foucault, Kuhn among others). The strength of the interdisciplinarity is the integrative approach.

The health sciences have had such a strong disease orientation that it becomes difficult to look beyond this approach. A typical example of this problem is the use of the quality of life concept in health and medical research. After its introduction, there was a brief period of a broader understanding of the quality of life concept but it is now dominated by the so called "health-related quality of life" research, actually evaluating the effect of medical interventions on people's quality of life. This is good and relevant research but it should rather be called disease-oriented quality of life research, as the concept of positive health has been lost.

2.6 Welfare as a Prerequisite for Well-Being

Welfare within the industrialised world after World War II was increasing at a stable rate until the early 1970s. Material living conditions also improved for the majority of the population. In sociology, the negative effects of economic growth raised the question of other welfare measurements besides the gross national product (GNP) per capita.

Although concepts such as the standard and level of living have been used since the early twentieth century, they were not defined before the UN published a report on "International Definition and Measurement of Standards and Levels of Living" (1954). This report stated that the best way of defining the level of living in a population is to quantify clearly defined aspects, or parts of the individuals' life situation, correlating to the objectives of the UN Charter. The UN attempted to find a composite measurement to describe components of different life spheres of the population. The components chosen represented the aims of the different UN organisations. Standard of living was later defined as:

> The level of satisfaction of needs of the population assured by the flow of goods and services enjoyed in a unit of time or…the extent to which the overall needs of the population are satisfied.
>
> (Johansson 1970)

The first studies using these measures were conducted in the UK and West Germany, where indicators such as the extent of ownership of TV, cars, telephones etc., were used. The UN has later been criticised for the over-emphasis on the importance of consumer goods.

The OECD in Europe developed a system of measuring social development. This activity has later been combined with similar activities within the UN. The economic recession in the mid-1970s increased the interest to develop compound social indicators. These were developed through a process of, firstly by developing a list of social concerns, secondly by developing indicators and thirdly by field testing. The first list of indicators was published in 1973 (List of Social Concerns Common to Most OECD Countries) and was revised in 1982 (The OECD list of Social Indicators 2009). The latter includes the following indicators:

1. General Context Indicators
2. Self-sufficiency Indicators
3. Equity Indicators
4. Health Indicators
5. Social Cohesion Indicators

In the Nordic countries, Sweden was the first to apply studies on the level of living. The emphasis was on finding and describing the living conditions of the general population with special focus on low income groups. The perspectives used were distribution of resources and individual control, and the level of living standards were defined as:

> The individuals' disposition of monetary resources, goods, knowledge, physical, mental energy, social relations, security …, which enable the individuals to control and consciously influence the conditions. The components that were considered relevant in the late 1960s

> in Sweden were: health, nutritional patterns, housing, conditions of upbringing, family relations, education, employment, working conditions, economic resources, political resources, leisure time and recreation.
>
> (Johansson 1970)

The Swedish study influenced subsequent Norwegian, Finnish and Danish national studies of living conditions. Completed in 1975, the Finnish study was a comparative Nordic study, which also explicitly uses the term of quality of life. The study, entitled "Having, Loving and Being", defined welfare as: *"a state where people are able to satisfy their central needs"* (Allardt et al. 1980).

Allardt et al. (1980) described two dimensions of welfare: the material and the non-material. The level of living is set by the degree of satisfaction of material needs while well-being is defined by satisfaction of non-material needs. The dimensions of standard of living and quality of life are given in Table 2.1.

The level of living (having) is defined in material (objective) resources and the individuals' satisfaction with these (subjective). Quality of life (loving and being) is defined by the individuals as satisfaction of non-material needs in relation to other people, society and nature.

In the United States a somewhat similar tradition developed. The focus of interest was perceived satisfaction in respect to different spheres of life. Campbell defined quality of life as a subjective measure describing how people experience their lives (Campbell et al. 1976). Objective conditions of life were considered less important. The central concepts in Campbell's research were satisfaction and happiness.

A combination of both subjective and objective data was introduced by Andrews and Whitney developing measures of "perceived life quality" (Andrews and Whitney 1976). Life is divided into different roles (working life, housing, family, companionship) and different values (success, beauty, freedom, happiness) and a combination of the above. Statistical analyses resulted in 12 factors important to the individual's quality of life: the individual's experience of: (1) self-concept, (2) family life, (3) economy, (4) life enjoyment, (5) housing, (6) family activities, (7) disposition

Table 2.1 "Welfare" having – loving – being

	Objective indicators (needs)	Subjective indicators (wants)
Emphasis on the material and impersonal	Level of living: objective measures of material or impersonal resources	Dissatisfaction: subjective feelings of satisfaction – dissatisfaction as regards the material living conditions
Emphasis on the non-material and social	Quality of life: objective measures as regards people's relation to 1. Other people 2. Society 3. Nature	Happiness: subjective feelings of happiness

Allardt et al. (1980)

of personal time, (8) leisure time activities, (9) government, (10) local access to goods and human services, (11) health, (12) occupation. Originally 100 different spheres were analysed and about 5,000 people were interviewed.

In the Nordic countries, as a critique to Allardt and Johansson the Swedish sociologist, Swedner, developed a model he calls "Take-Have-Give" where both qualitative and quantitative methods are used to describe the social reality of people (Swedner 1983). According to this model, "health" is something the individual achieves and maintains (have). In order to be able to accomplish this, resources are actively taken from the immediate surroundings (take). Quality of life is defined within the activity arena (give) (love, self-respect, appreciation, self-realization). This model considers individuals as social beings. A good quality of life is achieved when social networks are functioning and psychological needs are fulfilled.

To achieve a high standard of living the individual has to be satisfied within the following life areas: physical capability, ability of social contact, knowledge, working skills, influence on physical environment, power, ability to reach set objectives. These resources can be used to reach certain objectives both on the individual level (happiness or joy) and on a group level (companionship, security, solidarity). These life objectives are considered to be the qualities of life, which describe the existence of an individual or a group (Swedner 1983). Do people who live in welfare states perceive they have a high state of mental health or well-being? This question is difficult to answer.

Subjective well-being has such a strong cultural component. However, one can see that the welfare states have provided dimensions that improve physical and social well-being and Denmark and Sweden, with well established welfare states, rank repeatedly among the first in the world in relation to happiness or subjective well-being. Whilst it is impossible to talk about direct causal relationships, there is evidence that interventions at community level improve and increase mental well-being. The strongest evidence comes from the WHO healthy city project where a controlled intervention in a city proved that providing multilevel resources increased levels of satisfaction and optimism of the population (de Leeuw 2003).

In social science, quality of life has been included in the concept of "welfare" to describe mainly non-material human needs or perceived well-being or "loving" and "being". Human activities or "doing" and "giving" in the sense of self-realisation and self-respect and respect for others have later been introduced as quality of life concepts.

There are some additional theoretical aspects that can be useful in this context of finding coherence for systems. They have served as inspiration but are not further explored in this chapter. These are the concept of "habitus" by Bourdieu (Bourdieu 1993) (which relates to a common collective consciousness), and Bronfenbrenner's ecological development model (combining micro, meso and macro systems) (Bronfenbrenner 1979).

Some concepts have recently come to the fore within health promotion research. These are the concepts of social capital and empowerment. Social capital identifies the social resources of a person in terms of human relationships. Social capital and networks have always been difficult to study and quantify empirically. While Diderichsen and Whitehead make a distinction between vertical and horizontal social capital (Whitehead and Diderichsen 2001).

Horizontal social capital relates to people's intimate and immediate human relationships. In terms of health, horizontal social capital seems to promote mental and psychological well-being and the individual's self-esteem. Vertical social capital refers to how the individual relates to horizontal social capital and other social levels such as neighbourhood, local community, city, region and nation. This notion is similar to the concept "connectedness" used in resilience research in school age children. Connectedness seems to promote both physical and mental health and school success. The instrument is developed by the United Nations Children's Fund (UNICEF) and has been tested in over 60 different countries with similar positive results (Blum,[1] personal communication, 2001).

The next concept central to the health promotion process itself is the principle and theory of empowerment (Freire 1970; Rappaport 1987). Freire used empowerment as a way of learning, focusing on populations that have difficulties in acquiring learning in ordinary institutions. He was working on the reduction on inequity by learning and mobilising the uneducated. He was for a period expelled from his country, Brazil, because his government became afraid of the revolutionary component in his learning philosophy regarding redistribution of power. Empowerment is about giving people control and mastery over their own lives; similar to the enabling process in health promotion. It is about the development of abilities and coping skills and endowing people with the ability to enable and to work for active critical consciousness-raising. It is also a democratic concept looking at the structure of power and a process of professional activity and a relinquishment of the professional power.

2.7 Can Learning Be Conducive to Mental Well-Being?

Like empowerment, the learning process itself can promote well-being, if it is carried out according to the principles of health promotion. Learning, in its broadest context, is the interaction between a person (the actor) and the world (the structure) and mediated by activity or other people producing coherent knowledge. The way people are treated by others in learning situations will affect their well-being. The science of learning is complex not easily transferable due to its strong associations with culture and traditions. For instance, the way mothers in Bali socialise their children by completely neglecting the child if it expresses its demands through aggression or crying would, in a Western context, be an indication of severe neglect. Another comparison between countries with students with a similar high level of mathematical skills, found different teaching methods were used. In the Netherlands, teachers tended to provide students with models for solutions, while in Japan the teachers first let the students try to find their own solutions. In both countries, students have excellent mathematical skills, yet it doesn't necessarily follow that the

[1]Professor Robert Blum, Department of Population, Family and Reproductive Health, Johns Hopkins Bloomberg School of Public Health.

Dutch students would become even better if the teachers adopted Japanese learning strategies. This is because the teachers' learning methods are indicative of the countries' individual cultures (Stigler,[2] personal communication, 2003).

Learning can be superficial, particularly where people are taught simply to memorise, without real understanding. Some have better skills (genetic or acquired) to memorise than others, however people tend to forget details after only a short period of time. Therefore, if teaching is to be effective, sustainable and correlated to mental well-being, superficial learning corresponding mainly to cognitive intelligence is not recommended as a learning principle for health promotion.

The effects of learning are also related to the micro-culture of the student, i.e. social class and belonging. If these facts are not considered, learning can be ineffective and exclusive. Most schools are constructed around a non-differentiated learning model where the ones who come from a family background and social class with "school intelligence" are favoured as these children already have a "learning culture" to do well in schools. Schools could therefore unwillingly increase social and health differences (Rutter 1980; Nutbeam 1993; Nilsson 2003). Another approach is so-called in-depth-comprehension or deep-learning. In deep-learning there is a focus on connecting what is taught to the background and culture of the ones who are learning. In addition, deep-learning not only favours cognitive intelligence but also responds to the other qualities of intelligence (Gardner 1991).

Effective learning is related to the contents, the methods of delivery, the setting (context) including the emotional climate, the quality and relationship between learner and teacher and finally to the form of evaluation or outcome. Today it is considered that it is more effective to let students construct their own knowledge and integrate that into their value-system rather than being fed with ready-made facts. "Evidence based learning" exists in several forms and has to be adapted according to several of the factors mentioned previously creating wholeness, coherence and mental well-being (Lindström and Nafstad 2003). Effective learning is stimulated via a variation of methods, which should be shaped and defined through constant evaluation.

2.8 Positive Concepts of Mental Health Within Social Psychology

More than 40 years ago Marie Jahoda presented a report "Current concepts of positive mental health" (Jahoda 1958). The task was given by the US Joint Commission on Mental Illness and Health to find an evidence base to support decisions regarding the reconstruction of mental health services in the US. The report concluded that the most common definition of mental health is the absence of mental illness. Another approach was to use normality, either as a statistical normal phenomena or as a

[2]Professor Stephen M. Stigler, Department of Statistics, University of Chicago.

normative idea of how the human being should function. Jahoda voiced scepticism about both approaches, pointing out the danger of cultural definitions of normality such as those prevalent in Nazi Germany (she herself had been forced to flee Austria because of the German Anschluss).

Jahoda's report included six topics (all of which individually, or in combinations, were thought to serve as criteria for mental health):

1. Attitudes of the individual towards herself
2. The development of self-esteem
3. The degree of the integration of personality
4. The level of individual autonomy
5. The sense of reality
6. The ability of the individual to adapt to the environment

She then postulated what conditions characterise a state of good mental health. There is a need for: a positive self-concept; an ability to be active and to develop individual talents; to be an integrated person; to be able to take individual decisions and actions without isolating oneself from other people; to have an adequate perception of reality and good emphatic skills; and finally to be able to create deep and lasting relationships to other persons (at least one to a person of the opposite sex). However, there has been little use of Jahoda's work in practice.

The Norwegian psychologist, Siri Naess, created the concept "inner quality of life" equal to mental well-being (Naess 1974, 1987, 1979). The criteria for a good inner quality of life are based on a normative value system structured around a theoretical analysis. According to Naess the inner quality of life increases when the individual:

1. Is active
2. Has good interpersonal relations
3. Feels self-esteem
4. Has a basic mood of joy

These concepts are defined as:

1. *Active in the sense of*: being interested and engaged in something outside yourself (hobby, work, politics, religion, art) which you experience as meaningful, having an appetite for life.
2. *Self-esteem in the sense of*: knowing yourself, feeling good as a human being, being aware of your skills, feeling useful, satisfied with your achievements, morally valuable and reaching set standards.
3. *Good interpersonal relations in the sense of*: having a close, mutual and warm relationship to at least one human being, having an active satisfying sexual relation, finding friendship and loyalty and a feeling of participation and belonging (to friends, neighbours, working companions, friends).
4. *Joyful state of mood in the sense of*: having rich intense feelings of beauty, feeling close to nature, open and receptive, secure, harmonious, the absence of worry, anxiety and restlessness, a state of joy and compassion, finding life rich and rewarding, the absence of emptiness, depression, pain and discomfort.

The values are not ranked hierarchically but are all considered equally important (Naess 1974). Naess (1979) argues that society as a whole benefits more from allocating resources to children than to other population groups. This is because children have a long life ahead of them and they will be able to influence their own children who again will have children. On a population basis, the middle-aged group probably has the greatest resources available while the elderly have least resources at their disposal. Hypothetically, a society could use this argument and allocate such resources to increase the quality of life in the elderly. This intervention enhances the quality of life of the elderly but they can never reach the level of the general population. Sooner or later, the quality of life of other groups would decrease. Schools and day-care services for children would suffer, which would have a negative effect on the general quality of life of the population in the long term. Therefore investment in children would provide the best value for money.

Obviously, Naess' value system can create strong individuals or groups that have little solidarity towards society as a whole. A further development of Naess' ideas towards a system considering both the inner quality of life concept and external factors has been made by Kajandi: *"In spite of all, man is a social being, living in a social context in groups and societies out of the simple reason that this promotes survival and welfare. A central component of the quality of life is thus the sense of contribution to the best of the group and society by individual labour"* (Kajandi 1981). As a consequence Kajandi added the external conditions of life where work, the personal economy and housing are the central concepts. Thus, three spheres of life are included in Kajandi's model: external conditions (work, economy, housing), interpersonal relations (intimate relationships, friendships, family relations), inner psychological conditions (activity, self-concept, basic mood). The inner psychological conditions include: activity, self-image and basic state of mood (joy). These concepts are almost identical to the model that Naess created and are therefore not repeated here.

To conclude, quality of life in psychology was initially used to set objectives for people's mental well-being, based on theoretical analyses and normative value systems. Quality of life is described in life spheres where the psychological dimension represents the personal sphere (Naess et al. 1979), the interpersonal sphere describes social relationships and the external sphere socioeconomic conditions (Kajandi 1981). The model was developed further by Lindström for public health and health promotion including four life spheres as seen in Table 2.2 below (Lindström 1994).

This quality of life model is a development of Naess' and Kajandi's models. Naess (1974) described a value based model for "inner quality of life" using mental and social components. This was related to a socioeconomic context by Kajandi (1981). Here the model is expanded into four life spheres: The global, external, interpersonal and personal sphere. These components can be adapted universally to any human context: every person has a physical, mental and spiritual dimension representing the personal sphere. This is experienced in a context of social relationships and support, i.e. the interpersonal sphere which again has a socioeconomic context, i.e. the external sphere.

Finally there is a macro level including a society and its culture in a geophysical context, i.e. the global level. This general quality of life model needs to be further operationalised for the individual or population approached. This model has

Table 2.2 A general quality of life model, life spheres and dimensions

Spheres	Dimensions (objective/ subjective)	Examples
Global: ecological, societal and political resources	1. Macro environment 2. Culture 3. Human rights 4. Welfare policies	Physical environment, respect for human rights, equity, resource allocation
External: social and economical resources	1. Work 2. Income 3. Housing	Education, employment, economy, standard of housing. Satisfaction with these conditions
Interpersonal: resources in social relationships and support	1. Family structure and function 2. Intimate friends 3. Extended social support	Size of family, friends, intimate relationships, support from neighbours and society. Satisfaction with above
Personal: personal resources	1. Physical 2. Mental 3. Spiritual	Growth, activity, self-esteem and basic mood, meaning of life

Lindström (1994)

recently been suggested as an instrument in the evaluation of the effectiveness of health promotion (Raphael 2002).

Another model of similar value is the Canadian model: "Being, belonging and becoming", which has a clearer process orientation (Raphael 2002). Quality of life is here considered as a dynamic, holistic and complex multidimensional phenomenon, based on a deep and equal respect for the individual and his/her own expression, which is the outcome of interactions between the person and the environmental context. Hence the quality of life developed by the Canadian Centre for Health Promotion is:

> ... the degree to which the person enjoys the important possibilities of his or her life. (Rootman et al. 1992)

2.9 Methodological Problems in Assessment of Happiness, Well-Being and Quality of Life

There are many problems involved in the assessment of quality of life, subjective well-being or happiness. According to Heal and Sigelman cited by Shalock there are four major ways in which methods for assessing well-being can differ (Shalock 1990). Firstly, measures can be objective and/or subjective. Secondly, they can be absolute or relative, i.e. either directly index people's quality of life or compare it to an optimum standard. Thirdly, quality of life can be reported directly by the subjects of study or assessed by someone else (by an informant or a proxy such as a relative, friend or by the investigator). This method is used when it is difficult to get a direct reply from the subject because of developmental reasons or communication difficulties.

Finally, the measure can be generated by the investigator or by the subject of study. Measures can be objective, i.e. focus on conditions (such as standard of housing, income and level of education) or subjective, i.e. focus on perceived satisfaction with life in general or with specific conditions of life. Objective measures can be evaluated externally while the subjective ones need an internal evaluation.

Historically, in quality of life studies, only objective measures have tended to be used but today subjective or combined subjective-objective measurements are more common. There are several difficulties involved in the interpretation of the subjective dimensions and the perceived quality of life. Individuals, cultures and nations have different levels of aspirations and also different ways of expressing satisfaction. This means that people can express higher or lower levels of satisfaction with exactly the same objective circumstances. Generally people with low incomes and low education or older people tend to idealize their conditions, i.e. express more socially desirable levels of subjective well-being (de Maio 1984). However the effect on self-reported assessments has been shown to be small (Atkinson 1982; Crowne and Marlowe 1964), and the use of anonymous questionnaires also reduces this tendency (Naess 1987).

On the individual level there are people who tend to agree or disagree with whatever is being asked (so-called yay- or naysayers). It has been shown that subjective well-being measured as an overall life satisfaction on a national level is fairly consistent. Nineteen countries participating in a survey on life satisfaction, repeated over 10 years, kept almost the same rank order over time. Denmark and Sweden held the top positions (Ingelhart and Rabier 1985), while Japan and Greece ranked the lowest. No developing countries participated in the survey.

On the individual level, longitudinal studies have shown that subjective global well-being (or basic mood) is fairly consistent in spite of intermediate negative or positive life events. Life events have a time-limited effect on the subjective wellbeing (Veenhofen 1991). People tend to readjust to base levels quicker when positive, rather than negative life events have occurred (Lazarus and Lannier 1979).

In studies where several subjective measurements are used they have been found to correlate more strongly to each other than to the actual objective indices of quality of life (Mastekaasa et al. 1988). Children create a special problem in the assessment of subjective well-being, because their responses tend to be more inconsistent over time (Shalock 1990).

The measure of quality of life can be generated by the investigator or by the subjects of investigation (Campbell et al. 1976). Campbell used this latter method asking the population what areas of life were perceived as most important using about 100 alternatives and through various statistical methods ended up with 12 areas later used in interviews. Flanagan (1982) asked people of different socioeconomic and age groups about critical life incidences that had enhanced or worsened their life and arrived at five general dimensions of quality of life: physical and material well-being; relations with other people; social activities; personal development and recreation. Naess (1979) used a philosophical argumentation approach to design an instrument for the measurement of "inner quality of life". This method represents a value-based method which was also used by Kajandi (1981) but in combination with external life conditions.

A major decision in the study of quality of life is the choice between the individual approach and the population approach. Most quality of life research is based on individuals where their personal needs, functions and preferences are assessed. One of the limitations of the individual approaches is the difficulty of generalizing the findings to a whole population group. The population approach defines general characteristics of a group of people, and assesses the quality of life conditions that are important for this population. Thereby a standard or norm for such a population is formed. Each quality of life indicator is standardized on the basis of what is good or bad for the population (Shalock 1990). In this process a base value has to be set for each variable.

In welfare studies such base values or "floor values" have mainly been used to register problems, e.g., the number of children living in poverty (Allardt et al. 1980). The quality of life approach focuses on people's resources, thus the quality of life base values measure how well people are doing. It is possible to use life-enhancing mechanisms such as in the salutogenic approach, i.e. defining general resistance resources of a population (Antonovsky 1979, 1987).

Thus, if the objective is to establish an acceptable base level for the population, it is less interesting to describe groups that do extremely well or extremely badly. According to Mastekaasa the increase of a certain variable, such as an increase in economic resources, is not always positively correlated to quality of life (Mastekaasa et al. 1988; Naess et al. 1979). Up to a certain level the increase can have a positive influence on quality of life but this is not always constant. Sometimes a further increase can have no, or even a negative effect on quality of life (Ventegodt 1995).

It is possible to weight variables depending on their presumed importance. However, weights have seldom been used since it is difficult to find objective weighting criteria. One way to reduce this difficulty is to avoid variables that represent people's preferences and concentrate instead on variables that give people choices (Ringen 1988).

Finally, people in different societies live under different conditions and have different requirements. Therefore, the base values vary depending on what society is studied. Nevertheless, the framework as such can be applied and in those societies with strong similarities, common base values can be used to form a quality of life standard.

2.10 The Concept of Resilience

The concept of resilience stems from psychology and is a way of explaining how people can manage life and live well in spite of adverse situations. As a scientific concept it was first developed for children and young people and has later been expanded into adulthood. The evidence base on the concept of resilience includes over 40 years of data from a longitudinal study (Werner and Smith 1982, 2001). In addition, Rutter has presented a historical development of the concept of resilience which has been defined in a number of ways (Rutter 1985). At first it was a question of demonstrating how negative life events produced developmental delays and psychiatric disorders as was demonstrated in the mental health movements of the early twentieth century. Resilience was put on the agenda again after World War II through Bowlby's studies of separations and negative factors leading to psychiatric disorders (Bowlby 1979). Later the focus was on the conceptualization of various types of life events and their effects and how personal losses or environmental threats lead to psychiatric problems. According to Rutter, the risk potential of different life experiences varied in their impact on cognitive and behavioral development.

More recently, it was demonstrated there were many children who, in spite of these extreme conditions in their environment, still managed to develop normally. It was not only a question of the quality and quantity of life events but of factors related to the individual and the context. This lead to the concept of invulnerable children or Gidden's concept of "steel dolls", i.e. children who were constitutionally so tough they could endure almost any external pressure (Dencik 1989). However, it was later demonstrated that resistance is relative depending on both the environment and the constitution. Further, resistance is not a stable quality but varies over time and circumstances. It also became evident that there were factors that could ameliorate the impact of life events which again leads to the search for protective factors, which modify or alter a person's response to an environmental hazard.

The longest prospective study related to resiliency is a study from Kauai in Hawaii where consecutive generations have been studied over four decades (Werner and Smith 1982; Werner and Smith 2001). Fonagy et al. (1994) however, argue in a paper on the theory and practice of resilience that the first and most important key to resilience in childhood is based on the reflective dialogue, the person being confirmed, seen and respected for what she is by a trusted person or a significant other. The literature on resilience is difficult to review as it has so many entry points. In principle this research is looking for factors that enable people to develop normally in spite of adverse life conditions. Firstly, factors related to the individual (genetics, age, developmental stage, gender, constitution, life experience and life history). Secondly, the context (social support, social class, culture, setting) Thirdly, the quantity and quality of life events (desirability, controllability, magnitude, clusters, time-duration and long-term effects).

In adolescence there has been a focus on how well the social arenas of the young, the family, the social and geographical context, cultural and historical context, the learning systems, finally, the work place or daily activity, are connected. Evidence shows that the connectedness of these arenas has a major impact on resilience, life success and well-being (Resnick et al. 1997). This has been studied in different ethnic, social and cultural groups in over 60 countries. The conditions and skills to manage are different over different time periods and cultural contexts. This fact is important in the application of resilience theory. If it is a question of developing competence and a new repertoire to reach one's life goals, it is important to understand that competence applied yesterday perhaps is not functional today because the conditions have changed. This underlines the fact that in the post-modern times characterized by its rapid changes and turbulence, many of the traditional structures and functions of societal institutions, such as family and school, have been undermined and are no longer of such importance. In addition, values and structures have become less coherent as new players such as the market systems, media and new information technology move into the arena. We thus have to look for more flexible models of resilience. This is why the salutogenic model (see later in this chapter) has such strength – it does not deal with development, specific structures or protective factors.

Both Rutter (1980) and Antonovsky (1979, 1987) emphasize at the relativity of concepts; protective factors in one context can be risk factors in another and vice versa. One can easily be seduced by the idea of the resilient child or person but in a humanistic perspective it is first of all important to consider the issue of ethics, equity, sustainable human settlements and ecology rather than admiring the survival of the strongest and most competitive individuals. It would be much more important to develop societies and life conditions where individual resilience is not fundamental but rather focus on creation of settings where we all have the opportunity to live well. However, the knowledge gained from research on resilience can be used for this purpose.

2.11 The Salutogenic Framework

More than 20 years ago Aaron Antonovsky introduced his salutogenic theory, "sense of coherence", as a global orientation to view the world and the individual environment as comprehensible, manageable and meaningful, claiming that the way a person views life has a positive influence on their health (Antonovsky 1979, 1987). The sense of coherence (SOC) theory explains why people in stressful situations stay well and even are able to improve their health. The SOC theory, integrating a stressor-resource concept, could be useful to help people manage all kinds of daily stressors and major life events and still remain healthy. Fundamental to the salutogenic theory is that health is viewed as part of the health ease/disease continuum. Health is here seen as a movement or a process, where people are always in some respects healthy and independent of existing distress and diseases. The paradigm shift from the pathogenic focus on risk factors for diseases to the salutogenic focus on the strength and determinants for health was introduced (Antonovsky 1979, 1987).

Previously stress was seen as a negative event that increased the risk of breaking people down. Over time the understanding became more relative where the nature of the stress agent, the abilities of the people involved and the environment played important roles. Both health and stress research initially considered the stress factors (or stressors) as problematic negative events in people's lives. In contrast, Antonovsky stated that diseases and stress regularly occur all the time and it is surprising that an organism is able to survive at all for such a long time. His conclusion was that chaos and stress is part of life and natural conditions (Antonovsky 1991). The interesting question is how we can survive in spite of this or how we can manage the lack of control over our life? In his world, health becomes a relative concept on a continuum and the really important research question is what causes health (salutogenesis), not what are the reasons for disease (patogenesis).

Conceptually, it seems Antonovsky seeks support from many other theoretical frameworks to synthesise the core concepts of salutogenesis. The fundamental new concepts are the generalised resistance resources (GRRs) and the SOC. The GRRs are biological, material and psychosocial factors that make it easier for people to perceive their lives as consistent, structured and understandable. Typical GRRs are money, knowledge, experience, social support, culture, intelligence, traditions, ideologies etc. If a person has these kinds of resources available herself or in her immediate surroundings there is a better chance for her to deal with the challenges of life. They help the person to construct coherent life experiences. What is more important than the resources themselves is this ability to use them, the SOC, the second and more generally known salutogenic key concept. The GRRs lead to life experiences that promote a strong sense of coherence – a way of perceiving life and an ability to successfully manage the infinite number of complex stressors encountered in the discourse of life. The SOC is the capability to perceive that one can manage in any situation independent of whatever else is happening in life. The SOC is a resource that enables people to manage tension, to reflect on their external and internal resources, to identify and mobilize them, to promote effective coping by finding solutions, and resolve tension in a health promoting manner. SOC is flexible and not constructed around a fixed set of mastering strategies (like the classic coping strategies) (Antonovsky 1993a).

In the original text the SOC is defined as "*as a global orientation that expresses the extent to which one has a pervasive, enduring though dynamic feeling of confidence that 1) the stimuli deriving from ones' internal and external environments in the course of living are structured, predictable and explicable; 2) the resources are available to one to meet the demands posed by the stimuli; and 3) these demands are challenges, worthy of investment and engagement*" (Antonovsky 1987).

People have to understand their lives and they have to be understood by others, perceive that they are able to manage the situation and, most importantly, perceive that it is meaningful enough to find motivation to continue. The salutogenic concept is a deeply personal way of thinking, being and acting, a feeling of an inner trust that things will be in order independent of whatever happens. The inner trust developed by internalising the SOC concept leads us to identify, benefit, use and re-use the general resistance resources from our surroundings. Three types of life experiences shape the SOC: consistency (comprehensibility), load balance (manageability) and participation in shaping outcomes (meaningfulness).

SOC is applicable on the individual, group and societal level and is fluctuating dynamically through life. Antonovsky postulated that SOC is mainly formed in the first three decades of life (Antonovsky 1987). Thereafter he thought that only very strong changes in life could upset and change the SOC. Speaking in general terms people who are approaching their fourth decade in life today have had enough experience of life to become independent persons with a job and an education, have enough experience of social structures and relationships and also formed a view of life. Antonovsky further boldly postulated the SOC was universally applicable to all cultures and ethnic contexts. At the time of his death much of the empirical evidence to either support or refute his theories was not available. A year before his death he published an article that summarised the evidence up to 1992 (Antonovsky 1993a). Until now nobody has really tried to pull all the knowledge together in a systematic way.

2.12 Contemporary Evidence on SOC and Especially in Relation to Culture and/or Mental Well-Being, Quality of Life and Health

To date, the SOC questionnaire has been used in 33 languages in 32 countries on more than 200,000 subjects in studies varying from large samples of the general population covering 20,000 persons to small samples of 10–20 individuals (Eriksson and Lindström 2005). Most of the studies are cross-sectional, though there are also some longitudinal and intervention studies. SOC is strongly and negatively related to anxiety, burnout, demoralisation, depression and hopelessness and positively with hardiness, mastery, optimism, self-esteem, good perceived health, quality of life and well-being (Eriksson and Lindström 2005, 2006). SOC seems to be stable over time, at least for people with an initial high SOC, including fluctuations of about 10%. Furthermore, SOC tends to increase with age over the whole life span. Gender differences are found, men usually score higher on SOC than women.

SOC seems to have a main, moderating or mediating role in the explanation of health (Eriksson and Lindström 2006). Furthermore, the SOC seems to be able to predict health. The results are more consistent in relation to factors that measure mental health. There is a strong negative association between SOC and anxiety, anger, hostility and depression, and a positive association with optimism, hope, learned resourcefulness and constructive thinking. One conclusion of this would be that SOC is analogous with mental health.

The positive relationship between SOC and health seems to be relatively clear for individuals scoring high on SOC. A high SOC protects health, but we have no clear indication of where the cut off point is and where SOC loses this protective effect. There are many scales measuring quality of life and well-being among different groups of chronically or seriously ill people, people with disabilities and their families, and older people. Most of them report an association between SOC and quality of life, life satisfaction and well-being. The higher the SOC the more satisfied people are with their lives, and consequently report a higher level of quality of life and general well-being. Independent of the instrument used for measuring quality of life, life satisfaction and well-being, the results supports the salutogenic theory as a health promotional resource. However, the direction of the relationship and the causality is somewhat unclear, therefore further research is needed.

What people are at risk of developing poor health? Social class and social conditions have an effect on the individual health (Lundberg 1997). As a sociologist Antonovsky knew very well about the impact of social conditions on people's health. Can the SOC concept be realized only by people with a high level of education, a good economy, a good social support, and social integration, an elite? We do not agree that SOC can only be the preserve of certain sections of society, and neither did Antonovsky. In a lecture at the Nordic School of Public Health in Gothenburg in 1993 he explicitly pointed out the responsibility of society to create conditions that foster the strengths of coping – that is, SOC. It is not question about a free choice of the person to cope well. The key lies in a society and in people who care about others (Antonovsky 1993b).

Maybe the empowerment concept, which is a supporting process whereby groups or individuals are enabled to change a situation, given skills, resources, opportunities and authority, could be seen as a tool for the enhancement of the individual SOC (Koelen and Lindström 2005). Unfortunately the association between empowerment and SOC has not been completely clarified. However, one example is the testing of a home-computing model for children with learning disabilities. It was found that such a model empowers both parents and children as well as strengthening their SOC (Margalit et al. 1995).

One of the most fundamental elements of the empowerment concept is participation of individuals or groups. This enhances peoples' understanding of what happens around them and shapes a sense of control of the situation. In health promotion activities and in clinical practice the empowerment of people could be accomplished through the practice of a clinical communication based on the salutogenic approach or a resource-oriented discussion as described by Malterud and Hollnagel (1998, 1999). This relates back to the discussion on learning earlier described in this chapter. One of the GRRs that generates the SOC is wealth, i.e. economy both at an individual and community level. SOC is clearly related to socioeconomic factors (Lundberg 1997). The higher the income level the stronger the SOC.

Antonovsky never asserted that SOC was the only and unique property to explain the movement towards health. There are other related concepts which contribute to the understanding of the health process such as hardiness (Kobasa), sense of permanence (Boyce), the social climate (Moos), resilience (Werner) and the family's construction of reality (Reiss) all mentioned by Antonovsky (Antonovsky 1987). Additional concepts which he did not discuss and which resemble SOC's connection to health are learned resourcefulness, (Rosenbaum 1990) flow, (Csíkszentmihályi and Csíkszentmihalyi 1998) theories on welfare/well-being, (Allardt et al. 1980) quality of life (Naess 1987; Lindström 1994) and theories considering people in their social and cultural context (Bourdieu 1993; Klein 1990; Swedner 1983; Bronfenbrenner 1979).

The last 25 years of research has provided strong empirical support for the SOC theory. The analysis of variance shows that SOC is strongly related to health, especially mental health. The rest of the variance is explained or accounted for by other factors like age, social support, and education. The interpretation could be that SOC is not the same as health but is still an important disposition for people's development and maintenance of their health (Eriksson and Lindström 2006). The salutogenic orientation provides no prescription for a good life in the moral sense of the term; it can only help us understand health and illness (Antonovsky

1995). Furthermore, the potential of the salutogenic concept lies in its implications for creating societies that adopt a healthy public policy, where the content and the structure of all services are salutogenic, rather than a healthy policy only for the health services. It is important to strengthen available resources and to create new kinds of general resistance resources to make it possible for the citizens to identify and benefit from them. Maybe it is also time to consider a change of the original WHO declaration on health and adopt the salutogenic perspective in a revised definition. The authors of this chapter would willingly contribute to such a discussion.

Public health has largely operated within risk reduction framework. Identifying causal factors for disease and, together with medical science, searched for logical interventions to eliminate them. The history of this approach is as long as the history of public health, successful in simple causal relationships but finding it increasingly difficult to deal with more complex problems, sometimes even failing to solve them (e.g. the HIV/AIDS epidemic). However, if one could identify public health interventions directed towards the post-modern mechanisms there are perhaps other solutions available. Out of the new theories on health and life management, two themes have evolved.

Firstly, the salutogenic approach which claims health is open ended and dependent on the skills to organise the resources available in society, the social context and self. This capability has been named the sense of coherence (Allardt et al. 1980).

Secondly, the theme of resilience claiming there are certain patterns of interaction between the individual and his social context that develop hardiness against stress and the ill-health that could follow (Campbell et al. 1976).

Both resilience and sense of coherence, it is claimed, are developed mainly in childhood. Resilience theory addresses the post-modern issue of abstract systems alienating the individual from trust in self and local context. The essence of the literature of resilience focuses on the development of the reflective dialogue between the child and its social context. Salutogenesis again addresses mechanisms that enable people and populations to develop their health and deal with the fragmentation and chaos of reality through their senses of cognitive and emotional perception, behavioural skills and motivation through meaningful frameworks based on culture, tradition and belief systems. The combination of the two could perhaps guide public health and the children of the post-modern society towards a positive synthesis. The effect is that public health could make progress in an area where it has been least successful addressing social and mental well-being in a long-term perspective by the focus on prerequisites for quality of life (Andrews and Whitney 1976).

The contemporary knowledge base in health science claims that what we perceive as being good for ourselves (the sense of subjective well being) also predicts our positive outcome in objective health parameters, in other words, if we create processes where people perceive they are able to live the life they want to live, people will not only feel better but will also lead better lives. From a public health perspective there is of course not only a pursuit of an individual's good life, but the good life of populations, including future generations.

References

Allardt, E. (1980). Att, Ha., Att, Älska., Att, Vara: Om välfärd i Norden. Borgholm: Argos.

Andrews, F. M., & Whitney, S. B. (1976). *Social indicators of well-being: The development of and measurement of perceptual indicators*. New York: Plenum.

Antonovsky, A. (1979). *Health, stress and coping*. San Francisco: Jossey-Bass.

Antonovsky, A. (1987). *Unraveling the mystery of health. How people manage stress and stay well*. San Francisco: Jossey-Bass.

Antonovsky, A. (1991). The salutogenic approach to family system health: promise and danger. In: *European congress on "Mental Health in European Families"*; p.9. http://www.angelfire.com/ok/soc/agolem.html cited May 2009.

Antonovsky, A. (1993a). The structure and properties of the sense of coherence scale. *Social Science & Medicine*, 36(6):725–733.

Antonovsky, A. (1993b). Some salutogenic words of wisdom to the conferees. In: *The Nordic School of Public Health in Gothenburg, Sweden*; p.3. http://www.angelfire.com/ok/soc/agoteborg.html cited May 2009.

Antonovsky, A. (1995). The moral and the healthy: Identical, overlapping or orthogonal? *Israel Journal of Psychiatry and Relative Science*, 32(1):5–13.

Atkinson, T. (1982). The stability and validity of quality of life measures. *Social Indicators Research*, 10:113–132.

Bauman, Z. (1989). *Modernity and the holocaust*. Cambridge: Polity.

Bourdieu, P. (1993) *The field of cultural production. Essays on art and literature*. Cambridge: Polity.

Bowlby, J. (1979). *The making and breaking of affectional bonds*. London: Tavistock.

Bronfenbrenner, U. (1979). *The ecology of human development – experiments by nature and human design*. Cambridge, MA: Harvard University Press.

Campbell, A., Converse, P. E., & Rodgers, W. L. (1976). *The quality of American life: Perceptions, evaluations and satisfactions*. New York: Russell Sage.

Crowne, D. P., & Marlowe, D. (1964). *The approval motive. Studies in evaluative dependence*. New York: Wiley.

Csíkszentmihályi, M., & Csíkszentmihalyi, I. S. (1998). *Optimal experience. Psychological studies of flow in consciousness*. Cambridge: Cambridge University Press.

de Leeuw, E. (2003). Nurturing healthy cities: research responsibility and accountability. In: Takano, T., editor. *Healthy cities & urban policy research*. London: Spon.

de Maio, T. J. (1984). Social desirability and survey measurement: A review. In: Turner, C. F., Martin, E., editors. *Surveying subjective phenomena*. New York: Russell Sage, pp. 257–282.

Dencik, L. (1989). Growing up in postmodern age: On the child's situation in the modern family and on the position of the family in the modern welfare state. *Acta Sociologica*, 32(2):155–180.

Eriksson, M., & Lindström, B. (2005). Validity of Antonovsky's Sense of Coherence Scale – a systematic review. *Journal of Epidemiology and Community Health*, 59(6):460–466.

Eriksson, M., & Lindström, B. (2006). Antonovsky's Sense of Coherence Scale and the relation with health – a systematic review. *Journal of Epidemiology and Community Health*, 60:376–381.

Flanagan, J. C. (1982). Measurement of quality of life: Current state of the art. *Archives of Physical Medicine and Rehabilitation*, 63:56–69.

Fonagy, P., Steele, M., Higgit, A., et al. (1994). The Emanuel Miller Memorial Lecture 1992. The theory and practice of resilience. *Journal of Child Psychology and Psychiatry*, 35(2):231–257.

Freire, P. (1970). *Pedagogy of the oppressed*. Harmondsworth: Penguin.

Gardner, H. (1991). *To open minds*. New York: The Perseus Books Group.

Giddens, A. (1990). *The consequences of modernity*. Cambridge: Polity.

Giddens, A. (1991). *Modernity and self-identity. Self and society in the late modern age*. Cambridge: Polity.

Ingelhart, R., & Rabier, J. -C. (1985). If you are unhappy this must be Belgium: Well-being around the world. *Public Opinion*, 8(2):10–15.

Jahoda, M. (1958). *Current concepts of positive mental health.* New York: Basic Books.

Johansson, S. (1970). *Om levnadsnivåundersökningen.* Stockholm: Allmänna Förlaget.

Kajandi, M. (1981). Allmän översikt över forskningsområdet. Livskvalitet – en litteraturstudie av livskvalitet som beteendevetenskapligt begrepp samt ett förslag till definition. Uppsala: Forskningskliniken.

Klein, J. (1990). *Interdisciplinarity: History, theory and practice.* Detroit: Wayne State University Press.

Koelen, M., & Lindström, B. (2005). Making healthy choices easy choices: the role of empowerment. *European Journal of Clinical Nutrition*, 59(Suppl 1):S10–S16.

Lazarus, R., & Lannier R. (1979). Stress-related transactions between persons and environment. In: Pervin, L., Lewis, M., editors. *Perspectives in international psychology.* New York: Plenum, pp. 142–156.

Lindström, B. (1994). The essence of existence. On the quality of life of children in the Nordic countries – theory and practice in public health (Doctoral thesis). Göteborg: Nordic School of Public Health.

Lindström, B., & Nafstad, A. (2003). On the origin of salutogenesis. In: *The 4th Nordic health promotion research conference* 10–13 June. Västerås, Sweden; 2003.

Lundberg, O. (1997). Childhood conditions, sense of coherence, social class and adult ill health: Exploring their theoretical and empirical relations. *Social Science and Medicine*, 44 (6):821–831.

Mahler, H. (1987). The role of schools of public health in the development of public health. In: Köhler, L., editor. *Public Health – a Nordic Perspective.* In Swedish. Gothenburg: Nordic School of Public Health.

Malterud, K., & Hollnagel, H. (1998). Talking with women about personal health resources in general practice. Key questions about salutogenesis. *Scandinavian Journal of Primary Health Care*, (16):66–71.

Malterud, K., & Hollnagel, H. (1999). Encouraging the strengths of women patients. A case study from general practice on empowering dialogues. *Scandinavian Journal of Public Health*, 27:254–259.

Margalit, M., Rochberg, Y., & Al-Yagon, M. (1995). Home-computing model and children with learning disabilities: A systemic approach. *Learning Disability Quarterly*, (18):68–75.

Mastekaasa, A., Moum, T., Naess, S. (1988). Livskvalitetsforskning. Oslo: ISF Rapport 88:6.

Naess, S. (1974). Psykologiske aspekter ved livskvalitet: om begrepet "indre livskvalitet" som mål for sosialpolitikken og om et forsök på å operasjonalisere begrepet. Oslo: Institutt for anvendt sosialvitenskapelig forskning.

Naess, S. (1979). Livskvalitet: om å ha det godt i byen og på landet. Oslo: Institutt for anvendt sosialvitenskapelig forskning.

Naess, S. (1987). Quality of life research: Concepts, methods and applications. Oslo: Institute of Applied Social Research.

Nilsson, L. (2003). The encounter between health promotion and schools in theory and in practice. In Swedish (Doctoral thesis). Örebro: Örebro University.

Nutbeam, D. (1993). Advocacy and mediation in creating supportive environments for health. *Health Promotion International*, 8:165–166.

OECD. (2009). *Society at a Glance 2009 – Organisation for Economic Cooperation and Development Social Indicators.* www.oecd.org/els/social/indicators/SAG cited May 2009.

Raphael, D. (2002). Evaluation of quality of life initiatives in health promotion. In: *Evaluation in health promotion.* Geneva: WHO.

Rappaport, J. (1987). Terms of empowerment/exemplars of prevention: Toward a theory for community psychology. *American Journal of Community Psychology*, 15:121–148.

Resnick, M. D., Bearman, P. S., Blum, W., et al. (1997). Protecting adolescents from harm. Findings from the National Longitudinal Study on Adolescent Health. *JAMA*, 278(10):823–832.

Ringen, S. (1988). *Approaches to the measurement of welfare.* Oslo: Statistisk Sentralbyrå.

Rootman, I., Raphael, D., Shewchuk, D., et al. (1992). *Development of an approach and instrument package to measure quality of life of persons with developmental disabilities.* Toronto: University of Toronto, Centre for Health Promotion.

Rosenbaum, M. (1990). *Learned resourcefulness. On coping skills, self-control, and adaptive behaviour.* New York: Springer.
Rutter, M. (1980). *Changing youth in a changing society. Patterns of adolescent development and disorder.* London: Harvard University Press.
Rutter, M. (1985). Resilience in the face of adversity. *British Journal of Psychiatry*, 147:598–611.
Shalock, R. L. (1990). *Quality of life.* Washington, DC: American Association on Mental Retardation, Special Publications.
Swedner, H. (1983). *Social work – a framework for thought.* In Swedish. Stockholm: Liber. 18. Swedner, H. (1983). Socialt arbete – en tankeram. Stockholm: Liber.
Turnbull, C. M. (1961). *The forest people.* New York: Simon & Schuster.
Turnbull, C. M. (1972). *The mountain people.* New York: Simon & Schuster.
Veenhofen, R. (1991). Questions on happiness. In: Strack, F., Argyle., M., Schwarz, N., editors. *Subjective well-being.* Oxford: Pergamon.
Ventegodt, S. (1995). *Livskvalitet i Danmark. Resultater fra en befolkningsundersögelse.* Köpenhamn: Forskningscentrets Forlag.
Werner, E., & Smith, R. (1982). *Vulnerable but invincible. A longitudinal study of resilient children and youth.* New York: McGraw Hill.
Werner, E., & Smith, R. (2001). *Journeys from childhood to midlife. Risk, resilience, and recovery.* Ithaca: Cornell University Press.
Whitehead, M., & Diderichsen, F. (2001). Social capital and health: Tip-toeing through the minefield of evidence. *Lancet*, 358:165–166.
WHO. (1986). The Ottawa charter. Geneva: World Health Organization.
WHO. (1946). Preamble to the Constitution of the World Health Organization as adopted by the International Health Conference, New York, 19–22 June, 1946; signed on 22 July 1946 by the representatives of 61 States (Official Records of the World Health Organization, no. 2, p. 100) and entered into force on 7 April 1948.

Chapter 3
A Theoretical Model of Assets: The Link Between Biology and the Social Structure

Michael P. Kelly

Keywords Lifecourse • Lifeworlds • Vectors

3.1 Introduction

In this chapter a theory that describes the assets that help to protect health is presented. Assets, and their opposite – the conditions which create vulnerabilities to ill health – are located in the lifeworlds of ordinary human experience and the health benefits and disbenefits which accumulate over the lifecourse (Kelly 2006). The life-world and lifecourse together are the bridge between social structure and individual human biology. Together they constitute the focal point where society and biology intersect and interact. The lifeworld and lifecourse are the mechanisms through which the social determinants of health produce biological outcomes in individuals. This is the vital link in the causal chain from the social to the biological and from society to individuals. Assets and vulnerabilities are the crucial mediating or intervening variables between the wider determinants of health and the human body and it is those intervening variables that produce individual differences in health (Lazarsfeld 1966; p. 157).

The theory begins with a consideration of the interaction between human behaviour and the structural forces which determine health. These structural forces are called vectors (Kelly et al. 2009). Four vectors of causation are described; population, society, organisation and environment. The theory developed in this chapter builds on the work done by members of the public health team at NICE to support the WHO Commission on the Social Determinants of Health (CSDH) as well as NICE's experience of developing public health guidance (Kelly et al. 2007, 2009; Blas et al. 2008).

M.P. Kelly (✉)
Centre for Public Health Excellence, National Institute for Health and Clinical Excellence (NICE), London, UK
e-mail: mike.kelly@nice.org.uk

A. Morgan et al. (eds.), *Health Assets in a Global Context: Theory, Methods, Action*,
DOI 10.1007/978-1-4419-5921-8_3, © Springer Science+Business Media, LLC 2010

3.2 Vectors of Causation

3.2.1 The Population Vector

The first vector is the population vector. This consists of factors which impact on the health of populations as a whole, at national, regional and supra national levels. These factors arise because of the direct actions of organizations like the European Union (EU), nation states, global and national financial and banking systems, corporations and businesses, regional governments, some civil society organisations, donor organisations, and health systems. The actions of these bodies and organisations produce: (1) economic structures and processes, productive arrangements and concomitant markets which generate wealth *and* structural inequalities within and between societies and between individuals; (2) the legal and regulatory frameworks which either value health or do not, protect the rights to health or do not and provide for labour, women and children's protection, or do not; and (3) the mechanisms to monitor and evaluate the health of populations (Blas et al. 2008). There is considerable evidence demonstrating that these actors and their actions have profound effects on health of individuals and within and between societies (CSDH 2008).

The sequelae of the ways these actors and their actions work within this vector have been described in detail in connection with the WHO Commission on the Social Determinants of Health (CSDH 2008). For example the negative as well as positive outcomes of the economic process of globalisation have been delimited very precisely (Labonte et al. 2007). The ways in which legal frameworks can protect women from political and economic marginalisation is another (Sen et al. 2007). The potential power of sound data collection systems, as the means of holding governments to account is yet another (Kelly et al. 2007). This evidence offers a starting point for understanding the causal mechanisms especially of the patterning of health at population level. The population vector is both the framework and the economic processes within which the overall patterns of health arise. At governmental level, the degree to which states are fragile or corrupt, are accountable through the rule of law and the democratic process, are fundamental to the way the framework and process support or negate health. It may be thought of as an interlocking system of laws, regulation, markets and politics (Blas et al. 2008; Bonnefoy et al. 2007).

To a very significant degree the ways in which this vector impacts on health for good or ill is a matter of political will and determination or of neglect (CSDH 2008). In other words organisations like corporations and governments act deliberately in what they do and their behaviour arises directly from human agency and intent. These actors in the population vector are goal oriented because men and women set the organisations up and run them in particular ways to achieve certain ends – corporations to make profits, donor organisations to provide relief, governments to govern and so on. Although of course they will always only be partially successful in their goals, and all of them are subject to the vagaries of unintended consequences, system dysfunctions and goal displacement, there is never the less deliberate human intent behind the goals and actions (Merton 1940, 1957). This is somewhat different to the next vector, society, where the same degree of deliberate goal orientation is much less obvious. It is also important because therefore solutions also lie within the power of human agency to do things differently and in ways that can promote rather than damage health if the will exists (Kelly et al. 2007).

3.2.2 *The Societal Vector*

The second vector is the societal vector. It is conceptually distinct from the population level vector. Society is probably one of the most used but least well understood concepts in the social sciences. It is best described as that group of social forces which arise as a consequence of human behaviour in all its forms, which in turn impinge, constrain, and organise human affairs in ways which for the most part are not a *direct* result of intentional human agency or intention (Giddens 1979, 1982, 1984). Society arises spontaneously from the billions and billions of human actions that take place every single second of every single minute. Politicians and governments always seek to control society, with varying degrees of success, and the regulations and legal frameworks described above in the population vector are manifestations of this. But societies are difficult to control because they have a reality sui generis independent of individual will (Hume 1748/2007; Smith 1776; Durkheim 1897/1952).

Society is made up of various elements, some of which will be touched on here. The building block of society is the dyadic interaction between two people (Simmel 1950; Homans 1951; Parsons 1951; Garfinkel 1967). Interaction can take many forms of course. But every human encounter tends towards one or other of two ideal types of human interaction – authority or power (Weber 1947). In the first ideal type person A is perceived by person B to have some legitimate reason to interact with them and to seek to ask them to do something. The process is reciprocal in that both have expectations of the other which are regarded as legitimate and both benefit from the interaction (Homans 1951). The prototype of such an interaction might be a simple purchase in a shop. The shop keeper or shop assistant expects the customer, to ask them for something and if the shopkeeper has it, for a legitimate transaction to ensue in which goods are exchanged for money. This type of interaction does not only occur in financial transactions or commercial arrangements. So a spouse asking their partner to make love, or in the work situation a line manager asking a colleague to perform a particular work related task, or a doctor asking a patient to remove an item of clothing in order to conduct a medical examination, all represent examples of the ideal type. The key idea is that the interaction is based on some notion (different in each of these cases) of the legitimate authority of one person over the other. The shop keeper, the partner, the work subordinate and the patient understand that the customer, the wife, the manager and the doctor all have a legitimate right to ask them to do what they are asking (May and Kelly 1982). It is important to note that the meaning attaching to the interaction, the legitimacy, is situation and role specific. So if the interaction and requests occurred in other circumstances, or perhaps the roles were reversed, then the legitimacy evaporates and interaction tends to break down (Garfinkel 1967).

The alternative ideal type is when the person who is asked or told do something, does not want to do it because they do not recognise the right of the person doing the asking to do so. They resist. In order get their way, the person doing the asking uses power or force. So someone going into a shop demanding the contents of the till, someone wanting sex from someone else who does not, someone bullying a work colleague or someone telling another to remove clothing when the other does not want to, are ideal type examples. If the powerful are to get their way, they will have to use force or coercion or the threat of it to do so. The relationship is not reciprocal, because only one party benefits. The demand being made is not legitimate and is not desired by the other party. So this relationship is one of power not authority.

Of course human interaction seldom fits neatly into these ideal types and is best seen as a spectrum between the two pure types of authority and power. Indeed much social life is made up of negotiating meaning and the consequent boundaries of legitimacy in human interaction and whether an action is about power or authority, or what mixture of each. It is out of this interplay at individual, group and organisational levels that society arises as a complex web of meaning, negotiation and social relations. It all gets more complex as we move from dyads to triads and then to larger groups (Simmel 1950), but the social forms which arise from human interaction all develop out of the basic dyadic structure.

In the context of this chapter, power relations are of particular interest. To a very significant degree the shape of society reflects struggles for power and competition for resources and alternatively the degree to which social relations are governed by legitimate authority. This definition of power includes actions which are outside of any formal political process and include such things as teenage gangs struggling for territory, and elitist social groups attempting to maintain exclusiveness by elaborate social rituals, language and dress codes. Sometimes power is played out as violent aggression, sometimes as legally sanctioned oppression and violence, sometimes as the micro politics of the office or institution. The structures of power and domination from the most benign to the most malevolent are intrinsic to the human condition and from the perspective of public health the effects, especially of the negative experience of power, domination, aggression and force, and the more benevolent forms of social control, have direct impacts on health (Kelly 2001).

Power plays out formally as politics in the population vector, but if we restrict the analysis to formal political systems, the important social structural consequences of power relations, viz. patterns of inequality, will be missed. Power struggles and the consequent patterns of social differences occur notwithstanding the intentionality of the actors involved. Formal controls of the economy belong in the first – population – vector, but the consequent social differences of the outcomes of economic power struggles belong to the second – social – vector. The social vector therefore includes social differences of all kinds. The important axes of social difference are class, gender, religion, caste, tribe, place of residence, and status (Weber 1948). Social systems may be conceptualised as existing on a spectrum from those which are very homogeneous to those which are much more heterogeneous. Sociologists used to argue that the process of modernisation was one in which as societies became more advanced they also became more complex and more heterogeneous (Durkheim 1933). This feature is true at a very macro level, but it is also true that even the simplest societies exhibited a division of labour based on age, physical prowess, and gender and so on (Lenski and Lenski 1971; Megarry 1995). Social differences and their consequences may be simple or they may be complex, but they are a real feature of social systems with very real effects on society's members.

Social difference, in whatever great variety of forms it may take, is a universal characteristic of human social systems. These differences have important consequences including health consequences because they determine access to and possession of assets and exposure to vulnerability. Social difference determines access to resources and therefore life chances (Weber 1948). And access to resources is fundamental to being able to cope with the travails of life. Resources in the sense used here can refer to money, social support, social capital, skills, psychological resilience and market position. None of these factors are distributed equally or randomly in the population. They are differentially distributed according to social difference and are the outcome of power struggles.

Social systems generate cultures (Archer 1996). Culture is where meaning is created, formalised and preserved. So culture is as intrinsic a part of society as the struggle for power and dominance. All human systems develop cultures which are more or less complex and consistent sets of beliefs, norms, ideas, religions, ideologies and so on. Societies have means of expressing these in verbal, written and musical forms. A critical aspect of culture is the judgements made by powerful gatekeepers about good culture and poor culture, usually defined as taste (Bourdieu 1977, 1986). These judgments tend to reinforce definitions of who is a full member of the culture and who is not and are powerful resources for generating meaning linked to power. Societies develop varieties of ways of regulating cultural expression, religious and political ideas. To be distinctively human is to live in a cultural universe. To experience and share the membership of particular cultural groupings is essentially human and cultural groupings are in turn defined with reference the sharing of particular cultural artefacts, understandings and meanings. Culture is inescapable. It is impossible to opt out. We are born into an existing cultural milieu and through socialisation will be immersed in it.

From a public health point of view culture acts as a mediator of meanings associated with health, justice and fairness. People make sense of the worlds around them, including the changes they witness in their body as a consequence of disease. They assess illness and disease around them. They use cultural meanings to make sense of what they see. As they suffer the consequences of power and oppression or as they enjoy the fruits of their wealth, they will draw on cultural ideas to make sense of what is happening to them and to others.

3.2.3 The Organization Vector

The third vector is organizational. The architecture of human life is the organisations and institutions in which almost all human conduct takes place. Institutions and organisations include hospitals, employing organisations, large and small, in the private and public sectors, schools, universities, clubs, societies, professional associations and religious groups. It also includes some aspects of civil society, in the form of social groups and social movements. Obviously certain nation state organisations like civil services, the military and the police, are institutions and organisations and appear at this level as well as the state level, as do local government and municipal bureaucracies of various types. This list is not in any sense exhaustive. What is important is that the structures and functions of these organisations mediate as well as have direct health consequences on individuals.

The study of such organisations has been grist to the mill of sociology and industrial psychology for many years (Etzioni 1961, 1964; Burns and Stalker 1961; Buchanan and Huczynski 1985) and we know a good deal about the way such organisations work. The degree to which they are fit for purpose is a mixture of the task they are supposed to perform and the structures within, and the degree to which organisations are based on principles of flexibility or rigidity and external relationships. Organisations and professions involved in the delivery of health care are a particular subset of organisations. They are interesting for a number of reasons. They tend to be large. They tend to be expensive. They tend to be powerful, and all of us rely on them especially at times of extreme stress and anxiety, when we ourselves or our loved ones are ill or dying. In modern societies they are an incredibly significant cultural symbol too.

Such organisations have a significant role in delivering health protection, disease prevention and health promotion. They provide relief from pain and suffering. The impact on quality of life through the management of chronic illness is potentially and actually profound. Modern drug therapy means that many conditions which were once either fatal or were highly debilitating are no longer so, and instead the person with the condition can live a full and active life. The drugs which control epilepsy, diabetes and angina, are cases in point. There are also drug interventions which significantly reduce risk of certain diseases like heart attack and stroke – statins and antihypertensives are good examples. There is the surgery which usually significantly improves quality of life like knee and hip replacements, cataract surgery. Even minor correctives to vision, using spectacles has enormous benefits on the quality of life. All of these interventions and many others account for about 40% of health improvement (Bunker 2001). This is probably an underestimate of the potential benefits which the system could deliver if inefficiencies and dysfunctions could be eliminated, if the service reached out effectively to those most in need and if the take up and use of services were completely equitable.

3.2.4 Environment Vector

The fourth vector is the environment. The environment consists of everything from microviriology to global warming. The fact is humans inhabit a physical universe which is ubiquitously stressful or at any rate ubiquitously full of germs, viruses, radiation, dust, noise, heat, ultra violet light, asbestos and many other potentially harmful physical things, And as if that were not enough, humans take risks, for the fun of it sometimes, or more mundane reasons. The result is a steady stream of mortality and morbidity from a variety of environmental causes.

The material world provides a constant source of pathogens and passages between the pathogens and the body. Some of these pathogens and toxins are unavoidable, or risk goes unrecognised. It is a reasonable assumption that there are hundreds, if not thousands, of things in our personal environment which as yet we do not know are dangerous. There are also newly mutating viruses a few of which may wreak havoc of epidemic or pandemic proportions. On the other hand much that threatens us in this environmental vector comes out of, or is a response to, direct human actions intended or otherwise and is potentially avoidable. So some environmental dangers like radiation, prions, drug resistant viruses, climate change, the residue of many industrial processes, are the result of present or past human conduct. There is, in other words, a relationship, an interaction, between many elements in the environmental vector and human actions which speeds the agent from its point of origin to the host of the disease.

3.3 Lifecourse and Lifeworld

Public health requires a mechanism which bridges the social/population/organisation/environment vectors and human biology. That mechanism is to be found in the conjunction of the lifecourse and the lifeworld (Kelly 2006; Kelly et al. 2009). The epidemiology and sociology of the lifecourse are very straightforward. Through numerous studies of birth and other cohorts (Kuh et al. 2003) and a consideration of the associations between insults and benefits in utero (Barker and Martyn 1992) and subsequent patterns in later life (Graham and Power 2004; Hertzman et al. 2001; Irwin et al. 2007), it is possible to show that from the moment of conception to the moment of death the human organism is subject to positive and negative forces originating in all four of the public health vectors. These accumulate during the lifetime to produce the health state of an individual at any one time. Sometimes earlier negative impacts will be cancelled out by later benefits and also previous benefits may be wiped out by some subsequent negative impact. However, mostly current health is a cumulative outcome of factors which impinge on the individual over their lifetime. The lifecourse sees health state at any given point in life as a cumulative health profit and loss account. The lifecourse attends to the fact that along life's pathway, there are often critical moments when particular directions are taken which will have short and long term costs and benefits (Graham and Power 2004). Sometimes the pathway choice is largely driven by social circumstances; sometimes it is a real choice. But consequences there will be. So the type of job entered may be entirely driven by local labour markets, decisions to start to smoke by peer pressure, whether to use a condom on first intercourse, or not, by the state of alcoholic intoxication at the time and even the decision to add salt to food by cultural habit. But each of these actions has potential short and long term health consequences. It is important also to note that the trajectory through the lifecourse is not uniform, nor strictly speaking chronological, because the velocity and shape of the lifecourse trajectory of a boy born to white middle class parents in say Guildford, a rich and affluent city, and that of a girl born to Bangladeshi parents in Tower Hamlets, a poor part of inner city London, will most assuredly be different. The accumulated health benefits and insults and the critical decision points and opportunities will also mean they may follow quite different paths.

The lifeworld is the personal experience of the lifecourse. It is a private psychological subjective space where conscious cognitive processes operate. It is where thinking takes place and where perceptions of internal and external sense experience are lodged. It is where the human makes sense of the social and physical world around them. It is also the place where mind, by mediating external sense experience interacts with others external to self (Schutz 1964, 1967, 1970; Mead 1934). It is where the world of pain and suffering is experienced, where feelings of disadvantage are noted (Kelly 1996, 2001, 2006). It is where the physical world is interpreted as malevolent or benign. In this sense, the lifeworld is also a physical space where interaction takes place, not just symbolic interaction (in the mind) but the real physical interaction between people and the self. It is the place where the insults and benefits of the lifecourse are both experienced and are mediated.

Lifeworlds consist of internal representation of external and internal sense experiences (Hume 1748/2007). External interaction critically depends on having an inner sense of self. It also depends on that self making the assumption, that others who come into their lifeworld, and with whom they interact, perceive and see the world, and more or less make sense of it, in much the same way that the perceiving self does (Schutz 1964, 1967). Such an assumption can never be proven, and this has been a considerable source of anxiety for some philosophers who have concluded therefore that it is impossible to prove the existence of the external world at all (Berkeley 1713/1996). However, empirical confirmation that others see and interpret the world in much the same way as the self does, comes from two sources. First the future and external others' behaviour tends to be reasonably predictable. Things on a day to day basis, on the whole, tend to turn out pretty much like the past of which we already have had experience. In that past others mostly behaved as if they saw things in the same way as self. Second the causal attributions which self makes tend to be confirmed by the way others see and understand and explain the reasons for events (Hume 1748/2007). Lifeworlds tend to consist of unexceptional confirmation that even though we know that things do change, mostly we live in a predictable world and that permits life to flow along without it needing too much philosophical speculation (Descartes 1997; Hume 1748/2007).

Of course things do change and people's lifeworlds are sometimes subject to seismic shocks, some of which may be predicable, some of which may not, and life does change all the time. However, it is the predictability that is of particular interest here. The predictability resides in the fact that lifeworlds although subjectively unique are also shared and have a shared predictability. That sharing is cultural and coping in the lifeworld is the keynote to understanding vulnerability and assets. Lifeworlds work because people routinely solve the problem of intersubjectivity, i.e. anticipating well enough roughly what others are thinking and feeling in order to interact with them. This is because even though each cognitive lifeworld is unique, it exists in a cultural and social milieu in which experiences and meaning are shared. Shared backgrounds, patterns of socialisation, and indeed the recurrent patterning of social life at the social level, mean that there are large amounts in localised lifeworlds that are similar. So families, workmates, friendship groups, the primary attachments of social life, have the characteristic, not of producing exact copies of each other's lifeworlds, but rather of lifeworlds where a great deal overlaps. Of course as people move through space and time their lifeworlds change and the potential malleability is large. But the coalescence of lifeworlds, the development of shared patterns of meaning and cultural assumptions produces a predictable patterning of everyday life and of interrelationships between different but overlapping lifeworlds. The patterning of disease at population level is a consequence of this. So because lifeworlds are shared among individuals who share social position, and who experience similar consequences of the social, population, environmental and organisational vectors, and their patterns of behaviour have high degrees of similarity, the individual disease pathways acquire a population level dimension.

Lifeworlds are the locus of experience, of pain and suffering, of discrimination and disadvantage, the place where the vagaries and the good fortunes of life as they are visited upon us and take their toll across the life course, have their direct effects. The social, environmental, organisational and population vectors produce individual level diseases through the lifeworld. Individual disease pathways manifest themselves and operate via the lifeworld of the individual. There are individual biological differences between individuals on account of genetics, nutritional status, previous disease exposure, indeed the accumulated benefits and insults of unique passages through the lifecourse. There are also differences in the assets with which people cope with their lifeworlds and along with individual biological differences, this produces individual health differences.

3.4 Coping in the Lifeworld

So far this essay has operated predominantly within what Antonovsky called a pathogenic approach (Antonovsky 1985, 1987). That is the assumption is made that bad outcomes have preceding bad or pathogenic origins or causes. Antonovsky famously observed that all of medicine and almost all of the social sciences have this orientation whether the purpose is to explain human disease or social pathology. Antonovsky's work in introducing salutogenesis as the opposite to pathogenesis was truly a paradigm shift in the social and medical sciences, at least conceptually. In very simple terms he insisted that in the health sciences in particular, but also the social sciences, the search for the origins of health should be at least as important as the search for the origins of disease. This he called the salutogenic or origin of health-approach.

His original insight came via two different observations. The first was of his early studies of health inequalities. He noted, in empirical investigations of American blue collar workers that although their rate of mortality was higher than white collar workers, when the greatly enhanced risks intrinsic to blue collar occupations, their poorer housing conditions and their greater poverty in old age were considered, the surprising thing was that their rates of premature death were not very much higher than they actually were. He reasoned that there must be protective factors at work which mediated the noxious effects of their lives. His second insight came from studying survivors of the holocaust. He was interested in people who had been imprisoned in Nazi concentration camps, survived and gone on to settle into ordinary and productive lives in post war Israel. The conventional (pathogenic) approach was to see the consequences of the appalling experiences of the concentrations camps as producing pathology in the form of subsequent severe psychiatric morbidity. The reality was rather different. While some concentration camp survivors were undoubtedly psychologically unwell as a consequence of their experiences, the majority were not. This was not to say that they were unscarred by their experiences but they had coped with them and returned to a new and ordinary life. Once again Antonovsky concluded that there must be some protective factor at work. He argued that both the American blue collar workers and the concentration camp survivors exhibited a similar underlying psychological resource which provided the key to their protection from noxious social conditions or produced equanimity in the face of extraordinary human suffering. He called this, the sense of coherence (SOC).

Antonovsky's work recalls an earlier literature on coping, adaptation and survival (Dubos 1980). What was proposed was an underlying ontology in which the human is seen as living in world which is intrinsically threatening, dangerous, risky, noxious and stressful but with which they cope (Lazarus 1976, 1980, 1985, 2001; Lazarus and Folkman 1984a, b; Lazarus and Launier 1978). The reality of the human condition produced by the four vectors and mediated through the lifeworld is precisely this. The stresses and stimuli are chronic, originating in the vectors, only interrupted by more or less occasional periods of acutely high levels of even more extremely stressful stimuli. In this regard, humans are all subject to stresses all of the time because ordinary human life is a life of routine aggravation and difficulty. From time to time these are overlaid by major life events like illness, death of loved ones, divorce and war. There are in this view of things, relatively few periods of calm and peace in the human condition. The lifeworlds of most people most of the time are routinely difficult.

However, in spite of the ubiquitous nature of problems, most people more or less get through, and some deal with these things better than others. Some seem to have more assets with which to cope. To return to Antonovsky's hypothesis, there must be something intrinsic to some people's lifeworlds which produces a greater ability to cope. Antonovsky sought to find the answer in the idea of sense of coherence which fundamentally he conceptualised as a psychological trait. But this is only part of the explanation. It is more helpful to think of these assets not as psychological traits but as skill based transactions between persons and their environment.

There are four assets or groups of coping skills which help to clarify the way people survive their own lifeworlds. These are technical, interpersonal, intrasubjective and intersubjective. These are the four different types of skills or assets with which we master the lifeworld in varying degrees and therefore mediate the stressors originating in the vectors.

The technical level is about the technical tool based skills which people use to deal with situations and people, things and the environment. Humans have evolved the ability to fashion and to use tools. Tools take many forms, and include the use of language to shape thought as the most basic tool of all. Our access to tools, and our ability to use them skilfully, including in particular occupational and professional configurations, not only determines our place in the labour market, but also in the wider world and within our own lifeworlds. Skills are the basis in evolutionary terms of survival; this is because they are the basis of being able to handle and deal with everyday life.

Many years ago Max Weber the German sociologist pointed out that the possession of skills for use in the labour market was a powerful determinant of life chances, by which he meant access to, or the means to exert power over others (Weber 1948). This is still fundamentally true – although extending Weber's ideas to skills to deal with everyday life, means we include not just professional market skills and qualifications but the ability to manage encounters with bureaucracy, handling money, to the technical skills which determine the ability to use devices and machines. This includes everything from using the internet, mobile phone, motor car, as well as reading writing and communicating. These tools allow for mastery of the lifeworld, and the ability to negotiate meaning and interaction. They are the principal mediator of life chances in the face of powerful others. They are, in other words, fundamental assets which allow persons to exercise control over the vagaries of their lives and in turn act as mediators against the negative forces which impinge on the person's lifeworld.

The second key component of managing the lifeworld, the second asset, is interpersonal. This is about managing relationships with others. The basis of human society is interaction. Human interaction is made up of two elements. The first is actual physical interaction, either face to face, or through some electronic means like a telephone – which happens in real time. The second is symbolic interaction. This means that as, we physically interact with others, or as we anticipate or reflect upon interacting with others, we are also rehearsing symbolically in our minds what the other person is thinking and will themselves do next in response to what we do and say. We put ourselves figuratively in the shoes of the person with whom we are interacting. This ability to more or less accurately take the role of the other is the core component of what makes interaction work. Our management of relations with others and our ability to successfully interact provides us with a fundamental means of being able to control our lifeworlds (Mead 1934).

Life is made up of routine skirmishes as well as smooth transactions with bureaucracies, retailers, local councils, tradesmen, neighbours, workmates, relatives and friends. Most people have the interactive skills to take the rough with the smooth although a few do not (May and Kelly 1992). Although some of these interactions may be deeply unsatisfactory, we can at least extricate ourselves from them and move on to other arenas, where we can escape the hassle and deal with other more satisfactory aspects of our lives. But for some people their lifeworld consists of chronically difficult ways of interacting with others, be they neighbours, in the domestic environment, work, community and officialdom of various sorts. These interactions are characterised by struggles for the claim to be taken seriously as a human being (in relationships governed by legitimacy and authority). These claims are denied by others acting in ways which seek to exert power over them. In other words some individuals spend much more of their time having others define what and who they are, rather than being self directed. So at this micro level the ability to control the lifeworld is undermined.

The next assets are called intra subjective – inside the subject. At the heart of our lifeworld is the emotional or intra subjective epicentre. This is the world of raw feeling and emotion, of sensibilities and sensitiveness, of fear and hatred, of love and empathy, of all those psychological states of which the human is capable. It is also the cognitive and calculating seat of thinking and feeling. Modern psychology classifies these things in a variety of ways and of course psychoanalytic approaches offer degrees of insight into the origins of these feelings. The task here is not to arbitrate between the various approaches that may be brought to bear to explain these aspects nor indeed consider the great philosophical debates from Descartes and Berkeley onwards, which have sought to reflect on these concerns. The point is rather more simple. It is to acknowledge that the human is a thinking being, that is sensitive to its external environment and stimuli in it and, is capable of manipulating sensations and ideas into highly complex patterns of reasoning and understanding. As well as being a reasoning calculating agent with a continuous sense of itself existing through time and space, it is also a highly volatile emotional creature capable of feelings of great passion and emotion.

Most germane to the question at issue here is that those emotions and feelings can be decidedly painful and indeed distressing to the point of psychological morbidity. As Antonovsky observed, some people seem a lot more resilient than others to the stressful external stimuli which assail the human. So too some seem better able to withstand inner turmoil and distress. It might be thought of as varying degrees of an inner toughness or psychological resilience. We might bring into play Antonovsky's sense of coherence, or some of the many other scales of psychological resilience and coping which abound in the literature. Whatever of these mechanisms turns out in the next generation of empirical investigation to be the better explanation remains to be seen. But the inescapable fact is that the individual feels psychological distress. That psychological distress is itself linked to somatic changes in the human body. The link between the emotional state of the person and underlying biology is real, although all the precise pathways remain to be fully elucidated. In a model which focuses on assets, what we have here at the heart of the lifeworld is either a relatively robust set of mechanisms that mediate stressors, or a relative vulnerability offering at least a part explanation of the link between the social and the biological mediated via the psyche. This is not the whole story and will apply in some but by no means all, causes of morbidity. On the other hand working towards the kinds of mechanisms that can help to produce psychological resilience at the heart of the lifeworld, through formal techniques like cognitive behavioural therapy, or working towards greater self efficacy, offer very promising approaches.

The final asset is called the intersubjective, a term deliberately borrowed from phenomenological philosophy. In that context intersubjectivity refers to shared meanings between subjects, between human actors. Interaction depends on intersubjectivity. The basic assumption, as noted above, on which most human actors work is that they assume that other people see and understand the world in more or less the same way that they do. In real time during interaction shared meanings are not only assumed, but tend to emerge and change through processes of negotiation and testing during the interaction. Shared meaning is important because it provides the way humans make sense of the world. As humans we are constantly engaged in a process, usually at quite a low level, of providing psychologically satisfying accounts of our own actions, the actions of others around us, and in general of other events in the world. One of the most difficult and shocking things for us to have to deal with is where the accounts of the world we carefully rehearse and then test in interaction are undermined by the actions of others or by other external events. Reappraisal is called for as we then repair our sense of who and what we are and our place in the scheme of things. The ability to provide satisfactory accounts is at the heart of being able to cope with things great and small. The inability to do so leads to an overwhelming sense of dread and failure and psychologically terrifying experiences.

3.5 Conclusion: Assets to Control the Lifeworld

The lifeworld is the bridge between the social, psychological and the biological. Lifeworlds are psychological, social and physical environments which are the locus of experience and the arenas of shared experience. The lifeworld is the cauldron of vulnerability and risk and as well as the bastion of resilience, resources and protection. If we are to help individuals and communities to build their assets from the inside in a way that is essentially bottom up, the place to begin is with the four aspects of the lifeworld where the critical skills of coping, the assets, are located.

So first it involves building skills, (the technical level). These skills should be all embracing, from those which are necessary in changing labour markets, to those which facilitate management of mundane everyday life. This is so very important, not least because many communities at the sharp end of deindustrialisation, poor urban planning, chronic unemployment, crime, drugs and deeply engrained intergenerational social and health problems, have been stripped of their skill base.

They have been disempowered. The response of the various well meaning agencies of support in social services and local authority services has frequently been to reinforce the dependency of such communities, by for example emphasising claimants rights, rather than fostering their skill base. The skill base begins in preschool education and continues in the school curriculum. But it applies more widely to a vast array of disciplined activities.

At the interpersonal level, assets will only be built if community members value each other as well as themselves. There are not infrequently strong social networks and some social capital to build on to develop the interpersonal skill base. But at the same time zero tolerance to individuals and families who wantonly disregard the interests of others, zero tolerance to casual violence and aggression in teenage gangs and assistance to the police to deal with the organised crime which preys upon such communities and sells them contraband tobacco and illicit drugs, is first base for the development of such skills. Trusting interpersonal relationships depend on a culture in which individuals feel safe and not under siege, and where tolerance does not mean ignoring or turning a blind eye to the fall out of drug misuse and vandalism and other forms of petty and more serious crime.

At the intrasubjective level the assets are built on the deployment of psychological resilience and self efficacy. These are not quite two sides of the same coin but are comparable as the core of psychological inner strength. The resilience plays out of comparable processes to Antonovsky's conception of sense of coherence. This is probably best conceptualised in terms of Lazarus' model of the stress coping paradigm. Here the cognitive processes involved in the holding things together in the face of stressors and adversity involve making an assessment of the nature of the threat from the external stimuli. The assessment that then needs to occur is whether the stressor is benign, irrelevant or even positive. It also involves determining whether the stressor is harmful that is it could lead to threat harm or loss. If the stressor is appraised as any of these, the next assessment is to determine what can be done about it. There are four lines of action viz. seeking information, taking some kind of action, doing nothing or worrying. It is possible to develop these ideas as a basic way of handling stressful circumstances and developing resilience. The self efficacy approach involves cultivating the view that the individual is basically on top of things and will be able to deal with them. There are a number of strategies all very well rehearsed by psychologists which outline the basic elements.

Finally, the intersubjective assets are about the sense that things are meaningful and make sense. It is perhaps the most difficult of all as it requires the skill to see the bigger picture and to see how one stands in relation to the whole. It is significantly linked to a perception that the social structure is predictable and reasonably fair. It is about a conception that the world is largely predictable, secure and continuous. The idea that Antonovsky had, that of sense of coherence, actually comes close to it. Intersubjectivity in its original phenomenological sense meant the cognitive process whereby meaning is generated between subjects – people – and is shared. In the sense used here it emphasises the importance not just of shared meanings or understandings between people, but is about the way of arriving at shared meanings which help make sense of a chaotic external reality and allow us to make sense of things in ways which ameliorate some of the deeply distressing and potentially destabilising external stimuli and internal stimuli. This has been a theme which perhaps the sociologist Emile Durkheim gets closest to in his conception of anomie (Durkheim 1897/1952, 1933). For Durkheim the anomic society was one which a plethora of competing values and norms, expectations and understanding vies for attention and destabilises familiar anchor points. He concluded that the transition from traditional to modern societies made this process more likely. Post modernist writers have picked up the same vein of multiplicities of competing values, ways of living and so on. Durkheim argued for the importance of strong civil society including associations, professions and the like as the bedrock of protection from the vicissitudes of a changing society. This has a very contemporary resonance in concepts like social capital. It is the small scale community organisations through to institutions which can be relied on like police, doctors, teachers, that produce the stability which makes navigation through the perils of modern life easier and more meaningful. So the asset base here in order to help to reinforce strong and resilient intersubjectivity is the basic building block at community level.

Assets can therefore be grouped into these four areas. They are potentially available to everybody, but they are only available to some and some people deploy them more skilfully. Like so many phenomena which originate in social behaviour they both arise out of the thinking acting human consciousness and then create the very environment which impacts on the behaviour in the first place. At least though in some degree, such assets are learnable through socialisation and education. And while they will never be universal, institutions and organisations from schools, medical services, social care, as well as almost all the public and private bureaucracies which provide support to people, can act in ways which nurture these skills rather than deny them, or worse offer rights based solutions which can never be realised in practice, since they are political aspirations, not rights at all. These assets, or vulnerabilities are important not only of course because they can be nurtured and even more easily destroyed and eroded, but because they are the intervening variables which mediate between the major vectors of causation of disease and individual health outcomes.

References

Antonovsky, A. (1985). *Health Stress and Coping*. San Francisco: Jossey Bass.

Antonovsky, A. (1987). *Unravelling the Mystery of Health: How People Manage Stress and Stay Well*. San Francisco: Jossey Bass.

Archer, M.S. (1996). *Culture and Agency: The Place of Culture in Social Theory*, revised edition. Cambridge: Cambridge University Press.

Barker, D. & Martyn, C. (1992). The maternal and foetal origins of cardiovascular disease. *British Medical Journal*; 46:9–11.

Berkeley, G. (1996). *Principles of Human Knowledge and Three Dialogues*. Oxford: Oxford University Press.

Blas, E., Gilson, L., Kelly, M.P., Labmte, R., Lapitan, J., Muntaner, C., et al. (2008). Addressing social determinants of health inequities: what can the state and civil society do? *Lancet*; 372:1684–1689.

Bonnefoy, J., Morgan, A., Kelly, M.P., Butt, J., Bergman, V., with Tugwell, P., et al. (2007). *Constructing the Evidence Base on the Social Determinants of Health: A guide*. Report to the World Health Organization Commission on the Social Determinants of Health, from Measurement and Evidence Knowledge Network, The hub coordinating the Measurement and Evidence Knowledge Network is run by: Universidad del Desarrollo, Chile, and National Institute for Health and Clinical Excellence, United Kingdom.

Bourdieu, P. (1977). *Outline of a Theory of Practice*. Cambridge: Cambridge University Press.

Bourdieu, P. (1986). The forms of capital, in Richardson, J. (ed) *Handbook of Theory and Research for the Sociology of Education*. New York: Greenwood.

Buchanan, D.A. & Huczynski, A.A. (1985). *Organizational Behaviour: An Introductory Text*. Engelwood Cliffs: Prentice Hall.

Bunker, J. (2001). *Medicine Matters After All: Measuring the Benefits of Medical Care, a Healthy Lifestyle, and a Just Social Environment*. London: The Stationery Office/The Nuffield Trust.

Burns, T. & Stalker, G.M. (1961). *The Management of Innovation*. London: Tavistock.

CSDH (2008). *Closing the Gap in a Generation: Health Equity Through Action on the Social Determinants of Health*. Geneva: WHO.

Descartes, R. (1997). *Key Philosophical Writings*. Ware: Wordsworth.

Dubos, R. (1980). *Man Adapting: With a New Chapter by the Author*. New Haven: Yale University Press. First published 1965.

Durkheim, E. (1933). *The Division of Labour in Society*. trans G. Simpson, New York: Free Press.

Durkheim, E. (1952). *Suicide: A Study in Sociology*. trans J.A. Spaulding & G. Simpson, London: Routledge & Kegan Paul.

Etzioni, A. (1961). *A Comparative Analysis of Complex Organisations: On Power, Involvement and Their Correlates*. New York: Free Press.

Etzioni, A. (1964). *Modern Organisations*. Engelwood Cliffs: Prentice Hall.

Garfinkel, H. (1967). *Studies in Ethnomethodology*. Engelwood Cliffs: Prentice Hall.

Giddens, A. (1979). *Central Problems in Social Theory: Action, Structure and Contradiction in Social Analysis*. Berkeley: University of California Press.

Giddens, A. (1982). *Profiles and Critiques in Social Theory*. London: Macmillan.

Giddens, A. (1984). *The Constitution of Society: Outline of the Theory of Structuration*. Berkeley: University of California Press.

Graham, H. & Power, C. (2004). *Childhood Disadvantage and Adult Health: A Lifecourse Framework*. London: Health Agency Development Agency. http://www.nice.org.uk/aboutnice/whoweare/aboutthehda/evidencebase/keypapers/papersthatinformandsupporttheevidencebase/childhood_disadvantage_and_adult_health_a_lifecourse_framework.jsp cited May 2009.

Hertzman, C., Power, C. Mathews, S., Manor, O. (2001). Using an interactive framework of society and lifecourse to explain self-rated health in early adulthood. *Social Science and Medicine*; 53:1575–1585.

Homans, G.C. (1951). *The Human Group*. London: Routledge & Kegan Paul.

Hume, D. (2007). *An Enquiry Concerning Human Understanding*. Oxford: Oxford University Press. Ed and intro P. Millican. First published 1748.

Irwin, L.G., Siddiqui, A., Hertzman,C. (2007). *Early Child Development: A Powerful Equalizer – Final Report of the Early Child Development Knowledge Network of the Commission on the Social Determinants of Health*. Geneva: World Health Organization. http://whqlibdoc.who.int/hq/2007/a91213.pdf cited May 2009.

Kelly, M.P. (1996). Negative attributes of self: radical surgery and the inner and outer lifeworld, in Barnes, C. and Mercer, G. (eds) *Exploring the Divide: Illness and Disability*. Leeds: The Disability Press.

Kelly, M.P. (2001). Disability and community: a sociological approach, in Albrecht, G.L., Seelman, K.D., and Bury, M. (eds) *Handbook of Disability Studies*. London: Sage, 396–411.

Kelly, M.P. (2006). Mapping the life world: a future research priority for public health, in Killoran, A., Swann, C., and Kelly, M.P. (eds) *Public Health Evidence: Tackling Health Inequalities*. Oxford: Oxford University Press. 553–574.

Kelly, M.P., Morgan, A., Bonnefoy, J., Butt, J., Bergman, V., Mackenbach, J., et al. (2007). *The Social Determinants of Health: Developing an Evidence Base for Political Action*. Final Report to the World Health Organization Commission on the Social Determinants of Health, from Measurement and Evidence Knowledge Network, The hub coordinating the Measurement and Evidence Knowledge Network is run by: Universidad del Desarrollo, Chile, and National Institute for Health and Clinical Excellence, United Kingdom. www.who.int/social_determinants/resources/mekn_report_10oct07.pdf cited May 2009.

Kelly, M.P., Stewart, E., Morgan, A., Klloran, A., Fischer, A., Threlful, A. Bonnefoy, J. (2009). A conceptual framework for public health: NICE's emerging approach. *Public Health*; 123(1):e14–e20.

Kuh, D., Ben-Shlomo, Y., Lynch, J., Hallqvist, J., Power, C. (2003). Life course epidemiology. *Journal of Epidemiology and Community Health*; 57:778–783. Available from: http://jech.bmj.com/cgi/content/abstract/57/10/778 cited May 2009.

Labonte, R. Blouin, C., Chopra, M., et al. (2007). *Towards Health Equitable Globalization: Rights, Regulation and Redistribution – Final Report of the Globalization Knowledge Network of the Commission on Social Determinants of Health*. Geneva: World Health Organization.

Lazarsfeld, P.F. (1966). Concept formation and measurement in the behavioural sciences: some historical observations, in Di Renzo, G. (ed) *Concepts, Theory and Explanation in the Behavioral Sciences*, New York: Random House. 144–205.

Lazarus, R. (1976). *Patterns of Adjustment*. 3rd edition, New York: McGraw Hill.

Lazarus, R. (1980). The stress and coping paradigm, in Bond, L.A. and Rosen, J.C. (eds) *Competence and Coping During Adulthood*. New Hampshire: University Press of New England.

Lazarus, R.S. (1985). The costs and benefits of denial, in Monat, A. and Lazarus, R. (eds) *Stress and Coping: An Anthology*. New York: Columbia University Press.

Lazarus, R.S. (2001). Relational meaning and discrete emotions, in Scherer, K.R., Schorr, A., and Johnstone, T. (eds) *Appraisal Processes in Emotion: Theory, Methods, Research*. Oxford: Oxford University Press.

Lazarus, R. & Folkman, S. (1984a). *Stress, Appraisal and Coping*. New York: Springer.

Lazarus, R. & Folkman, S. (1984b). Coping and adaptation, in Gentry, W.D. (ed) *Handbook of Behavioral Medicine*. New York: Guilford.

Lazarus, R.S. & Launier, R. (1978). Stress related transactions between person and environment, in Pervin, L.A, and Lewis, M (eds) *Perspectives in Interactional Psychology*. New York: Plenum.

Lenski, G. & Lenski, J. (1971) *Human Societies: An Introduction to Macro Sociology*. 3rd edition. New York: McGraw Hill.

May, D. and Kelly, M.P. (1982). Chancers, pests and poor wee souls: problems of legitimation in psychiatric nursing. *Sociology of Health and Illness*; 4:279–301.

May, D. & Kelly, M.P. (1992). Understanding paranoia: towards a social explanation. *Clinical Sociology Review*; 10:50–69.

Mead, G.H. (1934). *Mind, Self and Society: From the Standpoint of the Social Behaviorist*. Chicago, IL: Chicago University Press.

Megarry, T. (1995). *Society in Pre History*. Basingstoke: Macmillan.

Merton, R.K. (1940). Bureaucratic structure and personality. *Social Forces*; 18:560–568.

Merton, R.K. (1957). *Social Theory and Social Structure*, revised edition. New York, NY: Free Press.

Parsons, T. (1951). *The Social System*. London: Routledge & Kegan Paul.

Schutz, A. (1964). *Collected Papers: II Studies in Social Theory*. The Hague: Martinus Nijhoff.

Schutz, A. (1967). *The Phenomenology of the Social World*. trans G. Walsh & F. Lehnert, Evanston, IL: North Western University Press.

Schutz, A. (1970). *On Phenomenology and Social Relations: Selected Writings*. Chicago, IL: Chicago University Press.

Sen, G., Ostlin, P., George. (2007). *Unequal, Unfair, Ineffective and Inefficient: Gender Inequity in Health – Why it Exists and How We Can Change It*. (Final Report of the Women and Gender Equity Knowledge Network to the Commission on the Social Determinants of Health). Bangalore: Indian Institute of Management. http://www.who.int/social_determinants/resources/csdh_media/wgekn_final_report_07.pdf cited May 2009.

Simmel, G. (1950). *The Sociology of Georg Simmel*. trans K.H. Wolff, New York, NY: Free Press.

Smith, A. (1776). *An Enquiry into the Nature and Causes of the Wealth of Nations* (edited by R.H. Campbell and A.S. Skinner) Oxford: Clarendon.

Weber, M. (1947). *The Theory of Social and Economic Organisation*. trans A.M. Henderson & T. Parsons, New York, NY: Free Press.

Weber, M. (1948). *From Max Weber: Essays in Sociology*. trans H.H. Gerth & C. Wright Mills, London: Routledge & Kegan Paul.

Chapter 4
Asset Mapping in Communities

John McKnight

Keywords Asset maps • Citizens • Associationss • Systems

4.1 Introduction

Policy makers have tended to create hierarchical systems where a small number of people are in charge of the mass production of standardised goods. Clients/consumers in large numbers grow dependent on this cycle of production. Such systems create dependency rather than empowerment. The author argues that in creating maps to reflect the way in which these systems work we have tended to neglect the notion of "associational community"; where there is a dependence on consent, choice, care and citizen power. Systems are seen to exploit need in individuals, whilst communities, in contrast nurture existing skills and capacity. Systems identify with "the glass half-empty" approach, whilst communities with "the glass half-full". The service culture produces "clients", whilst the community culture produces "citizens".

This chapter explores the nature of the relationship between systems, communities and citizens, and looks at the shift, in developed society, from equal relationships between citizens and communities to a relationship where systems are dominant. The author argues that the move towards an increasingly "consumerist society" has marginalized the role of the citizen. In order to encourage and build healthy communities we must recognise and appreciate the unique capabilities that communities offer in developing, nurturing and caring for their citizens.

J. McKnight (✉)
Asset-Based Community Development Institute, School of Education and Social Policy, Northwestern University, 2120 Campus Drive, Evanston, IL, USA
e-mail: JLMABCD@aol.com

A. Morgan et al. (eds.), *Health Assets in a Global Context: Theory, Methods, Action*,
DOI 10.1007/978-1-4419-5921-8_4,

4.2 A Twenty-First Century Map for Healthy Communities and Families

Policies and programs reflect our response to the map we create of the world around us. Our map, like all maps, is simply a model of the territory it portrays; sometimes accurate and at other times inaccurate. We all know of the European map makers who described a flat earth without a western hemisphere. Their inaccurate map shaped the policies, plans and action of mariners, kings, nations and communities. As we plan to set sail into the second decade of the twenty-first century, it is appropriate to re-examine the map that is used in most of our current policy making, in order to see whether it will show the way to safe, wise and healthful communities.

If one listens carefully to the proposals of our current social policy makers, we can construct a map of the territory where they believe they operate. This territory has two principal areas. The first is a space filled with systems. Policymakers see systems or institutions as the principal tool for the work of society. Therefore, their policies and programs are about "system design", "system planning", "delivery systems" and "system reform." The second area in their map is filled with the individuals who are the object of the systems – clients and consumers. Graphically, Fig. 4.1 shows the prevailing map of social policy makers.

To understand more clearly the dynamics of the area called a system, it is important to describe its nature and relationship to the client-consumer beneficiaries. The nature of a system is clarified by a more detailed map of its structure. Most policymakers see systems as tools that organize people in the relationships, as defined by the graphic representation in Fig. 4.2.

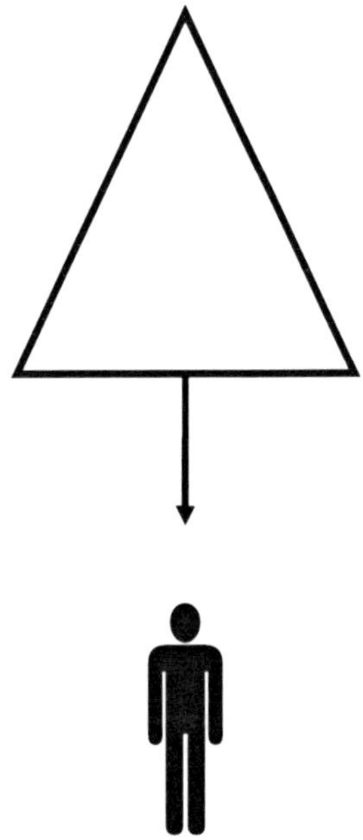

Fig. 4.1 Individuals and systems

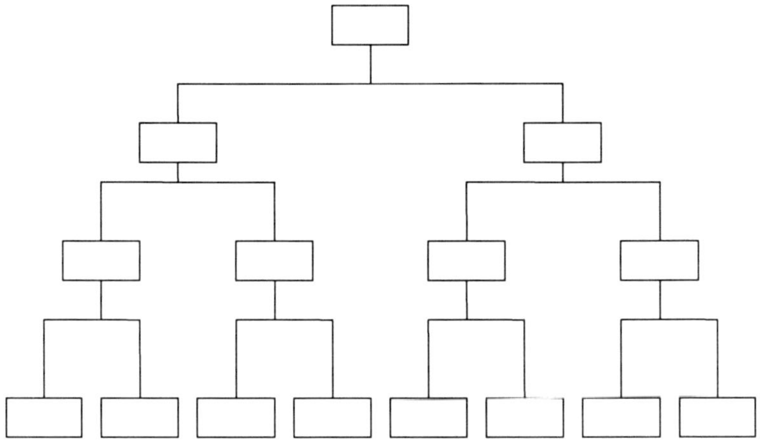

Fig. 4.2 The nature of systems

While there are limitless ways of organizing people to perform various tasks, this particular structure has several special features and purposes.

First, it is primarily a structure designed to permit a few people to control many other people. Its hierarchical order is a means of creating control. There are, of course, many advantages of a control system. For example, it allows the few who conceive a new automobile to ensure that the thousands who produce it will uniformly manufacture the same vehicle. Similarly, this structure is essential to the effective functioning of a modern airliner where we want one person, the pilot, to be in control with a clearly defined descending order of authority.

A second characteristic of a system is that its primary utility is its ability to produce a great deal of the same thing, whether goods or services. The hallmark of the hierarchical system is mass production – lots of the same.

The third characteristic of a system flows from the first two. If we are to create structures of control to produce great quantities of the same thing, the very proliferation of the product requires more users or users who purchase more of the goods or services. The current label for system users is client or consumer. It should be noted that the word client is especially appropriate for one who is the object of a system because the Greek root for the word client means "one who is controlled." Therefore, system growth or efficiency necessarily creates more consumption or clienthood and a consumer society emerges as systems grow.

In summary, the prevailing policy map is about the methods of organizational control that will proliferate uniform goods and services and increase the client and consumer activities of individuals. There are at least two obvious limits of this system tool. The first is its obvious lack of capacity for producing individualized outputs rather than mass standardized products. Therefore, policy makers who try to use this tool to create unique or individualized outputs, programs or services do not understand the nature or function of their own structure. This is why so many systems fail to meet individualized needs and their workers "burn out" in frustration.

A second limit is the fact that the power of the system is measured by the number of its clients and the amount of their consumption. This necessarily creates a growing relationship of client dependency upon systems. This is the reason that policy makers who attempt to use systems to empower people usually fail. They misunderstand, once again, the nature and function of their own structures.

Now that we have explored the nature of the current policymaking map involving systems and clients/consumers, we can examine its relationship to the territory it purports to describe. While it may not appear to be inaccurate, it is clearly incomplete because a space called "the community" does not appear to be present. It is, in this regard, reminiscent of the early maps that did not have the western hemisphere.

If we were to include the community, where would it be located and what would its functions be? Here, we have a historic explorer to help us answer the question. He was a French count who wrote the classic description of local American communities following his trip throughout the United States in 1831. He was, of course, Alexis de Tocqueville, and his map of our communities is described in his book, *Democracy in America* (de Tocqueville 1835).

He described a unique form of local structures and relationships. In Europe, he noted, decisions were made by elected officials, bureaucrats, nobility, professors, doctors, lawyers, engineers, etc. In the United States, however, he found critical decisions being made by the most common of people – every Tom, Dick and Mary. It was not their individual decision-making that he found unique. Rather, it was that they came together in small self-appointed groups to solve problems, create new approaches to production and celebrate the local society. It was he who named these groups "associations". This is graphically represented in Fig. 4.3.

The associations were small scale, face-to-face groups where the members did the work. The members were not individuals, clients or consumers. Rather, they were citizens. Acting together they were powerful tools of social and economic production. De Tocqueville noted that they involved citizens in three processes:

- Deciding what is a problem
- Deciding how to solve the problem
- Organizing themselves and others to implement the solution

As citizens engaged in these associational processes they created the power to build their local communities. It was the social space occupied by these associations that de Tocqueville first mapped as the centre of our communities. Today, this space is frequently called the civil society or the domain of mediating structures. Whatever the term, it was the structure and form of relationships that created the New World settlements and cities. Graphically, the community of associations might look like this (Fig. 4.4).

It is an informal network of groups of citizens creating and maintaining the centre of society. It also becomes a tool, which like a systems tool, is designed to perform vital functions. In order to understand the nature of the community tool, we can compare it with the system tool. The system tool is a mechanism of control. The community of associations depends on consent because it has neither money or grades to use to motivate people. Rather, it is the form through which people express their unique gifts, skills and talents in amplifying concert with their neighbours.

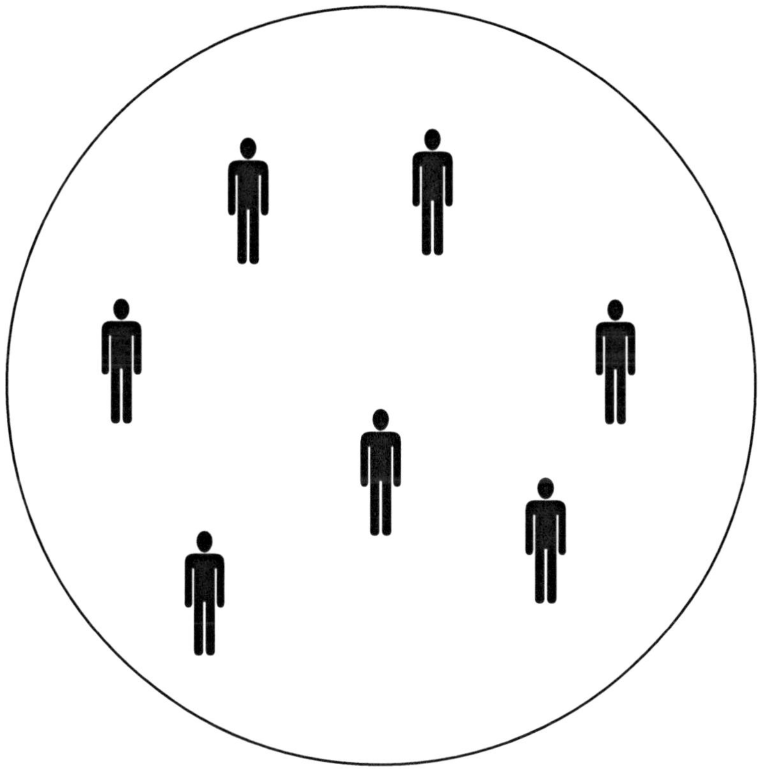

Fig. 4.3 Associations of citizens

The system tool is designed for mass production of goods and services. The community of associations is not designed to produce services. Rather, it is the context where care is manifested. Care, unlike service, cannot be produced. Care is the consenting commitment one has for the other, freely given. Care cannot be mandated, managed or produced as a service can. Indeed, one of the great errors in most policymaking maps is the pretension that systems can "produce care."

Care is the domain of the associational community. Where care is valued or necessary to achieve a societal goal, the appropriate tool is the community.

The system tool demands clients and consumers. The associational community requires citizens. Here, the critical difference is that "citizen" is the word for the most powerful person in a democracy. The contrast is the controlled person, a client. If we seek empowerment, the associational community is the appropriate tool. When we purport to empower clients, we are necessarily caught in a paradox where our best efforts will be no better than dependence on a more responsive system.

Thus, the map of the associational community is about the form of organization that depends upon consent in order to allow choice, care and citizenship. For these ends the community is the necessary, but not always sufficient, tool. Comparatively, systems provide control, mass production, consumption and clienthood. Associational communities depend upon consent and allow choice, care and citizen power.

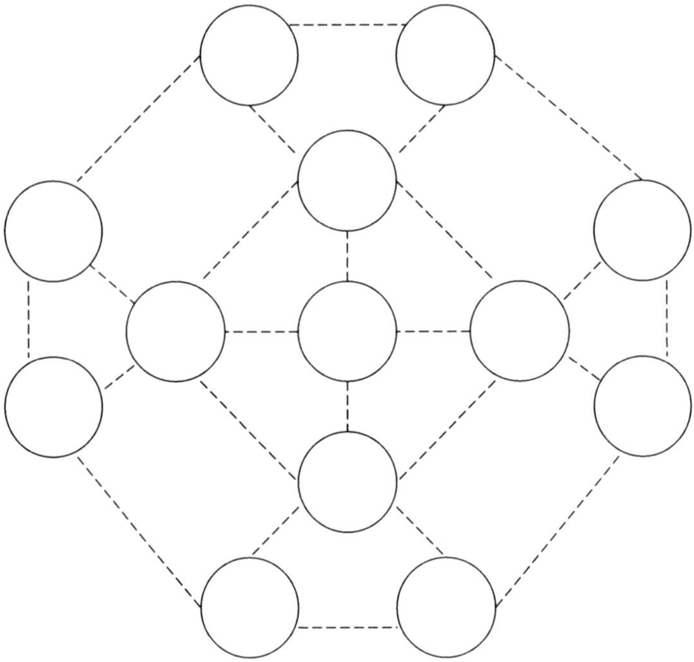

Fig. 4.4 Community of associations

There is one other distinction between these two tools that is critical in understanding social policies effecting communities and the families they encompass. Systems producing services depend upon a basic raw material. This raw material is the deficiency, inadequacy, brokenness or disease of people. When people have these attributes, they become eligible clients or consumers. The general term for these attributes is "need." In order for the system tool to be productive, it needs need. Therefore, systems create incentives and economies that focus people on their potential roles as clients and consumers.

In contrast, associational communities are structures that depend upon the capacities, abilities, skills and gifts of people. Therefore, they represent the critical incentive system for manifesting capacity rather than need. This fact is clarified when we recognize that a local person may have a heart ailment and carpentry skills. A needs system values his bad heart. The association that is building a community centre values his carpentry abilities.

In the symbolic example of the glass filled to the middle with liquid, the system needs the empty half while the community needs the full half. The service system needs a client. The community needs a citizen. When we recognize this difference, it becomes clear that communities are built through structures that mobilize the gifts and capacities of local citizens. Associational communities are the principal tool that identifies and mobilizes the gifts and capacities of citizens.

Having understood the distinctive nature and functions of the two tools, we can now map their potential relationships with each other. Whenever policy makers happen to recognize that there is a community territory, the map they draw usually looks like Fig. 4.5. Systems are represented by a triangle, while associations are represented by a circle.

This map is commonly described as a partnership. It suggests that each is an equal owner of or participant in an activity. However, the recent history of the actual system-community relationships suggests that the real territory is quite different. At least three kinds of alternative relationships are actually present in most cases.

The first alternative is a relationship of this form illustrated in Fig. 4.6.

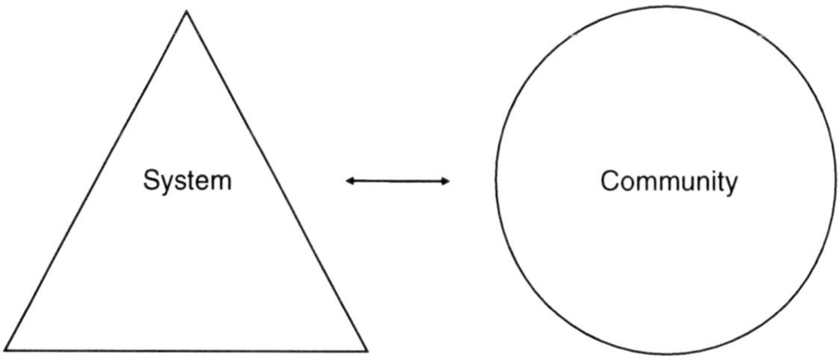

Fig. 4.5 Systems and associations

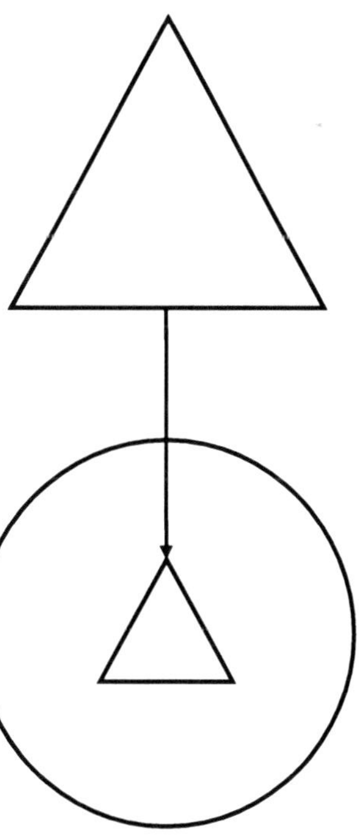

Fig. 4.6 Systems outreach

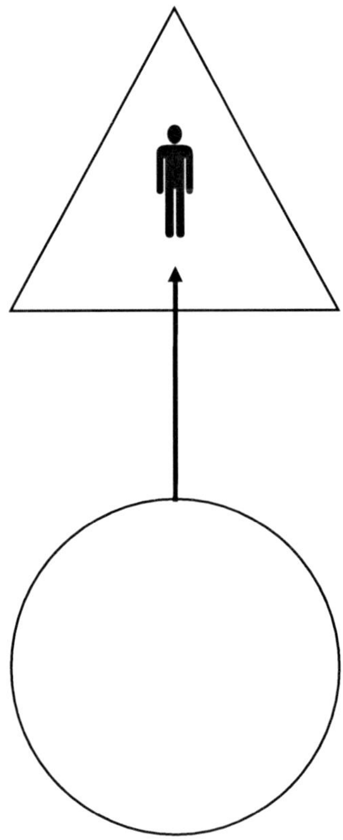

Fig. 4.7 Volunteering

In this relationship a subsidiary of a system is located in the associational community to assure access to local need. This relationship is most accurately described as system "outreach" rather than partnership.

The second form of relationship is illustrated in Fig. 4.7.

In this case the associational community is used as a source of unpaid workers for systems. The accurate name for this relationship is "volunteering" rather than partnership.

The third common relationship (shown in Fig. 4.8) is when a citizen(s) is chosen by a system to react to a system's plans. The citizen does not have authority or a vote but is advisory. The correct name for this relationship is a "citizen advisory group" rather than a partnership.

A genuine partnership is a relationship of equal power between two parties with distinctive interests. Each preserves its authority, distinct capacity and integrity but gains power through the partnership. It is difficult to find many examples of authentic partnerships of this nature between systems and associations. Instead, the actual power relationship is most often a system using a community of associations to foster its own ends.

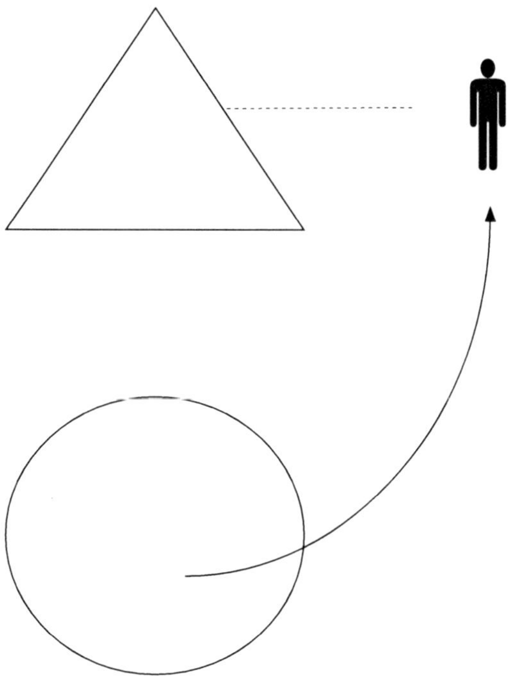

Fig. 4.8 Citizen advisory group

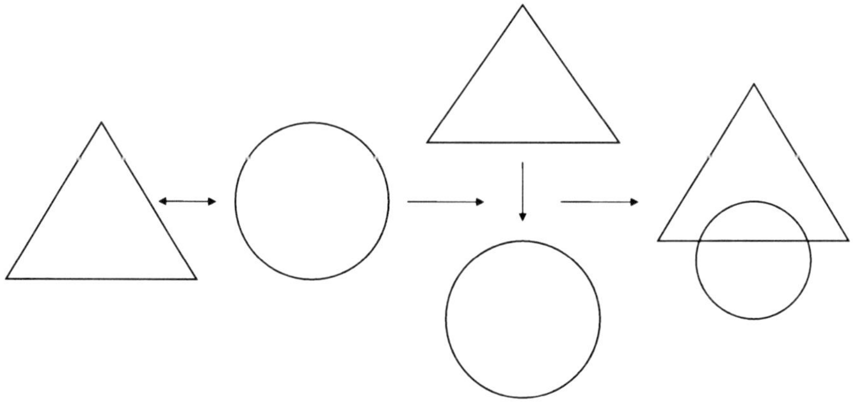

Fig. 4.9 Consumer society

Indeed, the principal history of the twentieth century relationships between systems and associations is the ascent of the system and the decline of the community of associations. The actual map of our era would chart this relationship chronologically as shown in Fig. 4.9.

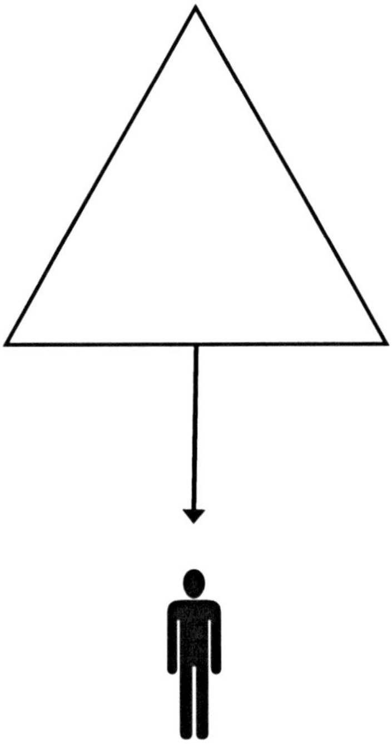

Fig. 4.10 Individuals and systems

The actual territory is one in which systems have moved from equality to dominance and then have generally eclipsed or pushed out the associations and their functions. This has happened as systems have commanded ever more authority, professional dominance, technology and public and private dollars. Another name for the result of this dominance is a "consumer society." It produces an unprecedented belief system and culture of its own.

Central to this belief system is the proposition that is embodied in the social policymaking map with which we began (Fig. 4.10).

That map indicates that systems produce our well-being. We understand that our health is located in and supported by health systems. Our safety is located in a criminal justice system. Our security is located in a pension system. Our learning is located in a school system. Our mental stability is located in a mental health system. Our justice is located in a lawyer. Our family stability is supported by the family service system. Our home is in the hands of the real estate system, and our meals are the product of McDonalds.

When this belief system becomes the dominant social construction of a people, their map of a good society is illustrated in Fig. 4.11.

One way of accurately describing this map is that it is a comprehensive, coordinated, wrap-around, inter-professional, multi service system.

Based upon this belief system, the most desirable map for strengthening families is illustrated in Fig. 4.12.

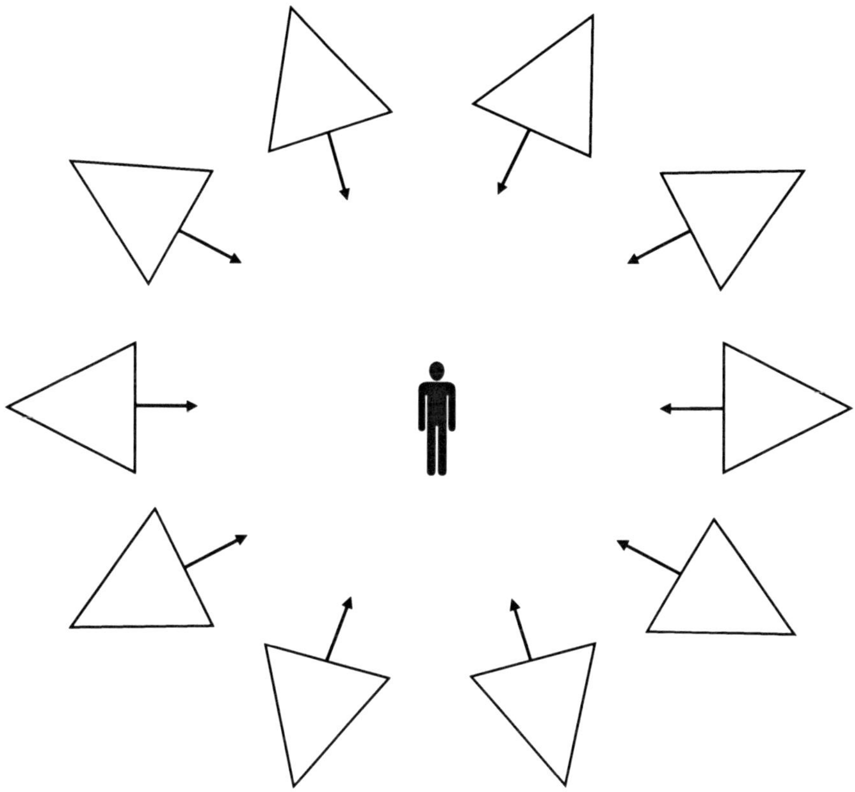

Fig. 4.11 Multi-service system

Those policy makers who believe in this map urge that its ability to produce evermore well-being for its client families depends upon two changes:

1. More money for the system
2. Better administration of the system

The result of these changes will be "systems reform" that will so effectively and comprehensively target families that our current social problems will be greatly diminished. It is this proposition and the map upon which it is based that we are asked to use in navigating the rest of the twenty-first century.

As magnificent as the map is, it has two inaccuracies. The first is a mis-mapping of known territory. The second is a great void like the Terra Incognito in the maps of old. The mis-mapping is clearly visible now. In this century we have greatly expanded the proportion of our gross national product for services such as medicine, social work, education, mental health, youth services, family therapy, legal services, recreational services, etc. And yet, the measures of social pathology are growing relentlessly. We need not rehearse again the social disarray that our media, professionals and social scientists are documenting and lamenting.

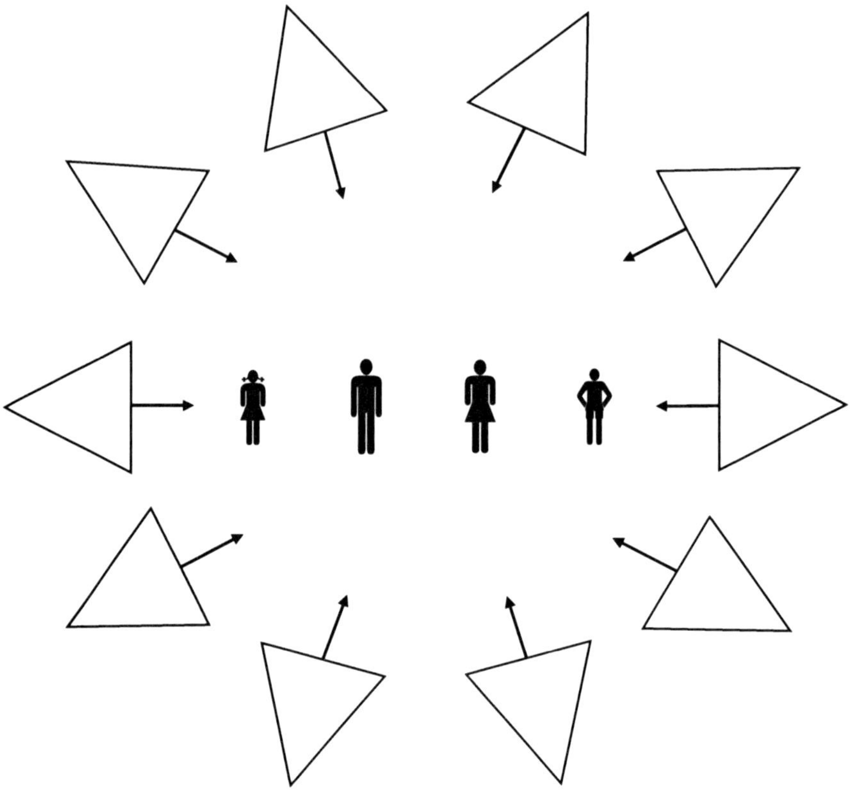

Fig. 4.12 Systems reform

The obvious question is whether even more dollars, resources, professionals, training and technology will finally stem the tide. It is clear that the public has grown dubious of this proposition. Increasingly, research scholars and foundation experimentalists are lending less and less support for the map of a family surrounded by expanding services.

Instead, basic questions are now arising as to whether the systems are actually one cause of the current social disarray rather than its principal solution. The answer to this question may depend upon whether we can draw a more accurate map that would show us a different way to proceed. We can begin by recalling the associational tools drawn by de Tocqueville (1835) and adding them to the social policy makers map with its great void between systems and individuals. This new map, shown in Fig. 4.13 would then have a different appearance:

In this map, we see families at the centre. They are further extended by kinship relationships. Then another circle of informal and formal associations provides a context for them to act through consent, care and citizen empowerment. Finally they are able to utilize system services when they will be benefited by control systems of mass production.

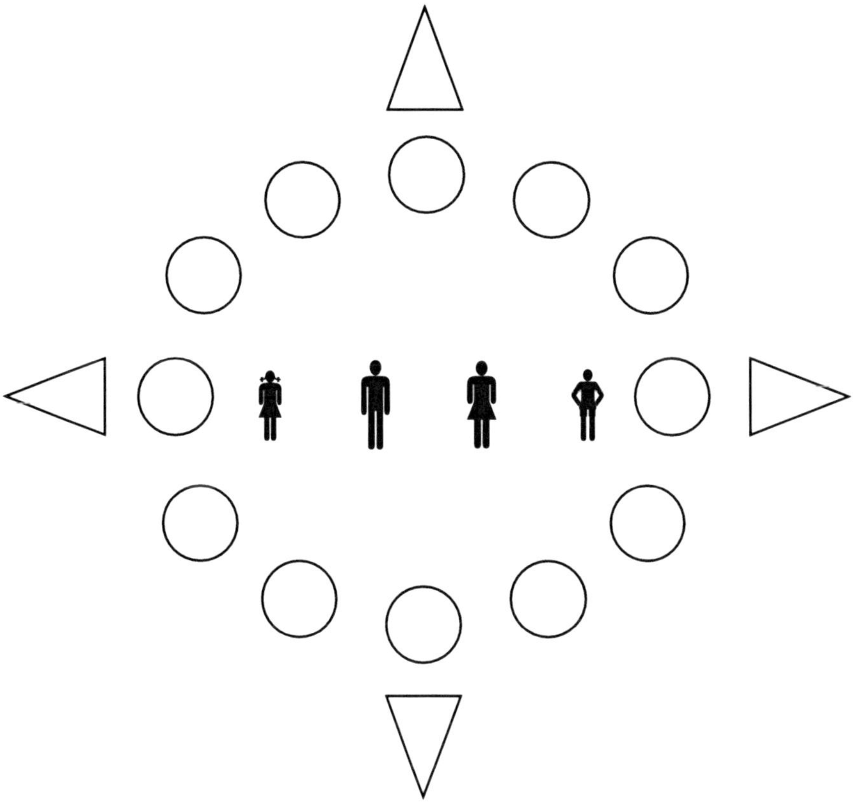

Fig. 4.13 Kinships, associations, systems

The problem with this map is that in many communities it is inaccurate because the system territory is very large while the associational community has been "crowded" into a very small space. As a result, the functions and capacities of associations are often underutilized or dormant. When this occurs we can consistently observe the parallel growth of systems and social disarray.

This apparent paradox is untangled if we examine the special capacities of associations. First, the associational community provides a network of care and mutual support that enables effective citizens to negotiate everyday life. Of more importance, however, is the support in times of crisis and stress that these networks provide.

This leads to a second community capacity which is the potential for a rapid response to local problems. Free of the time-consuming limits of bureaucratic regulation and protocol, local citizens are renowned for their ability to act in emergencies.

A third capacity is the individualization that is inherent in associational communities. This occurs when the community responds to the crisis of a particular individual in a particular way. It also occurs when each individual in an association contributes their unique ability or gift to the organization's work. Thus, the associational community is focused on the dilemma or gift of a particular individual and is able to tailor a response that is beyond the capacity of the system.

A fourth capacity of associations is their ability to recognize and utilize the unique gifts of each member. This provides a context for creativity that is critical to innovation in local problem solving. Indeed, most initial social innovation has been generated at the associational level of society and American institutions were uniquely spawned by associations.

The fifth special function of associations is to provide citizens experience in taking responsibility for society. In systems, people are ultimately fulfilling the responsibility of a manager. In communities, people are able to define and fulfil actions of their own design. It is this function that is at the core of the empowering function of associational life.

Related to this function is a sixth opportunity provided by associational life. The associational sector is often labelled civil society because it is the arena where the citizen function can be performed. A secondary aspect of this citizen function is voting. Its primary manifestation, as de Tocqueville (1835) noted, is the collective problem solving activity of local associations taking responsibility for the common good.

A seventh function of the associational community is the diverse and numerous contexts provided for leadership. While hierarchical systems are designed to provide definitional leadership to a few, the proliferation of associations provides a constant seedbed for multiplying leadership experiences and abilities.

Eighth, the network of local associations has also been the historic seedbed for the growth of local enterprise. We misunderstand economic development if we believe it grows from programs involving the creation of business plans. The soil that has nurtured enterprise and a burgeoning economy is the experiences, relationships and culture of a rich local associational community life.

Finally, and most basic, the community association is the powerful engine mobilizing the capacities of local people. It is this "half-full glass" that is the basic molecular unit of the structure of an effective society. Paradoxically, this power depends upon ignoring the empty half of the glass. It is a power grown from ignoring needs as resources. It is the power that mobilizes a person with a heart problem to use carpentry skills to build a community centre.

In summary, an associational community provides the context for:

- Care and mutual support
- Rapid response to local problems
- Individualized response and mobilization
- Creative social innovation
- Empowering responsibility
- Citizenship functions
- Leadership development
- Enterprise development
- Capacity mobilization

These functions, in combination, represent the unique role of the community understood as a network of local informal and formal associations. Where these functions atrophy, the resulting social disarray cannot be corrected by systems and their services or interventions. The reasons are those we have already explored, i.e., systems and associations are distinctive tools with unique capacities and neither can substitute for the other. Because the dominant social policy map does not recognize the associational community, it is a fatal guide to the twenty-first century. It will lead us to the shoals of a serviced society surrounded by a sea of social failure.

The map we need to navigate our future will look like the graphic in Fig. 4.14. It charts the centrality of kinship, association and enterprise and the secondary role of systems and their "inputs".

We are faced, however, with a critical dilemma. Is it possible that we can grow the community while the world of systems continues to expand? Or is it the case that inevitably, growing service systems will crowd out and ineffectively replace the functions of associational communities?

This is a historical question and its most searching exploration has been done by two great social historians. In their primary works, Jacques Ellul's Technological Society (Ellul 1964) and Karl Polanyi's The Great Transformation (Polanyi 1944),

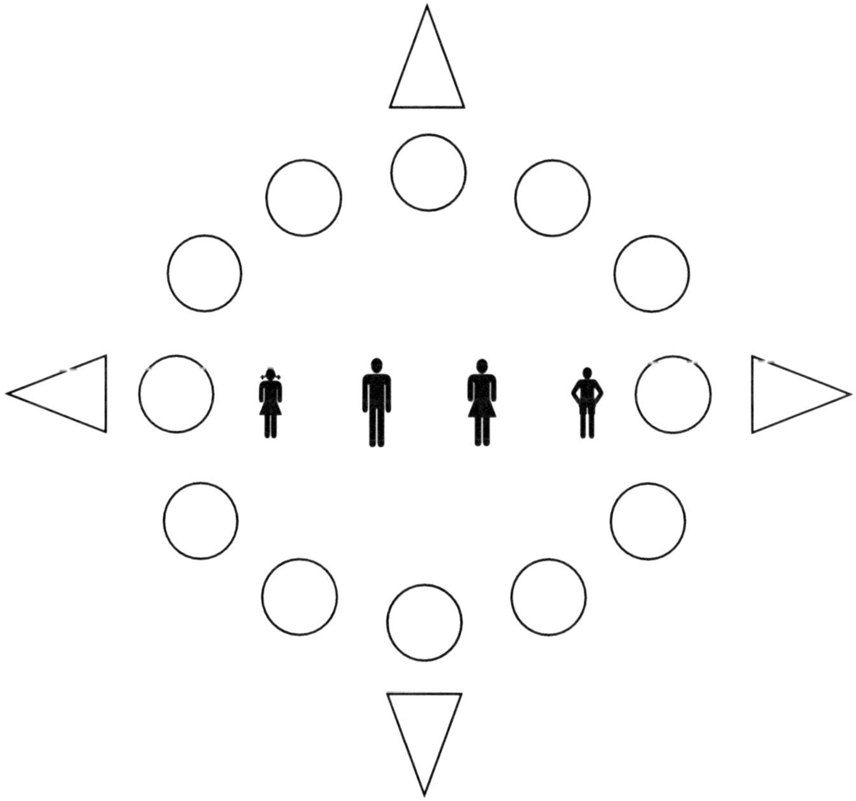

Fig. 4.14 Kinships, associations, systems

each describe from different perspectives how the form we call "modernization" in western society is a manifestation of the contraction of communal relations resulting from the growth of systems and their related tools. Their work suggests that we are in a competition between association and system. For one to win, the other must lose. It is essentially a zero sum game.

If this history is predictive, then the basic shift necessary for an effective twenty-first century map is a contraction of service systems in order to provide the territory and incentives for community structures to expand. Such a change is not really a "system reform". It is a different map, a paradigm shift.

To successfully navigate the future, policy makers will have to move in different directions. To reach their destination, they will need to enhance community power while diminishing system authority. As we undertake this journey, there are three basic principles that can guide us into a future where families and communities will flourish and social problems diminish.

First, funding priorities will shift. Over the last 50 years we have significantly increased the dollars committed to the vulnerable and disadvantaged. However, the increase has been largely allocated to service systems so that, for example, more than half of all the funds for the poor now go to systems rather than those with inadequate income.

The navigating principle here is a shift in the economics so that income and enterprise are the primary goals enhancing individuals and communities in the centre of the map. Therefore, resources will be diverted from secondary service systems to provide choice making income for individuals who are especially vulnerable. The pre-purchase of services will become a policy investment of last resort.

At the same time, other policy investments will be primarily focused on enhancing and expanding the enterprise capabilities of local associations and individuals. Community economic development, rather than remedial or compensatory services, will receive priority.

The second principle will be to recognize the nature of associational space, remove barriers to its functions and provide incentives for the community structures to assume new economic and social functions. The emerging associational map will chart the complex, diverse, interrelated array of local informal and formal associations. The purpose of the map will not be to seek associational assistance or advice to systems. Nor will it be in order to create partnerships. Rather the map will be needed to better understand the centre of local neighbourhoods, civil society and the mediating structures of locality.

From this map will be derived a set of enabling policies that remove barriers and provide support and incentives. While some may be tempted to prescribe these policies, their basic priorities and design will be developed by the local associations in concert. It cannot be expected that the associational community will assume new authority and power through the powerful directives of systems. Rather, the power must grow as their territory is recognized, barriers removed and appropriate support provided.

The third principle will be a legislative and planning focus that sees the community territory as the principle asset for investment (Kretzmann and McKnight 1993). This will require a shift from primarily focusing on needs. We will have a new compass pointing toward the capacities of individuals and families and the resources of local communities and their associations as the primary beneficiary of system authority and resources.

An asset focused family policy will be especially important in the new directions for policy makers. The principal family policy questions will be:

1. What are the necessary economic resources for an effectively productive family?
2. How can the local community of associations support the family's productivity?
3. What uncontributed gifts, capacities, skills and abilities do the family and all its members have to offer the community?
4. How can secondary systems support families so they can make these social and economic contributions?

In regard to young people who are members of families, these new principles will understand youth as assets rather than people in special need or individuals preparing to be members of society (Kretzmann and McKnight 1993). Practices will assume that:

1. Every young person has a gift, talent, knowledge or skill ready to be given, contributed or marketed now.
2. Every community is in need of these capacities if it is to be a healthy place to live.
3. The primary method to meet this need is for a local community to be organized to seek and use the capacities of youth in the productive centre of society.
4. To be in the productive centre, youth will be systematically connected to the productive work of adults and the associations at the centre of society. In this way they will become the beneficiaries of all of the functions of the associational community described earlier. Most important, they will be at the centre of care, capacity and citizenship rather than the artificial and ineffective substitute called service.

In order for these four landmarks to guide us toward a community of productive, useful, empowered young people, we will necessarily change a basic practice of most youth serving systems. We will end the age segregated bias of "youth programs" that isolate young people from the productive adults and associations at society's centre. Instead, we will seek continuing local connection of citizens of all ages in common daily experiences of productive social, civic and economic activity.

We have explored the nature of systems, clients and consumers. We have rediscovered the capacities of individuals and the associations that mobilize their abilities. We have seen the distinctive role that each must play in an effective community. We have envisioned a new map that incorporates all the known territory of the social universe. And we have charted the new policies necessary to travel the twenty-first century territory.

We should proceed, however, with a few cautions. The associational community, like systems, is a means – a tool. It has no inherent values. Therefore, as we have seen the Nazi's turn systems to their evil purposes, we have seen in Bosnia and Burundi that local communities and their associations can be turned to evil purposes. The critical issue is the continuing struggle for a culture of civility.

Another caution is that our twenty-first century map does not include an explicit space for spirituality. Nonetheless, it is clear that communities with mechanistic or individualistic cultures are missing this foundational resource. The result is still an arid space without the culture of soul that lifts citizens to a higher vision.

Finally, we must emphasize again that the local economic capacity for choice and sustenance is the threshold policy issue. For we have economically abandoned far too many communities and left at sea those citizens who have remained. It is these fellow citizens and their economic dilemma that is the first policy issue of the twenty-first century. For it is these fellow citizens who we need to contribute if our communities are to become powerful once again.

References

de Tocqueville, A. (1835). *Democracy in America.* Library of America.

Ellul, J. (1964). *The technological society.* American edition. New York: Vintage Books. (French edition published 1954).

Kretzmann, J.P. & McKnight, J. (1993). *Building communities from the inside out: A path toward finding and mobilizing a community's assets.* Chicago: ACTA Publications.

Polanyi, K. (1944). *The great transformation: The political and economic origins of our time.* New York: Farrar & Rinehart.

Chapter 5
Assets Based Interventions: Evaluating and Synthesizing Evidence of the Effectiveness of the Assets Based Approach to Health Promotion

Marcia Hills, Simon Carroll, and Sylvie Desjardins

Keywords Assets • Social capital • Evaluation • Evidence synthesis • Effectiveness framework

5.1 Introduction

As more and more evidence is collected that the determinants of population health (as opposed to "population illness") are related to a series of fundamental "assets" or "capacities" that individuals and communities have or don't have access to, it has become equally apparent that there are two basic research lacunae: the first is a lack of a positive or "salutogenic" approach to understanding patterns of health directly analogous to the traditional epidemiological approach to studying patterns of disease in populations; the second is the paucity of intervention research and evaluation on actions aimed at strengthening and supporting health assets as a way of producing healthy communities and individuals.

This chapter is focused mainly on the second lacuna, or gap. Just as there is a need to re-think traditional epidemiological assumptions in order to produce a new evidence base for which assets contribute to producing health rather than which deficits contribute to producing disease, there is a need to re-think traditional assumptions related to evaluating the effectiveness of health interventions aimed at strengthening health assets as opposed to eliminating or curing diseases. Working from a concrete example of a 4-year collaborative project in Canada aimed at developing a framework for evaluating the effectiveness of community interventions to promote health and build community capacity, we will introduce a series of profound methodological challenges that this type of evaluation research presents, along with a discussion of the attempt to use a "realist synthesis" approach to addressing these challenges.

M. Hills (✉)
School of Nursing, University of Victoria, Victoria, BC, Canada
e-mail: mhills@uvic.ca

A. Morgan et al. (eds.), *Health Assets in a Global Context: Theory, Methods, Action*, DOI 10.1007/978-1-4419-5921-8_5,

This chapter is organized into four sections: an overview and critical assessment of the implications of the "assets based approach" in relation to the field of public health and health promotion; a discussion of specific issues related to the evaluation of assets based approaches; a discussion of specific issues that the assets approach raises in relation to synthesizing evidence for the effectiveness of health promotion interventions; finally, a discussion of some lessons from a concrete example of a 4-year collaborative project in Canada aimed at developing a framework for evaluating the effectiveness of community interventions to promote health and build community capacity.

5.2 The Assets Based Approach

The assets for health and development framework was initiated as part of the broader "investment for health" (IFH) approach as put forward by Ziglio et al. (2000). This approach is underpinned by two reciprocal research discoveries: (1) the greatest improvements in people's health have come mainly from social and economic progress, rather than from traditional bio-medicine or narrowly defined public health. (2) healthier populations are also more productive populations, in need of less support by the health care and welfare system (Blane et al. 1996). The IFH approach is based on the idea that investing in health assets will both improve health outcomes and advance social and economic progress. Health "assets" can be defined as any "collective resource that could be used to promote health and gain more control over the determinants of population health" (Ziglio et al. 2000). Assets can include such things as: supportive family and friendship networks; intergenerational solidarity; community cohesion; environmental resources for promoting "physical, mental and social health"; employment security and opportunities for voluntary service; affinity groups; religious toleration; lifelong learning; safe and pleasant housing; political democracy and participation opportunities; and, social justice and equity (Ziglio et al. 2000). The crucial conceptual distinction is between health promotion interventions that focus exclusively or primarily on health "needs" or "problems" and those that focus on assets. If the primary objective of the IFH approach is to strengthen health assets, then an intervention that failed to reduce health needs would not necessarily be thought of as ineffective. Ziglio et al. put forward a two-dimensional conceptual grid, where both asset maximization and need reduction are taken into account. It is possible to improve health assets without an immediate reduction in health needs; conversely, it is possible to reduce health needs while at the same time damaging health assets. Above all, the IFH approach is concerned with advancing sustainable and ethical health promotion strategies. Any investment for health must mobilize community resources in an equitable and participatory process that works with and strengthens, rather than bypassing and diminishing, existing community resources.

What will be called the "assets based" approach in this chapter is actually a specific, and perhaps more comprehensive, public health approach that reflects a variety of disparate influences derived from a vaguely common concern. This common concern is not limited to internal self-reflections within the field of public health, but applies more broadly to social interventions in general. What has been seen as a generic concern is that the overwhelming focus of research on how and where to intervene in order to improve social and health outcomes is on the "problems" that individuals and communities have, rather than on what capacities, strengths and assets are available in these communities to tackle what are acknowledged by all to be significant obstacles to well being.

Perhaps the most persistent and consistent voice raising this concern has been John McKnight, who for over 30 years has been arguing that the exclusive focus on "needs", "deficits" and "problems" by researchers and "caring" professionals has often disabled and disempowered communities, replacing potential community driven solutions with an intensive "service environment", wherein helpful agencies and programs are funded in order to address community "needs". As Kretzmann and McKnight put it succinctly, in response to desperate situations:

> well-intended people are seeking solutions by taking one of two divergent paths. The first, which begins by focusing on a community's needs, deficiencies and problems, is still by far the most traveled, and commands the vast majority of our financial and human resources. By comparison with the second path, which insists on beginning with a clear commitment to discovering a community's capacities and assets, ...the first and more traditional path is more like an eight-lane superhighway (1993; p. 1).

The reason to start with this quote is that it sets up nicely the generic issue or concern, which the "assets based approach" to public health has to tackle in relation to its own specific set of problems. Within the public health field, the "superhighway" has been what is fairly described as orthodox epidemiological research. This includes even the more innovative and sometimes radical "social epidemiology", with the latter focused on more complex "social pathologies" as opposed to the restrictive physiological and environmental foci of its more traditional parent discipline. In other words, most public health science, with some exceptions, is entirely focused on the pathological generation of disease, as opposed to looking at the positive mechanisms that generate health. Many, particularly in Europe, would call the latter emergent approach, the "*salutogenic perspective*" (Chap. 1). It should be noted of course, that this shift of perspective to a focus on health rather than disease, is also the foundational tenet of the health promotion movement.

As there are many other chapters in this book that outline the assets based approach in detail, the rest of this section will focus less on explicating the overall perspective and more on a series of conceptual and methodological difficulties that are posed by making this switch in perspective. The reason to do so is that, when considering the assets based approach in relation to the issues of evaluating and synthesizing evidence on intervention effectiveness, it is these conceptual and methodological problems that come to the forefront. This somewhat distinguishes our set of problems from the type of issues that confront a community organizer trying to implement an assets based mapping exercise like the ones advocated by Kretzmann and McKnight (1993). There are two reasons for this divergence in problems. First, the problem confronting the community organizer is often a directly political one of convincing other members of the community and local authorities that an assets based approach is preferable to the normal, top-down, needs-based approach offered by existing services. We confront a different problem, in that what we face is an existing paradigm of research that is being challenged in terms of its appropriate scope, its relevance and its adequacy. Questions of "evaluation", "synthesis" and "evidence" are directly *scientific* questions that no doubt have profound political implications, but nevertheless require a rigorous confrontation with conceptual and methodological difficulties. Second, the assets based approach within public health acts at a much broader scale and scope and thus entails more complexity and more profound methodological problems than does the community assets mapping approach. As far as we are concerned, the type of "methods" developed by Kretzmann and McKnight (1993), while not perfect, are perfectly adequate to the task; what faces serious public health scientists in the task of shifting the public health research paradigm is a paucity of tools and methodologies rigorous enough to present a serious challenge to the reigning orthodoxy.

To begin, there is a very general problem that advocates of the assets based approach must confront. The fact is that the "normal" way of doing public health research is to do epidemiology. What this means is that, even when we are not doing research that would be termed "epidemiological", we are nevertheless held to the internal methodological standards of epidemiology as *the* public health *science*. While most researchers in the social sciences (with the possible exception of economics), as much as they may complain of "positivist orthodoxy", live in a world of quite extraordinary diversity in terms of philosophical approaches, methodologies and methods, public health sciences are dominated by a very well developed, coherent paradigm of research within epidemiology, which has its own internal rationale. Its focus on pathology is not exclusively due to a myopic obsession with needs, problems and deficits, but in fact has much more to do with core methodological issues than appears on the surface. Although "paradigm" is a badly misused term in much social science discussions, in this case, one can argue that its use is appropriate and relevant to the original sense given by Kuhn (1970). Arguably, one of the most challenging difficulties that a project of revolutionizing paradigms faces is that such revolutions are by definition not a "project"; rather, they tend to be "generational". First, it is only after an accumulation of anomalies confronts a discipline's ability to problem solve in the "normal" way that any serious consideration is given to radically different theoretical approaches. Second, the "alternative" has to gain some foothold in terms of credibility, and it has to be relatively coherent and consistent. Most crucially, it must offer clear methodological strategies and methods that can demonstrably produce findings that consistently "solve" existing anomalies (Kuhn 1970). As we will see in the rest of this chapter, we are only starting on the path to shifting perspectives within public health research.

Before moving directly to concrete problems in trying to evaluate assets based health interventions, there are several important conceptual and methodological issues to address concerning the overall assets approach. Let us start with the definition of health assets as offered by Morgan and Ziglio in Chap. 1: "as any factor (or resource), which enhances the ability of individuals, groups, communities, populations, social systems and /or institutions to maintain and sustain health and well-being and to help to reduce health inequities."

We find this to be an admirable definition and one that will surely offer some guidance to the field as it tries to develop research strategies to support the overall model. However, one can immediately see that the definition has two striking characteristics: one, it is remarkably *diffuse*; another, it implies enormous *complexity*. To say that this approach to definition runs against the grain of orthodox epidemiology would be an understatement. For most epidemiologists, and in fact, most scientists dealing mainly with quantitative methods, the values of parsimony and simplicity are the guiding principles for defining terms. Why? Because, for the purposes of mathematical representation and then measurement, terms have to have clear, unambiguous definitions. This is true no matter what theory of measurement one uses or what type of measurement scale. Even for a simple nominal scale, we have to be able to clearly identify exclusive units of the scale. Yet, what is a health asset and what is not? Think about what "any factor (or resource)" could mean. Let us look at a few of the possible assets listed above: supportive family and friendship networks; intergenerational solidarity; community cohesion. While all these terms have meaning and certainly, on an intuitive level, have enormous relevance to community health, they are also terms that are notoriously difficult to measure appropriately. Of course, there are many attempts to develop proxy indicators for these sorts of concepts, but the history of these attempts serve more as a salutary warning about methodological sloppiness, than as progressive steps toward a tidy solution (McQueen and Noack 1998).

To provide a more concrete example of the types of conceptual and methodological issues being referred to here, we offer a brief discussion of one of the more thoroughly studied concepts relevant to the assets approach: social capital. Other public health and health promotion researchers have offered critical reviews of how the concept of "social capital" may or may not be helpful to the field (Edmondson 2003; Labonte 2004). These latter references are important, but in order to dig more deeply into issues directly related to measurement, assessment and evaluation, an interesting tangential perspective can be offered by considering a tough-minded economic critique of the concept (Durlauf and Fafchamps 2006). We do this not in order to produce any original analysis of the concept of social capital, nor *a fortiori*, to offer anything substantive to the economic literature on this subject; instead what we intend is to explicate some of the analogous issues that pertain to the assets approach in general that can be found by considering this critique of the social capital concept.

Durlauf and Fafchamps' main concern is in relation to producing "rigorous empirical research" on the concept of social capital. They do not dispute the intuitive and theoretical relevance of the concept, no matter that it is currently enmeshed in all sorts of vagueness and ambiguity. They focus their argument on whether current research methods and approaches to social capital are adequate to empirically demonstrate the relationship between social capital and beneficial economic outcomes. They pay attention to both global aggregate outcomes, such as improved economic growth and development, as well as distributional outcomes such as wealth and income inequality. While these economic outcomes are not synonymous with public health outcomes, they are directly analogous: public health wants to see a relationship between health assets and improved overall health outcomes, as well as the relationship between health assets and more just or "equitable" distributions of health.

The basic premise of Durlauf and Fafchamps' paper is that, while social capital is a potentially powerful concept, and has some successful empirical applications, the vast majority of uses of the concept lack rigor and precision, employ circular reasoning, or make unwarranted assumptions in order to get off the ground. We will consider only two of their many trenchant criticisms, both chosen for their obvious relevance to concerns within public health and health promotion. First, we consider the problem of "non-triviality". That is, we need to be sure that our definitions of terms are not trivial, meaning, in this context, that they do not presuppose beneficial effects. Here is how Durlauf and Fafchamps put it:

> "The study of social capital is that of network-based processes that generate beneficial outcomes through norms and trust...By this definition social capital is always desirable since its presence is equated with beneficial consequences. This formulation is quite unsatisfactory from the perspective of policy evaluation (e.g., Durlauf 1999, 2002), if one denies the appellation of social capital to contexts where strong social ties lead to immoral or unproductive behaviors, there is nothing nontrivial to say in terms of policy."

As one can immediately discern, some of the same problems plague the health assets approach. Take for example, the use of "community cohesion" as a health asset. It is assumed in the definition that community cohesion (however it is measured) is *ipso facto* a beneficial "enhancer" for individuals, communities, groups, even whole societies to "maintain and sustain health and well being and to help reduce health inequities". However, if, by definition, it is not possible to have "community cohesion" affect the desired outcomes negatively, then what is the point of empirical investigation, never mind policy action? In fact, as Labonte points out, there is good reason to believe that "community cohesion" can have negative social exclusionary effects, and thus undermine at least the equity outcome named above (2004). A related issue when it comes to empirical work on aggregating and synthesizing data, is that such triviality in definition can actually lead to dangerous fallacies of composition. For example, if one wants to measure the effect of community cohesion on health outcomes, simply aggregating individual level data on health outcomes may ignore the distributional effect of some groups receiving large health benefits from community cohesion, while other more excluded groups are negatively affected. Thus, the aggregate data shows a positive effect on health of the population, yet some groups are actually suffering negative effects from community cohesion. Potvin et al. (2007), have been at the forefront of demonstrating this equity problem for public health, but this has been demonstrated formally elsewhere on a much more general level in terms of classical welfare outcomes (Durlauf and Fafchamps 2006).

The second problem with the concept of social capital, and by analogy with many proposed factors or resources that may act as health assets, is also tied to the problem of equity, and relates to the essentially *relational* aspect of these types of concepts. As Durlauf and Fafchamps point out, often some groups or individuals use social capital to get ahead of others groups and individuals in a competitive environment. While there is nothing to rule out universally beneficial outcomes from increases in social capital, to rule out potential conflicts between group and individual interest would be naïve. For these authors, the important point is to avoid importing unexamined conceptual assumptions into the methodology and measurement of social capital; however, their overall message applies equally to many related or analogous social science concepts and their place in building a body of empirical evidence. Needless to say, if the basic data collection is conceptually flawed, any attempt to synthesize results will be equally flawed, if not compounded by the false assumption that heterogeneity of results can be accounted for through statistical fixes, or other analytical approaches.

Finally, we can look to another source to emphasize the problem with the *relational* aspect of these types of social science concepts. Although increasingly referenced as an important theorist to consider for health promotion and public health theory, Pierre Bourdieu has been, with some exceptions, ignored when it comes to considerations of the concept of social capital. While Bourdieu certainly was not amongst the main protagonists in the Anglo-American literature on the social capital concept, and the roots of the concept are far removed from Bourdieu's specific set of theoretical concerns, his own conceptualization of the use of different forms of "capital" in structuring social hierarchies is highly relevant to the questions we have been outlining above. First, Bourdieu is quite clear that most of the forms of collective "capital" that we utilize to further our well-being are predicated on modes of *social distinction* (Bourdieu 1986). What this means is that the effectivity of certain forms of social capital derive their power by maintaining distinctions and conserving their value through scarcity of supply. Elite social networks and clubs are excellent examples of this process. These forms of social capital may demonstrably enhance the well being of their members and their offspring; however, a potential solution is not an additive one of simply increasing access for more people to these groups. This is because part (if not all) of their value is maintained *because* of their relational exclusivity, not due to any substantial identifiable and independent essential properties. In other words, the effectiveness or convertibility of these forms of social capital relies precisely on the fact that the symbolic power they exercise is based on the relational exclusivity of their memberships. While networks work differently in terms of maintaining boundaries, similar relational attributes apply. Being a central node in a social network loses its relative power in direct proportion to the level of equality in terms of density of ties between different nodes. The benefits of being a central node are partly determined by the fact that this level of connection is relatively rare. If everyone has the same level of connections, then the symbolic power of distinction is lost. This does not imply that access to social capital is devoid of positive non-relational benefits; what it does imply, is that in considering social capital and by analogy, health assets, we should not ignore this crucial conceptual advance made by Bourdieu.

What these conceptual problems in relation to equity reinforce is that we need to be very careful about our methodological strategies for empirical investigation in the area of health assets. There are two main lessons to keep in mind from our brief survey above. First, the candidate "health assets" that are routinely listed as the key factors or resources, have to be very carefully defined. Furthermore, their operationalization as variables and indicators needs to be built upon more careful ethnographic and observational research. It is not good enough to follow the conventional epistemology of psychometric validation. The theory of representation should be based on inherent validity derived from consideration of real world structural characteristics of the phenomena in question. In other words, measures, if they are possible at all, should take into account the complexity of the underlying concept, but should nevertheless aim at clarity over vagueness.

The second key lesson is that, whether "health assets" can be considered beneficial cannot be decided by a matter of definition, but must be understood in relation to the specific contexts within which such potential assets operate. This approach allows us to avoid the problem of triviality by understanding that the beneficial effect of different social factors or resources is a complex, non-reductive function of how they *interact* with other contextual factors. As we will see, for these reasons, a critical realist approach is helpful in untangling some of these more complex methodological problems.

5.3 Implications for Evaluation

The limited evidence of the effectiveness of health promotion initiatives is due, at least in part, to the inherent difficulties in evaluating assets based health promotion community interventions. As discussed in Chap. 1, historically public health and health promotion initiatives have tended to focus evaluations on a deficit perspective. "That is there is a tendency to focus on identifying problems and needs of populations that require professional resources and high levels of dependence on hospitals and welfare services" (Ziglio et al. 2000; Morgan and Ziglio 2006).

What is required is a total re-thinking and re-conceptualizing of evaluation that is appropriate for assets based health promotion initiatives. First, we need to emphasize an integrated approach to process and outcome evaluation, formative and summative approaches. Even in evaluations that are primarily focused on outcomes, issues of implementation context and complexity have to be considered. Second, these initiatives/interventions by their very nature, demand that empowering and participatory approaches to evaluation be used. Most orthodox approaches to evaluation are antithetical to the essence of assets based health promotion.

One of the most disappointing aspects of reviewing literature on evaluations of capacity building activities and health outcomes is the dichotomy between the type of evaluation approach that is seen as necessary for supporting effectiveness assessment and the type that is seen as more helpful for "formative" or "process" issues. In order to bring an evaluation focus to how enhancing health assets can lead to better outcomes, we need to move beyond this dichotomy. As was explained in the first section of this chapter, the type of phenomena represented by the factors and resources conceptualized as "health assets", is inherently complex and contextually determined. A phenomenon like "inter-generational solidarity" is not like a drug and does not act as a typical dose-response causal mechanism. Like many other potential health assets, inter-generational solidarity is multiply determined, tends to have causal effect in tandem with other interacting factors, and will in any case tend to have a non-linear relationship with positive effects on health, particularly through emergent, transitional thresholds. In order to capture these complex phenomenon and their causal effects on outcomes of interest, there needs to be an approach that integrates both data collection tools and analytical strategies to consider how particular health assets are internally structured, externally related to a set of interacting contextual factors and, finally, causally connected to positive health outcomes. In order to do this successfully, issues of process and implementation are not merely supportive after-thoughts for reviewers, or relegated to the periphery of reflective practice, but are *integrally* and *internally* related to the conceptualization of the evaluation of the "effectiveness" of health assets. For these reasons, there are three crucial advances necessary for the field: more subtle measurement approaches that capture the internal complexity of health assets; more attention to the socio-ecological contexts within which health assets operate; and, more innovative analytical strategies to match the complexity of the phenomena involved in assets based interventions.

Another important aspect that needs to be re-thought is the relationship between orthodox, non-participatory approaches to evaluation and the attempt to establish an assets-based approach. Orthodox evaluation because of its value and philosophical base, purposely does not allow practitioners that are engaged in implementing programs to conduct the evaluations because of the belief that these practitioners can only provide subjective evidence and that the results are not credible and are biased. It is time to question these assumptions if we are to begin to collect data that is relevant to assets based health promotion programs.

In orthodox evaluation an external evaluator is typically hired as a consultant to evaluate the community program. In essence, this evaluator collects data about the program, analyzes and interprets the findings and delivers a report with recommendations. This orthodox approach to the evaluation process, alienates those who care most directly about the program; it provides little or no opportunity to reflect, examine or learn from the data; it neglects opportunities for practitioners to develop data analysis capacity; and, it produces anxiety and cynicism about evaluation. As Reason describes,

> "Orthodox evaluation methods, as part of their rationale, exclude participants from all the thinking and decision-making that generates designs, manages and draws conclusions from the evaluation. Such exclusions treat the participants as less than self determining persons, alienates them from the inquiry process and from the knowledge that is its outcome, and thus invalidates any claim the methods have to a science of persons" (Reason 1988).

We need to challenge the assumptions that underlie orthodox evaluation by asking: What is the relationship between the evaluator and those delivering the program? What should be accepted as evidence upon which to base practice? What information do we need to explain program success and failure? For example, knowing the number of participants who attended a program can tell you about "reach", perhaps, but what does it tell you about what was learned or about what was changed? What caused the change? In our opinion, evaluators are not asking the appropriate questions that will help them explain causal relationships that lead to outcomes. For example, most practitioners who implement assets-based health promotion programs would agree that meaningful participation is critical to the success of these programs. However, there are very few examples, if any, of program evaluations that assess the impact of "meaningful participation" on program outcomes.

Perhaps, if we could begin to think about evaluation as "reflective practice" rather than program evaluation, we could begin to explicate the complexities that are inherent in these programs. After all, it is people that implement programs and the processes that they use directly impact the outcomes of that program. So, what actually makes one assets-based health promotion initiative work and another not?

It is beyond the scope of this chapter to describe alternative approaches to evaluation that are more consistent with the philosophy of health promotion, but many scholars are struggling with these issues and there is a recent emergence of several diverse approaches that provide some hope for future. (Hills and Mullett 2000; Minkler and Wallerstein 2003; PAHO 2004). The key point is that it makes little sense to utilize an evaluation approach that undermines the very strengths and capacities that it aims to evaluate. If we are trying to assess whether various health assets are being enhanced and what their relationship is to improved health outcomes, the real threat to validity is caused by a cynicism that negatively affects the assets we are trying to explore, generated by the lack of participation in the evaluation process we too often see in orthodox approaches.

Although there has been some move over the past few years to focus more on evaluating the impact of health interventions on positive assets and capacities in communities, most evaluation is still focused mainly on deficits and needs and how these are being addressed. Furthermore, there is a tendency to lump all focus on "capacities" into the category of "process" evaluation, which is dichotomously divided from "outcome" evaluation. This prejudice leaves communities in an awkward place because, in terms of reflective practice, process evaluation is seen as very important, yet, in terms of accountability to funding bodies, outcome evaluation is seen as paramount. The assets-based model opens a new opportunity to have an integrated evaluation approach that overcomes the old dichotomies between process and outcome evaluation, and between so-called "formative" and "summative" approaches. We need to start understanding improvements in specific health assets *as* intermediate outcomes in a linked chain of progress towards improving overall health and social outcomes.

It is crucial that we not underestimate the importance of letting a participatory approach to evaluation drive this new emphasis on assets. Communities, where all interventions eventually must have an effect, are naturally disposed to a focus on assets and strengths, as this perspective is also internally related to issues of empowerment and sustainability. Building on inherent capacities, even in the most vulnerable populations, is a way of ensuring both that communities can take prideful ownership of intervention processes, and that any gains made can be sustained.

Finally, it is equally important that a new and focused rigor is brought to bear on evaluation concepts and measuring tools that need to be developed to support the asset model. There is still too little work on well-designed indicators that can be integrated into evaluation strategies to assess the impact on health assets of health promotion and other public health interventions. We know that the importance of "context" in evaluating health assets is undeniable; yet, we have very little in the way of rigorous, consistent evaluation protocols and tools to collect evidence on contextual factors. These are areas that cannot be ignored if we are to deal with the intrinsic complexity of assets-based interventions and thus the complexity of their evaluation.

5.4 Implications for Evidence Synthesis

If there are major changes that are necessary in how we approach evaluation in order to be congruent with an assets-based approach to public health, this is equally, if not more true, in relation to the question of how to synthesize evidence from evaluation data to assess the effectiveness of assets-based interventions in general. In this section, we first try to distinguish between the concepts of "evaluation" and "effectiveness". We then move to consider the "realist" critique of existing synthesis approaches, and finally explicate the realist alternative.

5.4.1 Evaluation vs. Effectiveness[1]

"Evaluation" refers to a generic type of research, where a particular intervention or activity is examined to assess its "success" (or lack thereof) through the analysis of the processes and outcomes of that set of activities. Evaluations may provide information for a variety of uses, including: feedback to participants in the activities or projects; dissemination purposes; theory-building exercises; and, accounting for the benefit or worth of the activities in question in terms of effectiveness, efficiency, and equity etc. "Effectiveness", as implied above, is a much more specific concept. The goal of effectiveness research is to assess whether a specific *type* of activity (such as "community interventions") has the desired "effect" in relation to a specified objective or set of objectives (e.g. increased knowledge, awareness and improved health practices) (Tones and Tilford 1994). As mentioned earlier, evaluation is a broader research activity that has been an integral part of public health and health promotion since its beginnings; demonstrating effectiveness, on the other hand, is a more recent and much more demanding undertaking.

Evaluations are often concerned with *individual* interventions and their outcomes; effectiveness is concerned with the relationship between a *type* of intervention and outcomes that are observable across interventions. In other words, to

[1] It should be noted by way of caveat that often people understand the term evaluation to apply to the concept of effectiveness more generically. However, due to two developments in the literature, we want to emphasize this contrast: first, because of the rise of the systematic review, 'evidence review' or 'synthesis' are used more often in relation to questions of effectiveness; second, the types of methodological problems that arise in doing evidence syntheses are *sui generis* and need to be distinguished from the methodological debates within evaluation as a separate topic.

assess effectiveness, the researcher has to look *across* evaluations of a specific type of intervention in order to show that it works more generally. For example, it is possible to evaluate a specific community intervention in order to demonstrate that it achieved its goals in a particular setting; however, to show the effectiveness of community interventions, it is necessary to collect evaluation data from across many interventions in order to "test" the type of intervention as a generically successful or beneficial approach.

Although there are some superficial similarities in the methodological debates within the evaluation literature and the effectiveness literature, the latter's inherent demand for *comparability* means that the issues are different and are derived from a different historical and logical context. The effectiveness research debate centers around the increasingly urgent quest for evidence-based policy making (Pawson 2002a). Here the question is not so much about how to do evaluations (although it has large implications for the latter), but about how to do *systematic analyses* of previously collected evidence. As Pawson puts it concisely: "By building a systematic evidence base that captures the ebb and flow of program ideas we might be able to adjudicate between contending policy claims and so capture a progressive understanding of what works" (Pawson 2002a). In order to inform policy on the basis of evidence, some form of review of reviews is necessary or policy-makers are caught in a cycle of forever catching up with mountains of emergent evaluation data that never seems to offer direct guidance. Pawson (2002a) has argued that this is the crucial point that sometimes gets missed: "The case for using systematic review in policy research rests on a stunningly obvious point about the timing of research vis-à-vis policy: in order to inform policy, the research must come before the policy" (p. 158). For these reasons, we refer to this problem as one of "evidence synthesis".

Of course, depending on the approach taken to systematic review, what should count as adequate evaluation data (from the perspective of the effectiveness reviewer) looks very different, and this is where the two concepts converge. Evaluation approaches have traditionally been divided into two opposing views, either labeled "quantitative vs. qualitative" or "positivist vs. interpretive". There are many different and more specific categorizations of evaluation approaches; nevertheless, the more simple dichotomies referred to above are adequate to give a sense of what has been at the core of the debate. The two main streams of evaluation still fit under the broad categories of positivist and interpretive (Guba and Lincoln 1989), which equate roughly with the meta-analytical and narrative manners of conducting systematic reviews. There are two more recent approaches that are distinctive: the participatory evaluation approach; and, the realist evaluation approach, the one we propose to utilize here.

The participatory approach argues that both the positivist and the interpretive approaches are wedded to a notion that there is an "evaluation expert" that has special access to a form of knowledge that is superior to that of the people involved in the work of the initiatives being evaluated. The participatory approach recognizes the value of different types of knowledge and sees evaluation as a collaborative process of reflection-in-action, where researchers and participants work together to develop and implement evaluations (Hills and Mullett 2000; Minkler and Wallerstein 2003).

The realist approach argues, similarly, that the positivist and interpretive approaches are inadequate, yet for different reasons. The realists are inclined to agree with much of the interpretive critique of positivism, but are reticent about accepting the conclusion that evaluation can only be about "inter-subjective meaning". Realists are concerned to defend a position that can maintain "objective" standards of evaluation in so far as the reference of evaluative work is to *what is actually happening in the world*, as opposed to restricting themselves to what is *perceived to be happening* by particular groups of people. In other words, realists want to retain a distinction between what people think is going on and what is actually going on. So let us see how they criticize the positivist and interpretive views.

5.4.2 The Realist Critique of Meta-Analytical Systematic Reviews

Researchers tasked with performing a systematic review must rely on the type of evidence collated from the mass of evaluation data compiled by evaluation research. The dominant "meta-analytical" tradition of systematic review (in fact, often the definition of systematic review is conflated with meta-analysis) relies on evaluation data that has standardized, quantifiable outcomes. This approach considers the intervention itself a "black box", wherein what may or may not go on is of little methodological concern. The main issue is to abstract from each intervention outcomes data in terms of measures of impact (net effect) that is comparable across interventions, so that standard statistical methods can be applied in calculating the "typical" impact (mean effect). The level of analysis is usually aimed at assessing the effectiveness of "programmes" and their "sub-types" or methods of delivery. The implication for evaluation is that "good" evaluations are those that provide standardized outcomes measures (whether these are appropriate or not is left unexamined) (Pawson 2002a).

The meta-analytical approach suffers from some serious drawbacks. First, it reduces many different interventions to programme sub-categories that may or may not be comparable in terms of their basic theoretical perspective or their practical implementation. Often these categories simply lump together initiatives arbitrarily on the basis of professional specializations and bureaucratic distinctions. The point here is that meta-analyses do not investigate this issue systematically[2] and so cannot be sure that the categories they use compare like with like, a foundational requirement of any causal assertions.[3] Second, in terms of outcomes, meta-analysis often encourages the worst cases of what Alfred North Whitehead called the "*fallacy of misplaced*

[2]This is not the same as statistical measures of "heterogeneity" of data which tend to avoid the conceptual problem of identity and theoretical homology.

[3]Formally, if we cannot be sure that category X represents the class $x^1 \ldots x^n$, where all x's are equal, then X cannot be a putative cause of anything.

concreteness" (Whitehead 1997/1925). This is where abstractions, which may or may not have been useful and helpful in one context become employed in a second context as if they are fully concrete entities existing with a life of their own. Thus, the results from using measurement scales constructed for the purpose of identifying changes according to a particular psychological theory, become recruited and aggregated with other measures of psychological change as part of some more generic category of psychological change, which is then aggregated with other measures of even more general behavioral change as part of some "meta"-category of positive change, to arrive at what Pawson (2002a) calls "*means of means of means!*".

The desperate push to do respectable statistical analysis ends up with ghostly abstractions transubstantiating into flesh and blood measures of real performance. We are left with a "spurious precision" constructed through a rhetorically powerful masquerade of numbers (Pawson 2002a). Finally, and perhaps most glaringly from the perspective of its critics, meta-analysis squeezes out, if not eliminates, the context within which initiatives take place. This would not be such a serious concern if it was true that the context were not relevant to the outcomes; yet, it is a commonplace observation (in the very best sense of the term) that the success of many community initiatives depends on much more than simply the programme involved. Who is involved, how and in what circumstances are crucial factors in the success of any initiative (Labonte 1996; Pawson 2002a; Vingilis and Pederson 2002). The black-boxing of context in this case can lead to: Type I Error, where significant variations in outcomes are attributed to programme differences, when in fact they are due to confounding factors in the contexts of the interventions; Type II Error, where variations in outcomes are not significant enough to be attributed to programme differences, when in fact more significant differences would have been found if the confounding factors had been taken into account; and, Type III Error, where negative outcomes are attributed to programme failures when in fact they are due to poor intervention implementation. Much criticism has been leveled at meta-analysis for its cavalier attitude to these issues.

5.4.3 The Realist Critique of Narrative Systematic Reviews

The "narrative review"[4] approach to systematic review requires quite the opposite type of evaluation data. One could almost say that this approach starts with the maxim: "the more detail the better". In general, this approach to systematic review

[4]Pawson's term is, as admitted by the author, an umbrella concept that tries to capture a variety of approaches that meet up with similar methodological problems. "Meta-analysis" and "narrative review" are therefore not symmetrical terms; the former is a fully developed and standardized methodological approach, whereas the latter is simply a useful label for an array of differing and even mutually incompatible approaches. Furthermore, there have been recent advances in the narrative review approach that address some of Pawson's critique, particularly work by Jennie Popay and colleagues.

has developed in a number of directions, all of which are sensitive to the glaring inadequacies of the "meta-analytic" approach. These strands of research, often inspired by the interpretive paradigm of social scientific inquiry, attempt to pay much more attention to the process of interventions, detailing the key or significant aspects of each example in the hope that an accumulation of such data can be abstracted from to provide lessons about a program's effectiveness.

Narrative review can be characterized as a reaction to the fact that the technique of meta-analysis ignores, or at least does not take account of, much of what is available in the evaluation literature, never mind what could be made available. Its critique ranges from the gentle admonishment of meta-analysis's more arrogant extremes to a radical questioning of the entire program of meta-analysis. On the "gentler" end of the spectrum, critics suggest a more balanced approach to including data in systematic reviews to allow more detail of a qualitative nature (Dixon-Woods and Fitzpatrick 2001). At the "radical" end, there is a constructivist critique that tends to deny any sort of objective comparability at all (Dahler-Larson 2001; Guba and Lincoln 1989).

The first criticism of the narrative review approach is from the orthodox meta-analytical stance. Here it is argued that the narrative review approach is inadequate to the task of detecting small intervention effects, thereby leading to Type II error (false negative result), because of the heterogeneity of interventions, outcomes and contexts (Petticrew 2003).[5]

Whatever the merits of this particular criticism, a more fundamental one is that developed by Pawson (2002b), who argues that narrative review fails every time it attempts to move from in depth analyses of individual studies to a level of abstraction that is logically consistent and comparable *across* different studies. This is inadequate precisely because it merely churns qualitative data into countable indicators, without addressing the basic criticism of this procedure that underlies the original rejection of positivism. What is missing is a rigorous philosophical basis for an alternative approach. While the realist approach may suffer from equal difficulties in terms of concrete alternative empirical tools and method ological frameworks, as we will see, what it does have is a fully consistent philosophical alternative to the positivism inherent in orthodox meta-analytic approaches.

5.4.4 The Realist Synthesis Approach

Limitations to current approaches demonstrate the need to develop a new framework. Pawson's realist synthesis approach provides a foundation for such a framework (2002a, b). Pawson (2002a) argues that exposing exemplary cases has less to

[5]This is a somewhat ironic criticism, as the main thrust of the author's argument is that, meta-analysis tends towards a "stainless steel" law of review, where: "the more rigorous the review, the less evidence there will be to suggest that the intervention is effective" (Petticrew 2003: pp. 757–758).

do with reviewing evidence and more to do with testing submerged theories. Adopting a realist synthesis method enables the synthesis of evidence from different initiatives and programs and has the capability to link processes to outcomes by formulizing the interaction between a program's mechanisms, contexts, and structures (Pawson 2002b).

Pawson (2002b) argues that it is not the "programs" themselves that are generating change; it is the resources or reasons they offer to subjects. In order to successfully orchestrate evidence based practice, the emphasis on causality must be aimed at the basic processes of any initiative. These basic processes can then be broken down and analyzed and viewed as specific mechanisms. Determining whether the same mechanism yields similar results in diverse settings can draw meaningful comparisons; and both negative and positive results are equally important to consider (Pawson 2002b). This approach also points out that though some kind of systematic review is necessary to inform policy-makers, the timing of such a review is often not synchronized. To be successful at informing policy, it is crucial that research comes before the policy (Pawson 2002a).

Systematic reviewers, when dealing with a combination of mechanisms, need to sort through contexts that lead to successful outcomes from contexts that result in failure (Pawson 2002b). Contextual information can be taken into account as part of the underlying mechanisms, allowing comparisons across contexts. In the end, the systematic review should rest on "families of mechanisms", not on "families of programs" (Pawson 2002b).

The realist synthesis model offers great opportunity for growth in knowledge translation practice as it enables the synthesis of evidence across different programs and initiatives and provides a detailed formulation of the interaction between mechanisms, contexts, and structures of community programs in a dynamic model, linking processes to outcomes.

We now move to a concrete example of a research project that utilized a realist synthesis approach to guide the development of a framework for assessing the effectiveness of community interventions. As we will see, the much of the substantial elements of this project were concerned with community capacities and process that act as factors or resources that are health assets.

5.5 An Example: The Effectiveness of Community Interventions Project

In Canada, the Public Health Agency of Canada (PHAC) and Health Canada (HC) fund health promotion community initiatives that aim to promote health and enhance community capacity. These programs are based on a population health approach, and generally, they attempt to use an assets-based approach to bring about change. That is, they focus on the communities' resources and capacities to improve health. The project described in this chapter evolved from a need to gain a better understanding of the success of different community intervention approaches as well as their relevance in modifying different outcomes that lead to improved health. The basic driving force behind what has been called "effectiveness research" is the need for funding authorities, both public and private, to *account* for the utility of investments in specific forms of work and sets of activities. There is a continuing pressure on these funding authorities to ensure that the funds they expend are spent in the right areas and in the right ways. In other words, there is some return on their investment. In this context, in 2003, a 3-year collaborative initiative between the Canadian Consortium for Health Promotion Research and the PHAC was initiated entitled the "Effectiveness of Community Interventions Project" (ECIP).

This project focused on the development of a framework for assessing the effectiveness of community interventions to promote health. In particular, it concentrated on how to assess the evidence of the effectiveness of federally funded community intervention approaches that target three specific outcomes (increased awareness, knowledge and improved health practices). The project involved three main activities: A literature review on the effectiveness of different community intervention approaches that address awareness, knowledge and improved health practices; the design of a framework/tool for assessing the effectiveness of community intervention approaches in achieving their intended goals related to awareness, knowledge and improved health practices; an initial validation of the framework/tool (see Fig. 5.1) with selected Health Canada community interventions. The interventions were chosen from two strategic

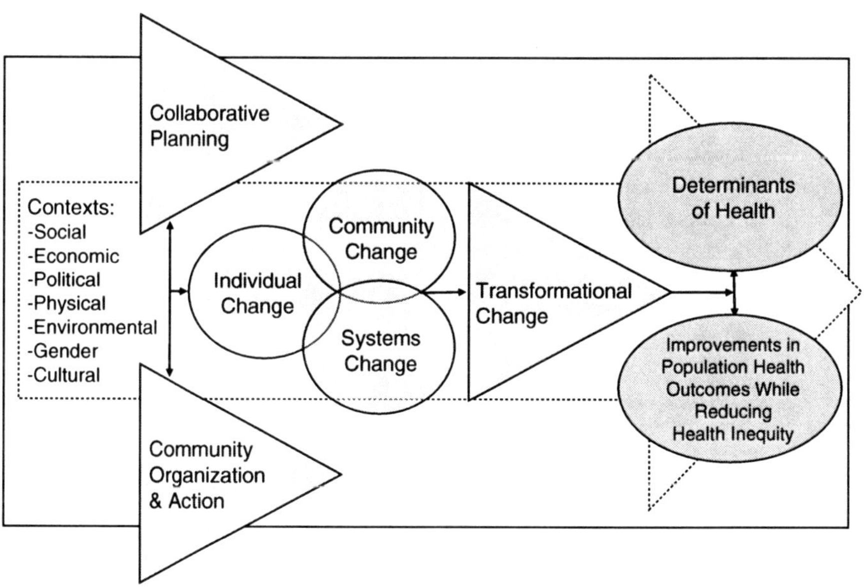

Fig. 5.1 Framework for assessing the effectiveness of community initiatives that promote health

areas (nutrition and HIV/Aids) and three programs (Canadian Prenatal Nutrition Program, Canadian Diabetes Strategy, and Canadian HIV/AIDS Program).

In acting as researchers on this project, the Canadian Consortium for Health Promotion Research proposed to use a modified "realist synthesis" approach as an alternative to the usual systematic review of evidence in order to address some of the complexity that was evident in trying to assess the effectiveness of the HC/PHAC programs.

In order to put this approach into practice, our first task was to identify a framework for assessing the effectives of these interventions, and as importantly to identify key mechanisms of action that were thought to be causally related to successful intermediate and long term health and health equity outcomes. The framework provided a logical basis for an analytic and synthesis strategy that related mechanisms, contexts, and outcomes. Thus, as Pawson argues, the "locus of comparison" is the mechanism(s), which may or may not be activated, and may or may not lead to the projected outcomes. For example, it may be that "Collaborative Planning" is identified as one of the basic processes that are necessary for successful community initiatives. The question then becomes: what mechanisms drive this process forward successfully? However, even if the correct mechanisms are identified, their *causal power* may not be activated in any particular circumstance, or even if the crucial mechanisms are activated (e.g. key stakeholders are involved), their affectivity may be counter-acted by other contextual mechanisms (e.g. political support is taken away). The issue here is that one can take account of important contextual information, without losing the level of abstraction that the mechanisms represent, and therefore maintain the basis for comparison across contexts. In this example, we may end up with "failure" in terms of outcomes; yet, because we can explain the reason the mechanism was not effective, the mechanism itself (involving key stakeholders) is not thereby discounted for its causal power. What we have then as the systematic reviewer's basic task is for any putative mechanism or a combination of mechanisms (M), to "sift through the mixed fortunes of the program attempting to discover those contexts (C+) that have produced solid and successful outcomes (O+) from those contexts (C−) that induce failure (O−)" (Pawson 2002b; p. 345). Of course, in order not to simply generate a list of positive and negative contexts, the contexts themselves must themselves be broken down into interacting processes thus preserving comparability for the purpose of policy making.

5.5.1 Components of the Framework

The five components in Fig. 5.1, represent either staged outcomes (proximal to distal) or parallel processes, depending on whether one is taking a static or dynamic perspective. The first two components are arranged in parallel to emphasize the interactive nature of the planning/action couplet. It has been noted by many researchers that successful actions are dependent upon an iterative process of reflection-in-action (Kemmis 1990; Heron 1996; Hills and Mullett 2000; PAHO

2004), where planning is improved by feeding back reflections from ongoing activities. The middle component represents, on the one hand, intermediate health promotion outcomes, including increased knowledge, awareness, and improved health practices; on the other hand, it represents a dynamic process of diffusion and adaptation in the wider local community. The third component, transformational change, focuses on promoting broader change that has an impact on societal norms and high level policy development. The final two components are again coupled, this time to emphasize the important causal relation between impacting the determinants of health and improving population level outcomes (e.g. smoking cessation is exemplary). These two last components represent broad population level changes and are more distal in terms of available outcomes.

5.5.2 Candidate Mechanisms of the Framework

The list below represents the candidate mechanisms the project has compiled, based on previous work in the field, a review of the literature (presented in details just after the list), an expert review panel, as well a first validation using six cases provided by PHAC/Health Canada (Hills et al. 2004a, b).

These mechanisms can be thought of as guiding principles or criteria for action that assist and promote individuals and communities to focus on their own assets, capacities and skills to bring about change that promotes health. The authors are in the process of developing and testing tools that help to capture the implementation of these mechanisms and their impact on outcomes.

5.5.2.1 Component 1: Collaborative Planning

1. Meaningful participation of all relevant stakeholders
2. Critical dialogue
3. Shared power
4. Project action planning and evaluation

5.5.2.2 Component 2: Community Organization & Action

1. Ongoing education and training opportunities
2. Evolving leadership
3. Sustained mobilization of resources
4. Critical reflection and systematic monitoring

5.5.2.3 Component 3: Transformational Change

1. Develop and attract champion
2. Generate publicity of project successes

3. Influence Public Policy and Decision-making Bodies
4. Work with relevant social movements and provincial and/or national advocacy groups

5.6 Conclusion

The most relevant lessons this very important collaborative research experience taught us about "assets based" approaches revolve around the disjunction that exists between the pervasive discourse about capacities, strengths, assets, and participation surrounding these innovative interventions on the one hand and the dominant approaches to evaluation and evidence synthesis on the other. Whenever we talked to practitioners or read informal accounts of what was most important to the success of these interventions and initiatives we invariably found reference to the key mechanisms we identified in the theoretical literature and in discussion sections of formal evaluations. However, when we looked for formal evaluation data on these key mechanisms, we looked in vain. So often, a formal evaluation report would focus on a set of traditional indicators, such as number of participants (reach) and individual changes in knowledge or behavior. The report would then conclude that there was insufficient evidence of changes related to the intervention, but would go on, in the discussion section, to note the many wonderful things that the intervention had an impact on but were never evaluated or couldn't be evaluated because there were no available indicators or tools to help document evidence of these changes; thus, we are left with more or less persuasive anecdotal accounts.

Another huge gap was in any available means to integrate contextual information into the analysis of effectiveness. There were neither data collection methods developed, nor were there ready-to-hand analytical techniques to synthesize and integrate into effectiveness assessment. Although the realist approach offers an excellent basis for philosophically justifying an approach that focuses on mechanisms and contexts, there is still much more work to do in the development of concrete methodologies and methods for collecting and analyzing data, and then the complex synthesis of these multiple sources of evidence.

As we hope to have shown, "health assets" in particular, are exactly the type of complex phenomena to require matching complexity, subtlety and innovation in methodological technique. Unfortunately, we have too often been left with the false dilemma of either accepting overly simplistic and rigid traditional methodology or being left with less than rigorous and vague references to how difficult this type of intervention research is for evaluators to handle. We have long since made important theoretical advances in understanding public health interventions as part of a complex, socio-ecological system, made up of many interacting parts. The assets based approach is entirely in line with this trend in theoretical understanding. However, we have found that we now need to go out and collect relevant data to test and refine these theoretical postulations. The assets approach will progress only if this key strand of its program is implemented and researchers actively collaborate with practitioners, policy-makers and community members to help produce this new world of evidentiary resources.

We are not the first ones to point out that evaluating phenomena such as participation, empowerment, social capital and other similar concepts is difficult. Yet, it is now time to stop fretting about how difficult it is and time to start developing innovative solutions. We firmly believe that success on this front is tied directly to how successful we are in developing collaborative, participatory approaches to both primary data collection and to evidence reviews. The former requires much closer collaboration between researchers, practitioners and community makers, while the latter requires much more close collaboration with policy makers, who are often the primary consumers of evidence reviews. We believe that the ECIP initiative in collaboration with the PHAC is one such collaboration, and many other successful collaborations have taken place in other jurisdictions. While it is justified to be very optimistic about the potential of the asset based approach, it will require a lot more groundwork in supporting the evidence base for the effectiveness of asset based interventions.

References

Blane, D., Brenner, E., & Wilkinson, R. G. (1996). *Health and Social Organization: Towards a Health Policy for the 21st Century*. London: Routledge.

Bourdieu, P. (1986). *Distinction: A Social Critique of the Judgement of Taste*. London: Routledge & Kegan Paul.

Dahler-Larson, P. (2001). From programme theory to constructivism: On tragic, magic and competing programmes. *Evaluation*, 7(3), 331–349.

Dixon-Woods, M., & Fitzpatrick, R. (2001). Qualitative research in systematic reviews has established a place for itself. *British Medical Journal*, 323, 765–776.

Durlauf, S., & Fafchamps, M., (2006). Social capital. In P. Aghion and S. Durlauf, (Eds.). *Handbook of Economic Growth*. Amsterdam: North Holland.

Durlauf, S., (1999). The case "against" social capital. *Focus*, 20, 1–4

Durlauf, S. (2002). On the empirics of social capital. *Economic Journal*, 112, 459–479.

Edmondson, R. (2003). Social capital: A strategy for enhancing health? *Social Science & Medicine*, 57, 1723–1733.

Guba, E. G., & Lincoln, Y. S. (1989). *Fourth Generation Evaluation*. Newbury Park: Sage.

Hills, M., & Mullett, J. (2000). *Methodologies and Methods for Community-Based Research and Evaluation*. Victoria: University of Victoria, Community Health Promotion Coalition.

Hills M., O'Neill M., Carroll S., & MacDonald M (2004a). *Effectiveness of Community Initiatives to Promote Health: An Assessment Tool Report*. Submitted to Health Canada on behalf of the Canadian Consortium for Health Promotion Research/ le consortium canadien de recherché en promotion de la santé.

Hills, M., Carroll, S., & O'Neill, M. (2004b). Vers un modèle d'évaluation de l'efficacité des interventions communautaires en promotion de la santé: compterendu de quelques développements Nord-américains récents. *International Journal of Health Promotion and Education. Hors série – 1, Supplement – Edición especial*, 17–21.

Heron, J. (1996). *Co-operative Inquiry: Research into the Human Condition*. London: Sage.

Kemmis, D. (1990). *Community and the Politics of Place*. Norman: University of Oklahoma Press.

Kretzmann, J., & McKnight, J (1993). *Building Communities from the Inside Out*. Chicago: ACTA.

Kuhn, T. (1970). *The Structure of Scientific Revolutions*. Chicago: University of Chicago.

Labonte, R. (1996). Community health promotion strategies. In PAHO (Ed.). *Health Promotion: An Anthology* (pp. 138–148). Washington, DC: Pan American Health Organization.

Labonte, R. (2004). Social inclusion/exclusion: Dancing the dialectic. *Health Promotion International*, 19, 115–121.

McQueen, D, & Noack, H. (1998). Health promotion indicators. *Health Promotion International*, 3, 117–125.

Minkler, M., & Wallerstein, N. (Eds.). (2003). *Community Based Participatory Research for Health*. San Francisco: Jossey-Bass.

Morgan, A., & Ziglio, E. (2006). Foreword. In Mel Bartley (Ed.). *Capability and Resilience: Beating the Odds*. London: Dept. of Epidemiology, University College London.

PAHO. (2004). *Participatory Evaluation of Health Municipalities: A Practical Resource Kit for Action (Draft): PAHO*. Washington, DC: PAHO.

Pawson, R. (2002a). Evidence-based policy: In search of a method. *Evaluation*, 8(2), 157–181.

Pawson, R. (2002b). Evidence-based policy: The promise of 'realist synthesis'. *Evaluation*, 8(3), 340–358.

Petticrew, M. (2003). Presumed innocent – Why we need systematic reviews of social policies – Commentary. *American Journal of Preventive Medicine*, 24(3 Suppl 1): 2–3.

Potvin, L., Mantoura, P., & Ridde, V., (2007). Evaluating equity in health promotion. In D. McQueen and C. Jones, (Eds.). *Global Perspectives on Health Promotion Effectiveness*. New York: Springer.

Reason, P. (Ed.). (1988). *Hum, Tan Inquiry in Action: Developments in New Paradigm Research*. London: Sage.

Tones, K., & Tilford, S. (1994). *Health Promotion: Effectiveness, Efficiency and Equity*. London: Chapman and Hall.

Whitehead, A. N., (1997). *Science and the Modern World*. Free Press, Simon & Schuster. (First published 1925).

Vingilis, E., & Pederson, L. (2002). Using the right tools to answer the right questions: The importance of evaluative research techniques for health services evaluation research in the 21st century. *Canadian Journal of Program Evaluation*, 16(2), 1–26.

Ziglio, E., Hagard, S., McMahon, L., Harvey, S., & Levin, L. (2000). Investment for Health. Paper presented at the Fifth Global Conference on Health Promotion, Mexico City, 5–9 June 2000.

Part II
Building an Evidence Base on Assets and Health

Chapter 6
Resilience as an Asset for Healthy Development

Mel Bartley, Ingrid Schoon, Richard Mitchell, and David Blane

Keywords Resilience • Diet • Capability • Health inequality

6.1 Introduction

This chapter examines positive adjustment and resilience as an asset, which can promote good health, even in adverse conditions. It presents a number of different models that have been put forward to explain how resilience works; compensatory, protective and challenge. Resilience is not a constant but is something moulded and shaped by the physical and social environment. Some people, depending on financial or social determinants, will have more freedom and capacity to make healthy choices.

A healthy diet is used as an example of a factor which can promote health resilience in some communities, even those where there are levels of socioeconomic disadvantage. Relative health inequalities in a number of Southern Mediterranean countries are used as an example of this. However, the authors argue that in these countries health advantage is conferred by a much more complex range of factors than diet alone. The role of social, religious and ethnic support following deindustrialisation is discussed. The paper concludes with an analysis of the largely unexplored impact of the contemporary removal of much unpaid female labour (both physical and emotional) from the domestic sphere and the untold impact of this on the physical and emotional development of the family. The changing roles and relationships of men and women within in the family have effectively, and perhaps unexpectedly, removed beneficial health assets.

As long ago as 1948, the World Health Organization defined health as a *"state of complete physical, mental, and social well-being and not merely the absence of disease or infirmity"* (WHO 1946; p. 28). Despite this affirmative definition of health, most subsequent studies over the past half century focused on health in terms of illness, disease, dysfunction and disability. A renewed call for attention to positive health

M. Bartley (✉)
Department of Epidemiology and Public Health, University College London, London, UK
e-mail: mel.bartley@btinternet.com

A. Morgan et al. (eds.), *Health Assets in a Global Context: Theory, Methods, Action*,
DOI 10.1007/978-1-4419-5921-8_6, © Springer Science+Business Media, LLC 2010

and well-being by the WHO Venice Office has given rise to a pioneering focus on assets rather than deprivation and on strengths rather than deficits. The early development of this programme of work was part of the inspiration behind the Economic and Social Research Council's (ESRC) Research Priority Network on *"Human capability and resilience"*. In this chapter, members of the Network set out some of the ideas that have informed our research, and some of the ways in which these may inform the further use of the "assets paradigm" in public health.

Most empirical studies of individuals and communities experiencing serious adversity, such as severe family disruption or persistent poverty, reveal that such adversity usually has negative consequences on health. "The poorer a community is, the greater will be their level of poor health and mortality", is a generalisation which holds largely, but not wholly, true, and which drives the dominant focus on deficits and risk in public health. However, the practices and processes by which some individuals and communities do adapt to adversity, and "cope" or even "thrive", despite it, are less widely observed and considered, even if they are usually admired when brought to our attention. Attempts by social scientists to understand this capacity are, however, relatively recent, and even more recent are attempts to extend this research into the field of public health. The founders of resilience research such as (Antonovsky 1979; Garmezy 1985; Werner and Smith 1992), turned away from an emphasis on illness or maladjustment among hazard-exposed groups and towards *"the strengths of risk-exposed individuals as well, both in terms of adjustment outcomes (competence in addition to symptomatology) and in terms of characteristics that promote positive adaptation – assets or protective factors as well as 'liabilities' or vulnerability-enhancing ones."* (Luthar et al. 2000a; p. 574).

Most of our present understanding of resilience is drawn from studies of children brought up in severe adversity who prove to be "hardy survivors" and go on to *"live well, work well, and love well"* (Werner and Smith 1992). In many of these studies, the definition of positive adaptation has been rather limited, often confined to the avoidance of addiction to drugs or alcohol and of criminal or violent behaviour and high-risk sexual behaviour. Such definitions unfortunately turn us away from focusing on the processes by which resilience can be achieved and the individual or community assets which foster these processes. A limited definition of resilient outcomes also diverts attention from the possibility that many might deploy resilience practices as a response to adversity, even if they are not successful in adaptation.

A recent review of the field distinguishes three models of resilience: compensatory, protective and challenge models (Fergus and Zimmerman 2005). The authors define "assets" as characteristics residing within the individual such as competence, coping skills, and self-efficacy. Factors external to the individual such as parental support, adult mentoring, or community organisations are defined as "resources". Others have used the term "resources" as a synonym for assets, referring to the human, social, or material factors utilised in adaptive processes (Masten and Reed 2002).

According to the compensatory resilience model it is the joint influence of different assets or resources, i.e. their cumulative effect which compensates or counteracts the effects of adversity. A cumulative resilience model assumes a direct effect of resource factors on an outcome, which can be independent from the risk factor (Fergus and Zimmerman 2005). The protective resilience model presupposes an interactive relationship between the protective factor, the risk exposure, and the outcome, whereby a protective factor shows its beneficial effects primarily for those exposed to the risk factor, but does not necessarily benefit those not exposed to the risk factor (Garmezy et al. 1984; Rutter 1985, 1987). The protection model of resilience assumes that the resource factors interact with (or, in epidemiological terms, "moderate") the risk factor and reduce the effect of a risk on an outcome. The third model of resilience, the challenge model, suggests that low or moderate levels of risk exposure may have beneficial or steeling effects, providing a chance to practice problem solving skills and to mobilise resources (Masten et al. 1999; Rutter 1987). The challenge model assumes a curvilinear association between a risk factor and an outcome, where the risk exposure must be challenging enough to stimulate a response, yet must not be overpowering (Garmezy et al. 1984).

Combining the existing approaches from social and developmental psychology with the new "health assets" approach requires some careful attention to terminology and definition of concepts. Fergus et al. conclude that: "A rich understanding of resilience processes ... necessitate including cumulative risks, assets, and resources studies over time." (Fergus and Zimmerman 2005; p. 13.9). In this way they create a clear link between the study of resilience and the increasing interest within social epidemiology in life-course processes in chronic disease (Kuh and Ben-Shlomo 1997), highlighting the need to examine the accumulation of both risks and resources or assets.

Up to the present time, life-course epidemiology has also tended to focus on the accumulation of "risk factors" only (Brunner et al. 1999; Bartley and Plewis 2002; Galobardes et al. 2004). Consideration of the possibility that health assets may also "accumulate", and that this may be expressed at certain times of life as resilience, requires more complex theoretical and methodological approaches (Schoon et al. 2002, 2003; Schoon 2006; Wiggins et al. 2004; Bartley et al. 2004).

Health assets are seen as being shaped by the social and physical environment. In agreement with this, Luthar and colleagues do not view resilience as a property of the individual, but as a set of conditions that allow individual adaptation to different forms of adversity at different points in the life course (Luthar et al. 2000b). Individuals are not born with resilience, nor do they develop it as a stable personal characteristic. On the contrary, levels of resilience may vary over time according to facets of the social environment (Schoon 2006). In this chapter we hope to show that resilient practices and processes may be regarded as health assets which need to be better identified and promoted by social and economic policies.

For example, research has consistently revealed the quality of social relationships, not just in the family but also in the school and neighbourhood, as promoters of resilience (Anonymous 2000; Masten and Coatsworth 1998). Having good-quality relationships with others is universally considered as being vital to positive health and optimal living (Ryff and Singer 1998). A full understanding of human health has to consider not only physical health but also psychological and social flourishing. Individuals with more positive social relationship histories show lower levels of allostatic load (defined by blood pressure, waist–hip ratio, cholesterol, haemoglobin, and "stress hormones" such as cortisol) – a stronger cardiovascular, metabolic and sympathetic nervous system (Ryff and Singer 2002).

The findings of the ongoing research of the Network is turning attention towards the importance of existing capabilities of individuals and communities who face adverse circumstances, even if these capabilities may be expressed in terms that do not fit with conventional ideas of "achievement". Young people growing up in harsh material circumstances and subject to negative attitudes may acquire a toughness that appears to middle class professionals as problematic behaviour in need of correction, when in fact these attitudes are protective given the realities of their lives. Ungar, in his book "*Nurturing hidden resilience in troubled youth*" (Ungar 2004) has challenged fixed boundaries between adaptive and maladaptive behaviours and emphasises the importance of experiences that enhance capacities, promote self-determination, and increase social participation. For example, young women in similar circumstances are more likely than their more privileged peers to become mothers early in life. These young mothers may not achieve as much in terms of education and later career success as their middle-class sisters, but early motherhood does not seem to damage their mental health over the longer term.

During the economic crisis of the 1980s, when mass youth unemployment emerged in the UK, suicide rates rose dramatically in young men, while they continued to decrease in young women, although rates of early motherhood increased. Research may reveal a range of "resilient practices" already embedded as health assets in communities which, if given support rather than discouragement, may be sufficient in themselves to meet a wide range of negative life events. It is better not to make assumptions about what is a "good" or a "poor" outcome over time. Such assumptions might, for example, enforce a definition of "living well" in terms of conventional career or family trajectories that might not be meaningful to all members of a population. This would be the equivalent to trying to force a river into a concrete channel that was pre-determined according to the interests and culture of a single interest group, which has been found to have suboptimal consequences. Rather, the research tends to indicate the importance of policies and services that leave open the maximum scope for different life-trajectories to be chosen without others being irrevocably shut off.

6.2 Resilience Capability and Freedom

Some of the literature on resilience seems to imply that the world might be a better place if no-one ever experienced adversity. And indeed, many of the case studies of, for example, extreme poverty, or alcohol or drug-related child neglect, describe circumstances to which no-one should be exposed. Does this mean that in an ideal world resilience would be an irrelevance? Not at all. Risk-taking is a normal and desirable feature of life for a very large number of individuals. Risks may be experienced involuntarily, but can also be voluntarily faced in order to follow a wider number of life choices, from the desire to exercise entrepreneurial skill to a wish to save the lives of others despite danger to oneself. By definition, any risk may result in a deterioration of life circumstances, whether this be financial, emotional or physical. The ability to adapt in the face of such negative change, and some degree of confidence in this ability, is therefore a major feature in the individual's perception of their own freedom to lead a valued life, that is, in Sen's sense, *"resilience increases capability"* (Deneulin and Shahani 2009). In turn, research also indicates that the more time an individual has spent in a capability-producing environment, the greater the resilience they are able to carry forward to meet the next challenge they may face. In order to understand how we think this works, it is necessary to look more closely at the relationship between capability and health.

Health itself has been characterised as a basic capability, in that good health enables a person to function as an agent, and thus freely choose a valued life (Tremblay 1999). In this chapter, however, which focuses on health issues as they exist in developed and emerging European nations, we need to take a step back from this position. Rather, we regard it as important for the individual to possess the freedom to pursue health itself, and therefore to understand in some detail the sources of limitation to that freedom. Examples of such limitations are wide-ranging but include being forced by financial necessity to accept hazardous or stressful working conditions; to live in polluted areas; and psychological challenges such as addictions, and the addiction-like behaviours referred to as "health risk behaviour". Both of these are problems faced by many individuals in developed nations.

6.3 Sources of Resilience and "Healthy Choices"

How might the freedom to pursue health ("make healthy choices") be increased for people facing such challenges? Of course, different threats to this freedom will require very different policy responses. Working conditions can only be improved by protective policies; the obligation to work or to live in unhealthy conditions can only be removed by adequacy of income for both those with and without employment. But psychological vulnerabilities such as addiction have their roots in the combination of individual life history and present life circumstances. In all of the (rather few) studies that have been carried out on this topic, there are no differences in knowledge about health hazards of diet and smoking between the more advantaged social groups and those less advantaged groups whose members are more likely to engage in health risk behaviour (Blaxter 1990; Shewry et al. 1992). If anything, the evidence is that those who smoke, for example, are even more aware of the risks than those who do not. Research points to the conclusion that the reasons for social inequalities in health risk behaviours (and thus the most effective preventive measures) are not to be found in beliefs or knowledge, but rather in features of the relationship between the individual and the social environment. It is clear that some forms of social environment increase the freedom of individuals to follow the health behaviours that they themselves regard as most desirable, and other forms reduce this freedom.

Forms of resilience will be important in the face of both physical and psychosocial hazards that are encountered later in life, but in very different ways. An individual who has had a healthy childhood will be better able to survive periods of hazardous employment should they indeed be forced to follow such a path or chose it consciously aiming for an improvement in their situation.

Research shows that physiological resilience is increased by having been born to a healthy mother after a normal gestation and brought up in a clean, safe, warm and dry home where income is adequate to needs (Skuse et al. 1994; Baxter Jones et al. 1999; Parker et al. 1999; Heim et al. 2001; Power 2002; Seguin et al. 2003; Hemmingsson and Lundberg 2005). These are conditions that would be desirable for all young citizens. However, such conditions are in fact more important to those who face later physical hazard even than to those who do not. Those who enter a psycho-social environment that increases the risk of addiction may similarly be empowered by a sense of self-esteem, good coping and social skills that have been facilitated in earlier life.

However, there are also wider influences of social norms and institutions that weaken the relationship between material disadvantage, social inequality and health-damaging forms of behaviour. We know that in a wider international perspective, socioeconomically disadvantaged conditions are not universally correlated to all forms of health-damaging behaviours (Kunst 1997; Mackenbach et al. 1997a). While not in any way wishing to use this as a justification for lack of policy action on socioeconomic disadvantage, it is instructive to examine the situations in which health assets are found among less privileged social groups.

6.4 Diet as a Source of Resilience: the Importance of the Social Context

A major comparative study of health inequality in the European nations (Kunst 1997; Mackenbach et al. 1997b) has found similar or greater inequalities (depending on age) between social classes in mortality in wealthy and egalitarian Nordic nations such as Norway and Sweden than it found in Italy, Ireland and Portugal. Even more surprisingly perhaps, inequalities in mortality during the 1980s were found to be larger in Sweden than in the United States in men aged 30–44 and no different in men aged 45–59 (Kunst 1997). Kunst reflected that:

> There were good reasons to expect that egalitarian socioeconomic …policies resulted in a substantial and lasting reduction in inequalities in health. However, comparative studies do not provide support for this expectation. Socioeconomic differences in mortality in countries with more egalitarian policies are not small from an international perspective. The potential role of some circumstances, for example cultural factors, has been ignored too long in health inequalities research (p. 142)

In the terms we use in this chapter, it seems that in some nations there was a source of resilience that enabled less socioeconomically privileged groups to escape the same degree of health disadvantage as that experienced by those in similar situations in other nations. The nations with the more resilient population groups were, broadly speaking, the Mediterranean countries.

The explanation favoured by many for this phenomenon is diet. Social class differences in the most relevant aspects of the diet: consumption of fresh fruit, vegetables, unsaturated fats and oils differed between nations as one might expect from the observed differences in health inequality, that is, very little. In those Southern

European nations, such as Italy, with relatively large income inequalities but long life expectancy and less health inequality, the diet followed by the majority of people was a healthier one (Kunst 1997; p. 206). "Having a healthy diet" was not some special "lifestyle" associated with cultural or economic privilege.

This study has provided us with data highly relevant to the notion of resilience as an asset for health. The radical difference in the association between social and economic advantage and diet seen in the Northern and Southern European nations is a prime example of a "health asset". Whatever the circumstances are that break the link between healthy eating and socioeconomic position need careful study. It seems that there may be two aspects to this asset. The first is quite simply the cost, quality and availability of food items. In countries where fruit and vegetables (and perhaps wine in moderate quantities) are cheap and plentiful, they form part of everyone's diet and are affordable to all. Quality of fresh food also tends to be higher, and products are more likely to be bought from markets and smaller shops rather than supermarkets in comparison to the USA and UK (Glitsch 2000). The good health of Southern European populations is therefore evidence of the importance of affordable supplies of high quality fruit and vegetables; the salutogenic impact could perhaps even be quantified. Such a health asset would be endangered if, for example, economic forces resulted in the run-down of local farming practices that provide cheap and healthy food, in favour of more imported and highly processed food.

However, we do not believe this is the whole story. Although far more careful studies of diet would be necessary for a better understanding of diet as a source of health resilience, it is likely that attention needs to be paid to food preparation. A sociological analysis of health assets would, we will argue, need to be centrally concerned with questions of gender inequality. Diet as a source of resilience against socioeconomic disadvantage provides us with the first example of how important this may be. It is likely that more elaborate food preparation is more widely carried out in situations where many women do not have paid employment and therefore have no choice but to spend larger amounts of time in domestic labour. In this case, the healthy diet might be regarded as a consequence of inequality in social power between men and women. In fact, it is striking that some of the developed countries with low health inequality are those which have retained more traditional family arrangements, low levels of access to highly paid jobs for women, and low divorce rates such as Japan and the Mediterranean nations (Esping-Andersen 1999).

In the USA and UK, where women are increasingly involved in employment with long hours of work, but also often with high financial and social rewards, a higher proportion of meals are eaten outside the home, and more of the food eaten at home requires minimal preparation. Under these social conditions, diet quality will be heavily dependent on both knowledge about healthy eating and household income levels. Ready prepared "healthy" foods are increasingly available, but at a high cost. Where the long hours are being spent in a well-paid job, there may be no harm to health as a healthy diet can be bought. Where they are spent in low-paid "welfare to work" jobs, the health effects on women and their families could be severe. With no time or energy for elaborate cooking, people on low income are reduced to eating the cheapest, lowest quality instant foods.

So, although we may have located an important health asset which constitutes a source of resilience against socioeconomic disadvantage, this discovery also raises serious problems. Although some might think it desirable to somehow reimpose the obligation on women to remain in the home, and on men to support sexual partners financially, there is no historical precedent for this: once divorce and separation have become socially acceptable, there is no way to turn the clock back. It takes a political catastrophe such as those that have occurred in Afghanistan and may currently be occurring in Iraq to remove from women the rights to education and de jure access to all sectors of the labour market which have resulted in increases in female employment. So that although there is strong evidence that diet is a health asset that should be quantified and treasured, this does not automatically lead, in any simple manner, to policy prescriptions as to how this asset may be preserved.

One rare example that shows how access to employment by women need not result in increasing inequality in diet may be taken from experiences during the World War II in the UK. Women were employed in large numbers in "war work" to substitute for men serving in the armed forces. However, due to a combination of rationing and the availability of communal kitchens and canteens, diet quality for working-class people improved to levels previously unseen, and socioeconomic inequalities in diet were greatly reduced (Zweiniger-Bargielowska 2000). This is a case where policy measures were designed to fit a situation where women were needed in the workforce, but at the same time the protection of population health was of high priority.

6.5 Deindustrialization: Health Risks and Resilience

A very different example of the importance of understanding the sources of resilience can be taken from the consequences of deindustrialisation in Great Britain. Beginning in the 1980s, there was a drastic decline in the numbers of jobs available for men with little formal education, or whose skills were attached to traditional heavy industries such as mining, shipbuilding, iron and steel and assembly line production of household goods and vehicles. Much attention (though arguably not enough) has been paid to unemployment and its consequences for health (Iversen et al. 1987; Voss et al. 2004; Mattiasson et al. 1990; Korpi 2001; Martikainen 1990).

However, in the 25 years since the beginnings of this industrial decline, many have found alternatives to conventional work. Although what should be termed "non-employment" is now seen as a major policy problem in Great Britain, it does not seem to have been always harmful. In fact, as the numbers exposed to industrial hazards fell, life expectancy in men rose during this period at a faster rate than in the previous era of heavy industry. We know that many of those who lost their employment in the traditional heavy industries remained outside of the formal economic activity. However, far less is known about any alternative forms of activity that took the place of the old jobs.

Economic inactivity grew rapidly during these years, in all of the affected areas of the UK, but so did self-employment, and we know very little about the activities of those whose lives may have taken a new path. Being unemployed is, of course, a long term risk factor for poor health in later life. But there is evidence to suggest that those who left employment early, as long as this was something over which they felt they had control, experienced an improvement in quality of life. Post-retirement activities have been found to include an increase in physical exercise and in further education and study. Some of these people will most likely have found a recipe for turning a smaller amount of money than they had previously earned into an amount of welfare that is at least equivalent – that is, of maximising the capability derived from their income. In former mining areas for example, coal was provided free of charge to those not working full time, equating to the means of keeping home and family warm in the winter. Evidence from one network project in fact showed that avoiding paid employment via claiming physical incapacity, or choosing not to take job offers was an important means of maintaining financial and community support.

Deindustrialisation seems to have had in some cases a far more severe effect on the health of younger men. Rates of both suicide and death by homicide in those aged 16–30 rose rapidly during the 1980s and have continued at a high level (Charlton et al. 1993; Crawford and Prince 1999). Such sustained rises in this kind of mortality illustrates that it was not only the circumstance of job loss and loss of prospects which adversely affected the younger adults in the 1980s but also that life as a young adult in the post industrial desolation during the 1990s and early twenty first century presents challenges. Boys in these areas present the education system with a series of intractable problems, and many leave school with no qualifications to help them take up the newer forms of employment (Nickell and Quintini 2002; Nickell 2004).

Addiction to hard drugs has become endemic in some pockets of the old industrial areas. Although the traditional manual jobs were extremely hard and hazardous, the availability of such jobs, and the community structures around them, seems to have provided young men with a significant health asset, whose disappearance has had serious impact on psychosocial well-being, but whose nature has never been fully clarified.

However, in one network project, in-depth studies of de-industrialised areas did find that not all of them experienced the adverse health consequences expected among younger people. It appears that whilst the original source of community coherence – a shared industrial experience and employment – was lost, the assets of close community cooperation established during the industrial era can sometimes be maintained in the post-industrial era where the common experience is now unemployment and a struggle against poverty. Those areas which retained a reasonably stable population in the wake of mine and factory closure, also sometimes retained their community structure and organisation. These assets have assisted such areas to build social stability, if not economic prosperity. In other areas, where community cohesion was founded on shared ethnic or religious identities, resilience to economic decline was also detected.

In some areas, such as the northern English town of Oldham, large numbers of people had emigrated from South Asia to fill a strong demand for labour in the textile industry. In the 1980s, this industry was one of those which declined sharply in the face of competition from countries where labour costs were much lower, and most of the textile workers, British and Asian alike, lost their jobs. In the Asian community, long-range social networks were revived in order to set up businesses that went on to thrive. In fact, some of the unrest and inter-ethnic conflict in towns such as Oldham has been attributed to the great differences in the ways in which British and Asian ex-textile workers responded to the economic crisis.

These social and demographic trends are being repeated in several European nations, and in the new Europe. Below we put forward some reflections on the complex implications that may be drawn from these trends for understanding health assets and resilience.

6.6 Capability and the Production of Well-Being

We do not see it as our role here to advocate resilience as cheerful acceptance in the face of poverty or other forms of hardship. What has been highlighted importantly in the work of Sen, however, is the error involved in directly equating commodity (such as money income) with capability. We would like to argue that as nations modernise, they may become subject to processes that actually lower the capability-producing powers of money, or to put it another way around, make it necessary to spend increasing amounts of money for the same levels of perceived life satisfaction. This dilemma underlies much of the anxious preoccupation in some branches of economics with "well-being", pointing out that large increases in income per capita have not been accompanied by parallel increases in reported well-being.

The question of "reproductive labour power" is of great and wide ranging significance for both mental and physical health. The feminist economist Esther Boserup (1989) estimated that women carry out some 60% of all the work that is done in developing nations. There has been less attention to the unpaid work done by women in developed nations. However, a list could contain the essential activities of maintaining the hygiene of the home, and the health of its occupants by the provision of food and emotional support. The skills of the cook will also have a major impact on household budgets by determining how much will have to be paid for food as a "finished article" or how much can be saved by buying basic ingredients that can be transformed. Modernisation first saw the steady change from the provision of clothing by home production methods as mass production brings down the price of garments and shoes. At the present time, however, this process is extending to small-scale domestic food production with major implications for health. Yet very few health promotion campaigns regard knowledge about food and cooking skills as a valuable "asset for health".

As legal and political change opens all sectors of the education system and labour market to women, inevitably there will be a shift in time-usage from the home to the workplace, particularly by women who do well in education. Whilst we do not mean to argue that these roles *must* be carried out by women, it has been women who were previously contributing an enormous amount of "value-added" to more traditional economies. The shifting of their efforts away from home production has never, so far, been taken seriously as a policy issue. Although many societies now more fully embrace the value of women in the workplace, there is general failure to equalise contributions to home production from men. Instead, several nations have indulged in moral panics around such issues as rising child obesity, the breakdown of relationship between pupils and teachers, and other similar issues, demonising children and childhood.

One may criticise current attacks on the behaviour of some children and youth. However, research shows that troubled young people often become troubled adults, with serious consequences for their own well-being and freedom of action. We therefore propose that the skills involved in the conduct of family relationships are a major neglected health asset. This conclusion is supported by research that indicates the importance of warm and supportive family relationships in child development, especially under conditions of relatively low material living standards (Schoon 2006). In other words, family relationships can both be health assets, and a source of resilience in the face of adversity.

It will not do, however, merely to advocate (in this case at least) the preservation of such an asset in its present form. Once social and legal norms have changed in such as way as to admit women to all sectors of the labour market, the genie cannot be put back into the bottle. The same could be said of the increasing promotion by advertising of "fast" foods with very poor nutritional content. Rather, the challenge is to preserve the asset of skilled domestic and emotional "reproductive" labour by spreading it further in demographic terms. We return here to the theme of freedom; women's freedom has no doubt been increased, (though perhaps not quite as much as might be imagined), by greater access to education and jobs. However, it is as important, we will argue, to increase the capabilities of both men and women to choose a way of life they can sustain themselves in terms of both physical and emotional self-care. One way in which this may be helped to happen would be by a revaluation of necessary skills. More careful attention to what is required for optimal growth and development, both physical and mental, and in both childhood and the adult years, would be a major step in this direction.

In Durkheimian terms, we might think here about yet further increases in the "Division of Labour", rather similar to the separation of more and more work from the home to the factory and office during the Industrial Revolution. Another way to look at these processes is in terms of what might be called the commodification of human relationships. We use this term here in a purely descriptive rather than an evaluative sense. As with many other important secular trends of modernisation, the commodification of relationships is largely a result of changes in the situation of women, and these are changes that have come about as a result of democratic processes. The domestic and emotional work previously done without payment by women in relation to husbands, sons and male co-workers was to a large extent constrained by women's inferior and less powerful economic and legal position. Once this situation changed as a result of political reform, however, the work involved did not begin to be shared more evenly by men and women.

As women began to work more hours in the formal economy, men only very slowly began to take up an appropriate share of domestic labour. As more women began to gain satisfaction from work that gave them power and influence, men did not rush to take up the roles previously played by subordinate women, either within the home or within organisations. And as marriage became a more fragile institution, in part for many of these same reasons, the emotional ties between fathers and their children also became less secure.

Among those who could afford it, quite a lot of this emotional and domestic labour could be bought in the marketplace in various forms such as domestic servants and nannies, smaller class sizes in private schools, professional therapists and life coaches etc. Much of the emotional and domestic labour that had previously been done without payment was thereby comodified, and now requires to be bought in the market place, in a process similar to the movement of the production of clothing, bread and cheese out of the household in the nineteenth century. For this reason, access to forms of social relations that lie at the basis of important aspects of human health and development has become increasingly socially unequal.

The disappearance of "free emotional labour" spreads its effects far beyond the poorer social groups however. Like the infectious diseases that prompted some of the great social reforms of the nineteenth century, the effects of impoverished family relationships are pervasive. Children from families affected by financial or emotional hardship require a far higher input from their teachers, for example, leaving less energy to be spent on more psychologically stable children. The families of the latter are therefore forced to consider the expense of moving away to a more socially segregated area, or of private education. The more privileged family will therefore have a double demand on its income, ample though it may be: expenditure is necessary to provide care for the home (and perhaps home care for the children as well); and yet more is required in order to avoid the disruption at school caused by the children of the less fortunate. By this process, in a manner similar to that proposed in the work of Wilkinson, Kawachi and colleagues (Wilkinson 1996; Kawachi and Kennedy 1997), social inequality is increased and at the same time the well-being of even better-off families is reduced.

Rather similar processes take place in neighbourhoods. Here the loss is not of women's unpaid labour, but of the very presence in public space of citizens who are neither tied to the workplace nor too poor to take part in community life. The loss of the "civilizing" effect of the presence of retired people, adults with parental leave from work to look after children, municipal workers and others has been lamented by commentators on neo-liberal economic reforms. As many public spaces become more threatening, resources must be used to protect and transport children (and adults) to alternative locations, and to protect these locations themselves. The need to compete in the property market in order to "buy" access to an acceptable residential area takes an additional toll on the income of middle class households.

As the economic disparities become further etched in space, social and demographic inequalities between neighbourhoods get wider and wider. The dialectic relationship between neighbourhood and household incomes and identities ultimately serves only to widen the gaps between the richer and poorer. Those who cannot afford a secure and calm domestic life, tend also not to be able to afford a secure and calm residential neighbourhood, and their children grow up and learn in more dangerous, more difficult surroundings. The need for resilience in the face of these adverse surroundings is then even greater, but the likely assets and capabilities of the young people to show resilience are reduced.

There are many aspects of human relationships whose vital role as assets for the health of both individuals and communities, because they are never given any monetary value, only become evident when they are lost. We do not think it would be accurate to characterise these assets as "social capital" (in any of the rather shifting meanings of this term). Rather, these assets arose from a historically specific combination of economic and social circumstances, some of which, such as the exclusion of women from many of the better paid and more influential forms of employment, have disappeared for very good reasons. The problem has been that the processes that produced these assets were never understood before being swept away, and their importance has only become evident in hindsight.

The WHO Assets for Health and Development programme seems to us a vital attempt to gain such an understanding, not in order to freeze history in its tracks, but to make sure that the development of these capabilities are pursued with the same amount of energy as economic and technological progress.

References

Anonymous. (2000). Resilience and protective factors in the lives of adolescents. *J Adolesc Health*, 27(1):1–2.

Antonovsky, A. (1979). *Health, stress and coping*. San Francisco: Jossey-Bass; 1st edition.

Bartley, M., & Plewis, I. (2002). Accumulated labour market disadvantage and limiting long-term illness: data from the 1971-1991 Office for National Statistics' Longitudinal Study. *Int J Epidemiol*, 31(2):336–41.

Bartley, M., Sacker, A., & Clarke, P. (2004). Employment status, employment conditions, and limiting illness: prospective evidence from the British household panel survey 1991-2001. *J Epidemiol Community Health*, 58(6):501–6.

Blaxter, M. (1990). *Health and lifestyles*. London: Tavistock.

Baxter Jones, A. D. G., Cardy, A. H., Helms, P. J., Phillips, D. O., & Smith, W. C. S. (1999). Influence of socioeconomic conditions on growth in infancy: the 1921 Aberdeen birth cohort. *Arch Dis Child*, 81(1):5–9.

Boserup, E. (1989). *Womens role in economic development*. London: Earthscan.

Brunner, E., Shipley, M. J., Blane, D., Smith, G. D., & Marmot, M. G. (1999). When does cardiovascular risk start? Past and present socioeconomic circumstances and risk factors in adulthood. *J Epidemiol Community Health*, 53(12):757–64.

Charlton, J., Kelly, S., Dunnell, K., Evans, B., & Jenkins, R. (1993). Suicide deaths in England and Wales: trends in factors associated with suicide deaths. *Popul Trends*, 71:34–42.

Crawford, M. J., & Prince, M. (1999). Increasing rates of suicide in young men in England during the 1980s: the importance of social context. *Soc Sci Med*, 49(10):1419–23.

Deneulin, S., & Shahani, L. (eds) (2009). *An introduction to the human development and capacity approach*. London: Freedom and Agency Earthscan.

Esping-Andersen, G. (1999). *Social foundations of postindustrial economies*. Oxford: Oxford University Press.

Fergus, S., & Zimmerman, M. A. (2005). Adolescent resilience: a framework for understanding healthy development in the face of risk. *Annu Rev Public Health*, 26:131–1321.

Garmezy, N., Masten, A. S., & Tellegen, A. (1984). The Study of Stress and competence in children: a building block for developmental psychopathology. *Child Dev*, 55:97–111.

Garmezy, N. (1985). Stress-resistant children: the search for protective factors. In *Recent research in developmental psychopathology*. Davids A. Elmsford, NY: Pergamon Press, pp 213–33.

Galobardes, B., Lynch, J. W., & Davey Smith, G. (2004). Childhood socioeconomic circumstances and cause-specific mortality in adulthood: systematic review and interpretation. *Epidemiol Rev*, 26:7–21.

Glitsch, K. (2000) Consumer perceptions of fresh meat quality: cross-national comparison. *Br Food J*, 102(3):177–94.

Heim, C., Newport, D. J., Bonsall, R., Miller, A. H., & Nemeroff, C. B. (2001). Altered pituitary-adrenal axis responses to provocative challenge tests in adult survivors of childhood abuse. *Am J Psychiatry*, 158(4):575–81.

Hemmingsson, T., & Lundberg, I. (2005). How far are socioeconomic differences in coronary heart disease hospitalization, all-cause mortality and cardiovascular mortality among adult Swedish males attributable to negative childhood circumstances and behaviour in adolescence? *Int J Epidemiol*, 34(2):260–7.

Iversen, L., Andersen, O., Andersen, P. K., Christoffersen, K., & Keiding, N. (1987). Unemployment and mortality in Denmark. *BMJ*, 295:879–84.

Kawachi, I., & Kennedy, B. P. (1997). Socioeconomic determinants of health. 2. Health and social cohesion: why care about income inequality? *Br Med J*, 314(7086):1037–40.

Korpi, W. (2001). Accumulating disadvantage: longitudinal analyses of unemployment and physical health in representative samples of the Swedish population. *Eur Sociol Rev*, 17(3):255–74.

Kunst, A. (1997). Cause specific mortality and occupational class in 11 Western countries. Cross-national comparisons of socio-economic differences in mortality. Den Haag: CIP-Gegevens Koninklijke Bibliotheek, pp 113–24.

Kuh, D., & Ben-Shlomo, Y. (1997). In *A life course approach to chronic disease epidemiology*. Kuh D, Ben-Shlomo Y. Oxford: Oxford University Press.

Luthar, S. S., Cichetti, D., & Becker, B. (2000). The construct of resilience: a critical evaluation and guidelines for future work. *Child Dev*, 71(3):543–62.

Luthar, S. S., Cichetti, D., & Becker, B. (2000). Research on resilience: response to commentaries. *Child Dev*, 71(3):573–5.

Mackenbach, J. P., Kunst, A. E., Cavelaars, A. E. J. M., Groenhof, F., & Geurts, J. J. M. (1997a). Socioeconomic inequalities in morbidity and mortality in western Europe. *Lancet*, 349(9066):1655–9.

Mackenbach, J. P., Cavelaars, A. E. J. M., & Kunst, A. E. (1997b). Socioeconomic inequalities in morbidity and mortality in western Europe – Reply. *Lancet*, 350(9076):517–8.

Masten, A., & Coatsworth, J. (1998). The development of competence in favorable and unfavorable environments. *Am Psychol*, 53:205–20.

Masten, A. S., Hubbard, J. J., Gest, S. D., Tellegan, A., Garmezy, N., & Ramierez, M. (1999). Competence in the context of adversity: pathways to resilience and maladaptation from childhood to late adolescence. *Dev Psychopathol*, 11(1):143–69.

Masten, A. S., & Reed, M-G. J. (2002). Resilience in development. In *Handbook of positive psychology*. Snyder CR, Lopez SJ. Oxford: Oxford University Press, pp 74–88.

Martikainen, P. (1990). Unemployment and mortality among Finnish men. *BMJ*, 301:407–11.

Mattiasson, I., Lindgarde, F., Nilsson, J. A., & Theorell, T., (1990). Threats of unemployment and cardiovascular risk factors: longitudinal study of quality of sleep and serum cholesterol concentrations in men threatened with redundancy. *BMJ*, 301:461–6.

Nickell, S., & Quintini, G. (2002). The recent performance of the UK labour market. *Oxf Rev Econ Policy*, 18(2):202–20.

Nickell, S. (2004) Poverty and worklessness in Britain. *Econ J*, 114:C1–25.

Parker, L., Lamont, D. W., Wright, C. M., Cohen, M. A., Alberti, K. G. M. M., & Craft, A. W. (1999). Mothering skills and health in infancy: the Thousand Families Study revisited. *Lancet*, 353(9159):1151–2.

Power, C. (2002). Childhood still matters for adult health outcomes. *Lancet*, 360:1619–20.

Rutter, M. (1985). Family and school influences on behavioural development. *J Child Psychol Psychiatry*, 26:349–56.

Rutter, M. (1987). Psychological resilience and protective mechanisms. *Am J Orthopsychiatry*, 57:316–31.
Ryff, C. D., & Singer, B. (1998). The contours of positive human health. *Psychol Inq*, 9:1–28.
Ryff, C. D., & Singer, B. H. (2002). From social structure to biology: integrative science in pursuit of human health and well-being. In *Handbook of positive psychology*. Snyder CR, Lopez SJ. London: Oxford University Press.
Schoon, I., Bynner, J., Joshi, H., Parsons, S., Wiggins, R. D., & Sacker, A. (2002). The influence of context, timing, and duration of risk experiences for the passage from childhood to mid-adulthood. *Child Dev*, 73(5):1486–504.
Schoon, I., Sacker, A., & Bartley, M. (2003). Socio-economic adversity and psychosocial adjustment: a developmental-contextual perspective. *Soc Sci Med*, 57(6):1001–15.
Schoon, I. (2006). *Risk and resilience: adaptations in changing times*. Cambridge: Cambridge University Press.
Seguin, L., Xu, Q., Potvin, L., Zunzunegui, M-V., & Frolich, K. L. (2003). Effects of low income on infant health. *Can Med Assoc J*, 168(12):1533–8.
Shewry, M. C., Smith, W. C. S., Woodward, M., & Tunstall-Pedoe, H. (1992). Variation in coronary risk-factors by social-status – results from the scottish heart health study. *Br J Gen Pract*, 42(363):406–10.
Skuse, D., Reilly, S., & Wolke, D. (1994). Psychosocial adversity and growth during infancy. *Eur J Clin Nutr*, 48(Suppl 1):S113–30.
Tremblay, R. E. (1999). When children's social development fails. In *Developmental health and the wealth of nations*. Keating DP, Hertzman C. New York: The Guildford Press, pp 55–71.
Voss, M., Nylen, L., Floderus, B., Diderichsen, F., & Terry, P. D. (2004). Unemployment and early cause-specific mortality: a study based on the Swedish twin registry. *Am J Public Health*, 94:2155–61.
Ungar, M. (2004). *Nurturing resilience in troubled youth*. Toronto: University of Toronto Press
Werner, E. E., & Smith, R. S. (1992). *Overcoming the odds: high risk children from birth to adulthood*. Ithaca: Cornell University Press.
WHO. (1946). Preamble to the Constitution of the World Health Organization as adopted by the International Health Conference, New York, 19–22 June, 1946; signed on 22 July 1946 by the representatives of 61 States (Official Records of the World Health Organization, no. 2, p. 100) and entered into force on 7 April 1948.
Wiggins, R. D., Schofield, P., Sacker, A., Head, J., & Bartley, M. (2004). Social position and minor psychiatric morbidity over time in the British Household Panel Survey 1991-1998. *J Epidemiol Community Health*, 58(9):779–87.
Wilkinson, R. G. (1996). *Unhealthy societies: the afflictions of inequality*. London: Routledge.
Zweiniger-Bargielowska, I. (2000). *Austerity in Britain: rationing, controls and consumption 1939-55*. Oxford: Oxford University Press.

Chapter 7
How to Assess Resilience: Reflections on a Measurement Model

Nora Wille and Ulrike Ravens-Sieberer

Keywords Mental health • Adolescents • Community • Resilience • BELLA study

7.1 Mental Health of Children and Adolescents Within the New Morbidity

7.1.1 The New Morbidity and Its Consequences for Our Understanding of Health Determinants

During the past century health of children and adolescents improved radically in Western industrialised countries. Nowadays we can hardly imagine that in the beginning of the past century infant mortality and malnutrition as well as infectious morbidity and epidemics were major health problems (Palfrey et al. 2005; Markel and Golden 2005; Razum and Breckemkamp 2007). However, these characteristics of the "classical paediatric morbidity" were replaced by problems of the "new" and later the "millennial morbidity" (Palfrey et al. 2005). Today children and adolescents in Western industrialised countries are more likely to suffer from problems related to mental health concerns such as social, emotional and behavioural difficulties. Associated problems of raising importance are school violence and injuries, suicide as well as alcohol and drug abuse (American Academy of Pediatrics and Committee on Psychosocial Aspects of Child and Family Health 2001; Palfrey et al. 2005). Today a child in the United States is more at risk *"to die from injuries or violence and suicide than from infectious disease"* (American Academy of Pediatrics and Committee on Psychosocial Aspects of Child and Family Health 2001; p. 1228).

N. Wille (✉)
Child Public Health Research Section, University Clinic Hamburg-Eppendorf, Hamburg, Germany
e-mail: n.wille@uke.de

A. Morgan et al. (eds.), *Health Assets in a Global Context: Theory, Methods, Action*, DOI 10.1007/978-1-4419-5921-8_7, © Springer Science+Business Media, LLC 2010

With respect to these current health problems, interventions to support healthy development of children and adolescents need to address a variety of factors that influence the morbidity in youth. The necessity to pay attention to children's and adolescents' living conditions was already recognised by paediatricians in the 1800s and led to a variety of community-based activities (Palfrey et al. 2005; Markel and Golden 2005). These efforts focused very basic preconditions for healthy development that were often related to poverty, e.g. clean water supply, improved housing for poor families, maternity benefits and promotion of breastfeeding (Palfrey et al. 2005; Markel and Golden 2005; Razum and Breckemkamp 2007). However, regarding the major health problems within the so-called new morbidity an even broader understanding of health determinants beyond such basic human needs is required. Most current health problems originate from a very complex and multifactorial process in which psychosocial aspects (such as characteristics of a child's personality, its family, and its further social surrounding) are highly important. However, socioeconomic status still plays an important role: poor mental health and its potential consequences such as teen pregnancies, sexually transmitted diseases, injuries or impaired school functioning are more prevalent among socioeconomically disadvantaged youth (Bradley and Corwyn 2002; von Rueden et al. 2006; Palfrey et al. 2005). Thus, efforts regarding prevention and health promotion have to consider different levels of determinants including societal structures and resources, socioeconomic circumstances of a child's family or community, social interactions within families, schools, and communities as well as characteristics of the individual itself.

In the following we will describe the importance of mental health promotion in children and adolescents against the background of the new morbidity. With respect to current knowledge regarding relevant health determinants, the importance of taking health assets into account will be pointed out. Afterwards we would like to introduce important concepts regarding the interaction of risks and resources in the context of mental health and resilience. The potential of population-based studies will be outlined and ways to operationalise risks and – most important – assets will be described. To end, an example from our own study will clarify how the theoretical concept of assets and their protective effects can be supported by empirical evidence in order to develop effective public health initiatives that address not only the individual child and its health problems but also its family and the community in which it lives.

7.1.2 *The Rising Importance of Mental Health Problems in Childhood and Adolescence*

Mental health problems in childhood and adolescence comprise a wide range of disorders such as depressive disorders, anxiety disorders, disruptive disorders or eating disorders, which are defined by diagnostic manuals (ICD-10: WHO 1992; DSM-IV: APA 2000).

Even though the assessment of mental disorders requires a diagnosis by a clinician, it goes beyond the resources of most large epidemiological studies to conduct comprehensive clinical interviews. Therefore available studies employ different methods (e.g. screening instruments and/or two stage designs) and apply varying case definitions to determine prevalence rates. Consequently, prevalence estimates of mental health problems range widely between 1 and 51% (Roberts et al. 1998). However, despite major methodological problems regarding the comparability of epidemiological estimates, the median of prevalence rates in different international reviews was similar (e.g. 14% in Roberts et al. 1998 or 18% in Ihle and Esser 2002) and the majority of studies indicate that at any given time between 10 and 20% of children and adolescents suffer from disabling mental health problems (WHO 2001a; Patel et al. 2007; Costello et al. 2005; Belfer 2008). This estimate further increases when – beyond single measurement points – life time prevalence rates are taken into account. By the age of 16 years 37% of youth had experienced at least one DSM-IV disorder (Costello et al. 2003).

While the high prevalence of mental health problems is undisputed, there are different opinions regarding an increase of youth mental health problems over the decades. Whereas Roberts et al. (1998) were not able to identify such a trend, other reviews state a substantial rise in psychosocial disorders in many western countries over the past decades, specifically referring to problems such as suicide, delinquency, addictive behaviours, and depression (Rutter and Smith 1995; Fombonne 1998; Prosser and McArdle 1996).

Even if an increase in prevalence rates is hard to confirm, the need to strengthen prevention efforts and to promote mental health in children and adolescents is evident. Not only the sizeable proportion of youth suffering from mental health problems emphasises the necessity of effective public health initiatives. Beyond, mental disorders in young age are highly persistent (Ihle and Esser 2002). Children and adolescents who developed a psychiatric disorder once have a threefold risk to suffer continuously or repeatedly from the disorder (Costello et al. 2003). Further, the high percentage of mental health problems in adults that had their onset in childhood or adolescence highlights the importance of primary prevention in these critical time periods (Costello et al. 2005, 2006).

Mental disorders are accompanied by considerable adverse consequences for the affected young person as well as for society. Since childhood and adolescence are crucial periods of educational and social development, mental health related impairments can disrupt important developments and hamper an adolescent to reach his or her full potential (Ford et al. 2003). Mental health problems can result in educational underachievement or even dropout from school (McLeod and Kaiser 2004) and thus affect later adult life by deteriorating future prospects regarding employment and individual socio-economic position. On a societal level it can therefore result in a loss of economic productivity and higher expenditures in social welfare (Belfer 2008). Furthermore mental health-related social incapacity can lead to poorer social life and lack of a social network. In the worst case pronounced mental health-related behavioural and social problems can result in delinquency or even criminal careers and destabilisation of communities, which is again associated with high costs for the society.

It is obvious that the individual's quality of life is largely reduced by such circumstances, and that furthermore a high burden is imposed on the direct social environment (Belfer 2008). But also the societal impact is large and contains costs beyond the health care sector, i.e. in the educational system, the social welfare system, and the criminal justice system (Belfer 2008). The adverse consequences of mental disorders were also impressively demonstrated by the Global Burden of Disease Study that identified Unipolar Major Depression as the fourth largest cause of disability-adjusted life years with growing importance (Murray and Lopez 1996; Murray and Lopez 1997).

Regarding the prevalence and the consequences of mental health problems outlined above it can be concluded that, firstly, regarding mental health problems in children and adolescents primary prevention is an important task and beyond, there is a need to buffer the adverse consequences potentially connected to mental health problems for the individual and their surroundings. Measures of mental health promotion and the availability of health assets may play an important role here. Secondly, the diverse potential consequences of mental health problems illustrate how the mental health status affects very different sectors. This is not only true in the case of mental disorders that might harm the individual's surrounding and the society. Beyond – as outlined below – mental health in its positive sense contains the capacity for contributions in diverse fields such as social cohesion and economic capital (WHO 2005).

7.1.3 Beyond Mental Ill-Health: The Importance of Positive Mental Health

Unfortunately, the focus on mental disorders (mental ill-health perspective) restricts attention to a small part of the whole picture of youth mental health. Even though the manifestation of mental disorders is of high public health relevance and should be targeted by prevention and intervention efforts, these problems indicate only "the tip of the iceberg" and partly impede the sight on the broader topic of mental *health* – instead of disease.

If mental health is not conceptualised as a dichotomous state (with two categories "healthy" vs. "sick") but as a continuum ranging from poor mental health to good mental health, it becomes clear that the mental ill-health perspective does not catch the majority of differences between mental health states. Within the mental ill-health perspective the term "healthy" refers exclusively to the absence of mental disorders. However, mental health can also be conceptualised based on a positive understanding, e.g. as "*a state of well-being in which the individual realises his or her own abilities, can cope with the normal stresses of life, can work productively and fruitfully, and is able to make a contribution to his or her community*" (WHO 2001b; p. 1) as it was outlined by the WHO.

This positively defined core concept characterises mental health as the basis for the functioning and well-being of individuals and also expresses the connection between individual mental health and the functioning of the community. It hints at the individual's mental health being an important resource for the closer surrounding (such as the family) or the wider community, where it can contribute in a material or immaterial manner.

The conceptualisation of mental health in this positive sense in addition to the concept of mental ill-health has implications regarding the approaches to improve health. Not only to prevent disorders but also to enhance positive mental health in all its facets then becomes a justified priority. In practice however, although theoretically distinct, actions and outcomes of mental health promotion and prevention necessarily overlap since both address determinants of the mental state in order to modify them (WHO 2005).

7.2 Risks, Resources and Resilience: Promoting the Capacity to Cope with Adversity

7.2.1 *Different Levels of Mental Health Determinants*

The opportunities for improving the young population's mental health and for reducing the burden caused by mental health problems can only be fully exploited if the multiple factors that can enhance or harm an individual's mental health are recognised (WHO 2005). These determinants of mental health are often beyond the control of individuals and can be found on different levels. There were different approaches to categorise levels of health determinants. One possibility of categorisation is to group them according to their "distance" to the individual on a *"distal-proximal continuum"* (Luthar 1993; p. 444). In the centre of such classifications (e.g. Bronfenbrenner 1979; Dahlgren and Whitehead 1991) stands the individual itself, with its biological or psychological characteristics. Then, crucial proximal determinants can be identified in individuals' so-called microsystems (Bronfenbrenner 1979). These refer to the immediate environments such as family and peers and corresponding material and social circumstances and behaviours. Beyond, distal measures such as the broader social context – the exosystem – play a role. For example some characteristics of the school, neighbourhood, parents' workplaces and community impact a child indirectly, even though it does not directly participate in these contexts. Similarly, the so-called macrosystem referring to the larger cultural context (e.g. national economy, laws) as well as the occurrence of events over the course of life (chronosystem) is important.

The strong interconnectedness of the different levels and factors is expressed not only by Bronfenbrenner's category of the mesosystem, which considers the fact that individual's microsystems (e.g. school and family) influence each other. Furthermore, distal measures of risk are mediated by proximal measures (Luthar

1993). E.g. poverty is the root of many important stresses which in turn are major risk factors for emotional disorders (Albee 2006). It was shown that economically disadvantaged children are exposed to more risk factors for mental disorders such as family conflicts or violence. Their children have an increased risk of exposure to perinatal stress, crowded homes, substance use, inferior schools and dangerous neighbourhoods with high rates of crime that lack supporting social networks (Evans 2004; Patel et al. 2007; Garmezy 1991).

Other factors are not easy to classify since they are based on interactions between the levels. E.g. at first glance social support seems to be a property of the individual's surrounding. However, since social relations are based on reciprocal actions of individuals, social support is also dependent on personality traits and was even linked to genetic factors (WHO 2005).

Consequently, beyond addressing several levels of mental health determinants interventions must take into consideration the interconnectedness of relevant factors and the accumulation of risks in specific subgroups. Even though macro-level determinants may be hard to address within the framework of mental health promotion programmes, interventions should always be concentrated not only on the individual's characteristics but also on the more proximal and distal environmental factors.

7.2.2 Findings on Risk Factors for Mental Health and Shortcomings of the Risk Approach

Previous research reported convincing evidence on the importance of diverse factors that put children's and adolescents' mental health at risk. Some of these risk factors are biological such as premature birth (Gardner et al. 2004) as well as smoking (Fergusson et al. 1998) or drinking (Williams and Ross 2007) during pregnancy. Recent research also showed the influence of genetic predispositions, however, particularly their interaction with environmental adversity and psychosocial factors as exogenous agents plays an important role in the development of mental disorders (Caspi et al. 2002; Caspi et al. 2003). Many psychosocial risk factors regarding poor mental health have been identified that are connected to stressful life events or circumstances. Whereas factors such as witnessing or being a victim of violence (Ward et al. 2001) or sexual molestation (Briere and Elliott 1994) are extreme examples of adverse conditions with detrimental effects on mental health, other risk factors are highly prevalent and almost "normal" such as conflicts between the parents (Jenkins and Smith 1991) and family breakdown (Amato 2001) or physical illness of a parent (Barkmann et al. 2007). Further risk factors are less prevalent but still affect a considerable proportion of children such as physical illness of the child (Hysing et al. 2007), parental psychiatric illness (Rutter and Quinton 1984; Hammen et al. 1990) or parental alcoholism (Díaz et al. 2008). Some of these and further risk factors (such as large family size and overcrowding in the home, Rutter et al. 1975) again lead to the topic of poverty and socio-economic disadvantage, which are well-established risk factors for mental disorders (Bradley and Corwyn 2002; Klocke and Lampert 2005).

In general, risk factors do not emerge isolated, but tend to cluster together and interact. It was shown in several cumulative models that particularly the summation of stressors place individuals at risk for the development of mental health problems (Forehand et al. 1991; Sameroff et al. 1997). However, in general it should be noticed that such "risk factors" do not describe causal processes and thus do not predict necessarily negative outcomes. When a child is "at risk", it belongs to a group which is defined by a circumscribed exposition that makes it only more likely to develop mental health problems. Thus, Rutter (1971) pointed out the distinction between "risk indicators" and "risk mechanisms". Factors such as parental separation are more likely risk indicators since the key risk does not derive from the separation per se but mainly from other adverse experiences associated with the separation such as ongoing parental conflicts. Due to the difference between risk indicators and risk mechanisms the presence of risk factors stands only in a probabilistic relationship with mental health outcomes. Furthermore it has to be taken into account that the vulnerability to risk factors is not only dependent on their sequential or simultaneous occurrence, but also varies with age and sex and duration of risk impact (Scheithauer and Petermann 1999).

To conclude, risk factor models were helpful in identifying indicators of harmful processes and thus children at risk for mental health problems. Nevertheless these models are of limited explanatory power as well as limited usefulness. Not all children who are exposed to adversity develop mental health problems. Furthermore, a lot of risk factors regarding youth mental health can hardly be reduced by public health initiatives. Thus, the question arises why some children in adverse conditions develop mental health problems while others do not, and, in a second step, if their capacity to develop successfully can be promoted in other children as well by preventive interventions. This basic idea – to identify factors promoting health instead of concentrating on risks – corresponds to the salutogenetic approach by Aaron Antonovsky (1987) as well as to research on resilience which will be described in the following.

7.2.3 How to Maintain Health Despite Adverse Conditions: Taking a Look at Resources

The area of resilience is of special interest to public health professionals since many forms of stress and adversity in children's environments can hardly be eliminated. With respect to the many children who thrive in spite of adversity it seems reasonable to take a closer look at the resources that contribute to successful coping and development.

There are two important theoretical frameworks that provide a conceptual basis for investigating positive developmental outcomes in the presence of adversity. One is the concept of salutogenesis which was developed by Aaron Antonovsky (1987).

After observations in female holocaust survivors Antonovsky became interested in the reasons for staying healthy, i.e. salutogenic factors instead of pathogenic factors. He then assumed that a developed sense of coherence – a strong confidence that demands of life are understandable, meaningful and manageable – plays a central role in organising resources and maintaining or retaining health.

The second theoretical framework derives from developmental psychology and focuses the concept of resilience. The term resilience includes the latin word *resilire*, which can be translated with "bounce back". It was introduced to describe the phenomenon of so-called high-risk children who thrive irrespective of great environmental challenges. Correspondingly, research in resilience does not address pathological responses of individuals to stress, but investigates health-protecting mechanisms, i.e. the ability of individuals to maintain good health despite considerable stressors. Thereby the concept offers a broader theoretical framework than Antonovsky's approach and will be dealt with in detail in the following.

Surprisingly, research on schizophrenia played an important role with respect to the investigation of resilience in children and adolescents. By the 1970s, Norman Garmezy observed in schizophrenic patients that the course of the illness was associated with different premorbid histories. In contrast to the patients with a chronic course of the illness, the patients who recovered after a short treatment period were characterised by competence regarding their professional, family and social lives. Thus, Garmezy hypothesised differences in patterns of adaptation in the presence of exceptional stress. Consequently, he investigated high-risk children (who had poor families or schizophrenic mothers) who adapted well in order to identify attributes of competence that distinguished these groups (Rolf 1999).

A landmark study in the research on resilience was the Kauai Longitudinal Study by Emmy Werner and Ruth Smith (Werner and Smith 1982, 1992). They described characteristics of 698 children who were all born in 1955 and exposed to a high-risk environment and were nevertheless doing very well. Similarly, the British psychiatrist Michael Rutter conducted the epidemiological "Isle-of-Wight" studies (Rutter et al. 1976) and found that the majority of children thrive despite many risk factors.

Afterwards further studies investigated the phenomenon of resilience in a variety of contexts including children who were challenged by poverty and socioeconomic disadvantage, parental mental disease, maltreatment and community violence, chronic disease or traumatic life events (Luthar et al. 2000). These efforts were characterised by *"the paradigm shift from looking at the risk factors that led to psychosocial problems to the identification of strengths of an individual"* (Richardson 2002; p. 309). Researchers concentrated on the identification of resilient qualities, i.e. particular strengths or assets that helped the high-risk children under study to "bounce back" in the face of a stressor. The goal was to identify attributes which differentiated well adjusted children from those who did not cope successfully in order to explain observed variations in individuals' responses to environmental hazard (Luthar et al. 2000). The search for such correlates of resilience – referred to as protective factors or developmental assets – that can modify a child's response to adversity was hoped to inform on characteristics that can be promoted in prevention programs.

First research efforts concentrated on personality traits and characteristics of the individual child such as being adaptable and achievement oriented or having high self-efficacy and planning skills. However, with ongoing research, further sources of health assets were increasingly recognised. Eventually, protective factors were assigned to a triad of resilience consisting of (1) the personality disposition of the child, (2) qualities of family life, and (3) the wider social environment (Luthar et al. 2000). The acknowledgement of these important external sources of resilient qualities is in line with early results from Werner and Smith (1982, 1992), who had also pointed out the importance of the caregiving surrounding both inside and outside the family (Richardson 2002). Similarly, Rutter (1985) had highlighted characteristics such as positive experiences in school and a close relationship with a supportive adult as protective factors.

A similarly salutogenetic perspective was adopted by the Search Institute that published *"forty building blocks of human development"* (Benson 1997; p. 27). These 40 developmental assets were identified from literature and do not only contain factors that promote resilience but also factors that promote healthy development in general and the avoidance of health-compromising behaviour. Briefly, health-protecting and health-promoting assets are addressed here, while the concept of resilience primarily focuses factors that buffer effects of adversity. Correspondingly to the categorisation of protective factors these assets are grouped into internal and external assets. Internal assets that support optimal function in life comprise commitment to learning (e.g. achievement motivation and bonding to school), positive values (such as caring, integrity, and honesty), social competencies (e.g. interpersonal and cultural competence), and a positive identity (such as self-esteem and sense of purpose). The external youth assets do not only include receiving support (by family, school, other adults) and clear boundaries and expectations. They also address responsibilities of the community with categories such as empowerment (e.g. community values youth and provides useful roles for youth) and constructive use of time (referring to participation in youth programs and creative activities). Continued studies including more than 250,000 public school students in 460 school districts confirmed the assumption of the authors that as assets rise in number, developmental outcomes improve (Benson 1997).

Research investigating protective factors is still forging ahead. A current study in adolescents from China and the United States observed cross-nationally comparable effects of protective factors (such as control and support by the family and wider social environment) regarding alcohol and substance abuse (Jessor et al. 2003).

7.2.4 Resilience: Some Further Conceptual Clarifications

There is a broad consensus that the term resilience describes the achievement of positive adaptation by individuals within the context of significant adversity or – as Masten (2001; p. 228) puts it – *"Resilience refers to a class of phenomena characterised by good outcomes in spite of serious threats to adaptation or development"*. Thus, besides positive adjustment, the exposure to stressors is an integral part of the definition of resilience. Only the presence of demonstrable risk justifies the difference between "competence" (referring to adaptive behaviours in general) and "resilience" referring to manifest competence despite significant stressors (Norman Garmezy in Rolf 1999). These two crucial conditions are also displayed in Fig. 7.1.

Furthermore, it needs to be emphasised that the theoretical framework of developmental psychology does not conceptualise resilience as a personal trait, but as being based on an interactive process involving a person's constitution as well as functional qualities of its environment. These conditions allow individual adaptation since they buffer against the negative effects of harmful living conditions. This dynamic process involving internal and external assets as well as significant adversity, furthermore takes place within developmental progression. Thus, with changing life circumstances and emerging, disappearing or cumulating risk factors and resources the absence or presence of resilient outcomes may also vary. Terms such as "resilient children" are therefore misleading. Similarly, confusion derives from the term "resiliency" and from the literature on "ego-resiliency" (Block and Kremen 1996) which refers to a set of (protective) personality characteristics.

Furthermore, the multidimensional nature of resilience has to be noticed. Positive adaptation can be observed in different domains such as work or school performance, psychosocial adjustment or physical health. However, many individuals display substantial heterogeneity in functioning across different domains. E.g. they may manifest competence by having very successful careers but exhibit large underlying emotional distress. Since in general, consistently positive or negative developmental outcomes across multiple domains are unusual, the observation of such heterogeneity does not question the construct of resilience per se. However, it suggests that the concept of circumscribed domain specific resilience is more useful than the idea of global or overall resilience (Luthar 1993). Thus, researchers should (and increasingly do) specify the particular domains of positive adaptation, e.g. by terms such as "educational resilience" or "emotional resilience" (Luthar et al.

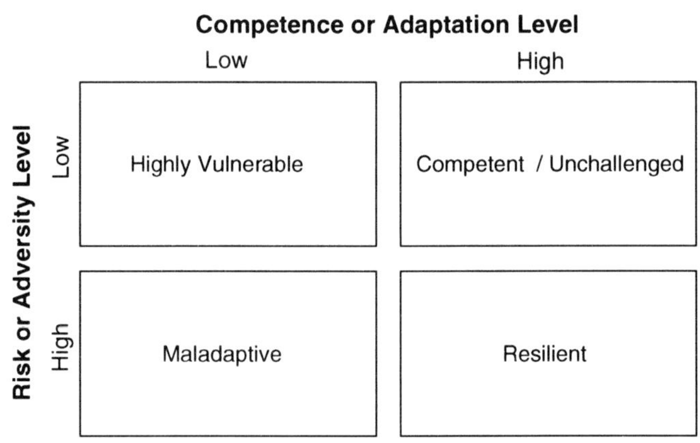

Fig. 7.1 Resilience in development (Masten and Reed 2002)

2000). Beyond this need of specification, all definitions of success need to be handled with care due to their normative character, presupposing universally valid criteria of success and failure.

A further conceptual challenge is the necessity to clearly distinguish resources from risk factors on a theoretical and methodological level. If resources are reduced to the opposite or absence of risk factors, supposed "protective" effects might be attributable to the lower burden by risks. The idea of bipolar risk factors that "*have a positive end associated with positive outcomes [...] as well as a negative end associated with negative outcomes*" (Masten 2001; p. 228) requires special attention here (e.g. the presence of good versus poor parenting). Furthermore risks and resources can be inversely related due to a third variable (Masten 2001).

7.2.5 Models of Resilience

Classic studies of resilience research such as the Kauai study by Werner and Smith (1982, 1992) employed person-focused approaches by comparing poorly and well adapted high-risk children with respect to their resources. Similarly, the other way round is possible by comparing children grouped according to their risks and resources with respect to their developmental outcomes. As person-based data analytic approaches developed, also discriminant function analysis, cluster analysis, and pathway models of resilience were applied (Masten 2001).

Although person-focused approaches are useful in order to detect specific patterns in the lives of "resilient children" they are not appropriate to analyse relationships between risks, resources, and developmental outcomes (Masten 2001). In order to achieve this goal variable-focused approaches are better suitable, since the application of multivariate statistics facilitates to test different models how assets work.

Garmezy et al. (1984) described three models of resilience to guide analyses of relationships between risk, resources and competence variables: the compensatory model, the challenge model and the protective factor model. The "compensatory model" suggests that different cumulating resources and risks compensate and counteract each other by exerting direct influence on the developmental outcome. These beneficial and detrimental effects are independent of each other and can be described by the application of simple linear multiple regression models or main effect models. The second model – the "challenge model" – conceptualises the connection between conditions of risk and developmental outcomes by presupposing a curvilinear association (modelled by a quadratic term in the regression equation). Within this concept a certain degree of stress serves as developmental asset since it poses a challenge to the individual and provides an opportunity to mobilise and develop its resources. However, if faced with excessive stress, the individual is overstrained and cannot longer maintain competence. A third model – the "protective model" – assumes that a protective factor modulates (i.e. buffers) the detrimental effects of stress. In the presence of a protective factor "*variations in stress will be less strongly reflected in variations in quality of adaptation*" (Garmezy et al. 1984; p. 102) than when the protective factor is lacking. In contrast vulnerability factors moderate the impact of stress by enhancing its effect. Such conditional relationships can be identified by means of adding interaction terms in the regression equation.

The last model particularly corresponds to the construct of resilience. Since protective factors primarily or exclusively reduce the effects of risk factors, their beneficial effects can primarily (or only) be observed in the presence of adversity. Several authors – among them Garmezy et al. (1984) – reserved the term "protective factor" for attributes that promote resilience by interaction effects (i.e. buffering processes against adversity) as outlined in the "protective model". Similarly, Rutter (1987) stresses the importance of a buffering effect as a precondition for assuming protective factors. The factor in question has to operate differently dependent on the given level of risk. That means either the protective factor is associated with lower rates of mental health problems only in youth experiencing adverse circumstances or the protective factor is linked to less mental health problems in all children, but significantly interacts with the risk factor and proves more effective in risk-exposed children. Therefore the examination of statistical interactions between present risk variable(s) and putative protective factors is crucial.

However, this terminology is not used consistently. In several classic and contemporary publications the term "protective" is also used with respect to main effect models. Furthermore, also with respect to interaction effects the terminology suggested by Garmezy et al. (1984) is imprecise. Against this background Luthar (1993) introduced more differentiated terms, e.g. "protective-stabilising" or "protective-enhancing" in order to specify if interaction results in maintenance or augmentation of competence in high-risk children. The term "protective" was suggested to be used in order to describe direct ameliorative (main) effects. Later, similar differentiations were suggested regarding vulnerability effects (Luthar et al. 2000).[1]

An appealingly simple terminology was applied by Steinhausen and Winkler Metzge (2001). According to them, there are risk factors and compensatory factors that have significant main effects on the likelihood of mental health problems by increasing or reducing it. These factors are distinguished from vulnerability factors and protective factors that display significant interaction effects due to intensifying or diminishing effects of the risk variable.

Considering theoretical and measurement problems, both, main effect models as well as interaction models have advantages and drawbacks. However, regarding the

[1]Problems with differences in terminology cannot only be found when it comes to the definition of the term "protective factor". There is further confusion regarding the use of words such as "assets" and "resources". While some authors use the terms interchangeably (Masten and Coatsworth 1998) others distinguish between assets as internal factors of the individual that help to overcome adversity and resources which are external to the individual (Fergus and Zimmerman 2005).

aim to draw conclusions with respect to prevention, both models can provide useful information. Main effects models can identify important key assets whose promotion might support a decrease in rates of mental health problems. However, since high-risk and low-risk children would gain from such assets to a comparable extent, their promotion cannot be expected to reduce health inequities, e.g. by being more beneficial to disadvantaged children.

7.3 Identifying Health Assets in Order to Foster Resilience

7.3.1 The Potential of Population-Based Studies

With respect to the high public health significance of mental health problems and many inalterable risk factors, to maximise resilience in the population of children and adolescents is a promising public health approach. Consequently, comprehensive knowledge not only regarding high risk groups but particularly regarding direct ameliorative as well as buffering protective factors is needed in order to inform policy makers from a salutogenetic perspective. In this regard large population-based studies that assess a variety of risks and resources can provide important insights that can guide the design of effective public health interventions.

As became obvious from the theoretical background of research in resilience, it is hardly possible to measure resilience directly. Although there are some attempts such as the Ego-resilience scale (ER89; Block and Kremen 1996) these efforts measure rather protective personal attributes (that are probably often involved in resilience) than resilience itself. Against the theoretical framework outlined above, assessment of resilience needs to focus the absence of mental health problems where they are expected due to considerable adversity. In order to derive implications for practice – at the same time – attributes that correlate with resilience need to be assessed, i.e. protective factors that might support the successful response to environmental hazards.

Population-based epidemiological studies have not only the potential to identify important (combinations of) key assets on a population level but – based on representative samples – can also point out their public health relevance and prevention potential. Large sample sizes furthermore facilitate analyses how specific assets may work differently in diverse subgroups at risk (e.g. children in poverty) and provide a scientific basis for particularly adapted interventions maximising assets in circumscribed risk groups to counteract health inequities. In this context, from an epidemiological and public health perspective it is not primarily important to investigate in detail the exact relationships among the individual and environmental factors and the processes underlying resilience. In order to promote public mental health and to tackle health inequities, the most essential task is to identify key assets that can modify or even eliminate the consequences of present risks on a population level. By focusing the potential to create and maintain health in disadvantaged groups this research paradigm also helps to overcome the deficit perspective.

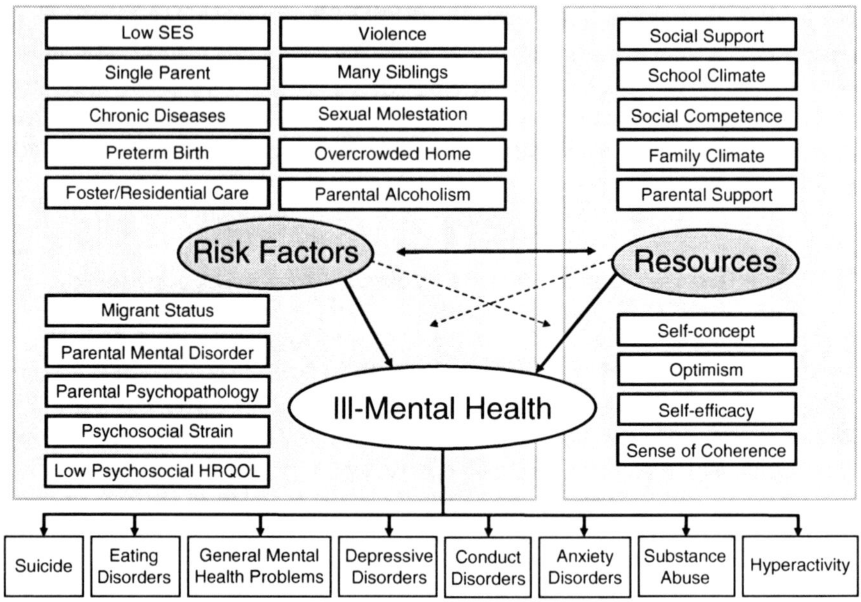

Fig. 7.2 Risks, resources and ill-mental health outcomes in the BELLA study

Despite the comprehensive body of literature examining risk factors or resources, studies including different kinds of risk as well as protective factors in representative population samples are rare (Kinard 1998; Masten and Reed 2002). In the following, an example how phenomenons of resilience and – most important – correlates of resilience can be assessed on a population level will be outlined. The descriptions of risks and resources as well as possible operationalisations refer to the BELLA study which is a module of the German Health Interview and Examination Survey in Children and Adolescents (Ravens-Sieberer et al. 2008a). This population-based epidemiological study focuses (the absence of) mental health problems in children and adolescents and associated risks and resources. Thereby, it considers internal personal factors as well as environmental factors specific to the child's family or to the broader social environment. However, the assessment of risk factors and resources as outlined in Fig. 7.2 serves only as an example and cannot claim to be exhaustive.

7.3.2 *Measuring Adversity: Risk Factors Assessment*

Some important risk (and mediating) factors are available from basic sociodemographic information such as age and gender of the child and family set-up. Regarding the latter, information on circumstances such as growing up with a single parent or with a step-parent or on the number of siblings can be drawn from the sociodemographic data. The age of the parents can be used to determine early parenthood (defined as one parent being younger than 18 years at the time of the child's birth) as a possible risk factor. Further interesting sociodemographic information is the migration status of a child as well as the family's socioeconomic status. Since the detrimental effects of poverty and social disadvantage were shown in several studies its measurement is essential despite of the co-occuring risk factors discussed above. In the BELLA study low socioeconomic status was determined by means of the Winkler Index which takes into account educational as well as occupational status and income of both parents (Winkler and Stolzenberg 1999). Moreover, inadequate living conditions were assessed such as living in a crowded flat, mildew infested rooms etc.

Several risk factors can be addressed by categorical questions in questionnaires or interviews with the parents. Within the BELLA study information regarding some important biological risk factors, such as smoking or drinking by the mother during pregnancy, perinatal complications and health problems of the child in the first 4 weeks after birth was available. In addition psychosocial risk factors were explored such as parents' alcohol consumption, unemployment or mental disorders, but also family conflicts, and conflicts between the partners. In order to identify high alcohol consumption, the interviewees were asked whether they ever thought about cutting down on their drinking and whether they were ever angry about being criticised for their drinking habits. Regarding unemployment, the parent's interview included a question asking whether the family had been affected by unemployment during the child's lifetime and whether this situation was perceived to be a burden. Similarly, current or former mental disorders in the interviewed parent or his/her partner were assessed. Furthermore, the parent was asked how well the family gets along and how happy the relationship between the partners is. Beyond, family conflicts during one parent's childhood and adolescence were asked after as well as presence of chronic diseases and circumstances such as the child resulting from an unwanted pregnancy or low social support received by the interviewed parent during the child's first year of life.

Other risk factors such as high parental strain or high parental psychopathology as well as low parental physical and psychological health-related quality of life were assessed using continuous measures. A high parental strain was studied using a catalogue of questions asking about the particular burden caused by various aspects of daily life, including household, tending a family member in need of care, job, financial worries, and lack of recognition from others. High parental psychopathology was determined by using a short form of the Symptom Checklist-90-R: the 9-item SCL-K-9 (Brähler and Klaghofer 2001) that considers dimensions such as somatisation, depression, anxiety, hostility, paranoid ideation, and psychoticism. Parental physical as well as psychological health-related quality of life was determined by means of the SF-12 (Ware et al. 1996).

Further questions referring to risk factors such as experience of violence and sexual molestation were assessed by children's and adolescents' self-report. Unfortunately, we did not acquire information regarding fear of violence which might be an important stressor as well when growing up in an unsafe environment.

7.3.3 Measuring Resources: Protective Factors Assessment

The resources that were assessed in the BELLA study can be attributed to three broader categories: personal/individual resources, familial resources and further social resources. Personal resources describe features of the child's or adolescent's personality such as high self-efficacy or pronounced optimism. High self-efficacy is conceptualised as a stable trait of personality and describes the firm belief in personal competence to manage stressful situations efficiently (Schwarzer 1994). Different studies provide evidence for the association between high self-efficacy and fewer mental health problems (Schwarzer 1994). In contrast, optimism describes a general positive outcome expectation – irrespective of the belief in one's own personal competence (Scheier and Carver 1985). In the BELLA study these resources were assessed by means of self-report scales developed for children and adolescents that directly target self-efficacy and optimism (Schwarzer and Jerusalem 1999; Grob et al. 1991) by items such as "I can find a solution for every problem" or "My future looks good". A positive self-concept was assessed by a global self-worth scale (Asendorpf and van Aken 1993) that enquires for example, if children are happy about themselves, about the way they are and the things they do. Moreover, overall perceptions of and satisfaction with one's health and one's self were assessed (Starfield et al. 1994/1997/2000). An aggregate score of personal resources was calculated from a five-item scale developed in the pre-test phase of the survey which included selected items deriving from different personal resources scales. There are many further personal characteristics that were discussed to be of importance such as intelligence, creativity, humor, good coping abilities or social skills (Werner 1993; Wolin and Wolin 1993; Barbarin et al. 2001; Cederblad et al. 1994). However, due to practical reasons, only an assortment of possible factors could be assessed.

Also familial resources such as parental support, authoritative child-raising, and good family climate or cohesion were discussed as important resources (Darling 1999). Earlier research showed that children raised in authoritative homes (characterised by warmth, involvement, support of autonomy as well as clear rules and expectations) show less psychological and behavioural dysfunction (Lamborn et al. 1991). Supportive and consistent parenting styles and a positive parent–adolescent relationship are protective and connected to lower levels of depression and less impaired functioning (Juang and Silbereisen 1999; Forehand et al. 1991; Graham 2004; Jessor 1998). The family has great potential to support resilience in a child and even very early life experiences play a major role here. A recent study showed that an intervention of 1 h home visits weekly enhancing interactions between mother and child had considerable effects on outcomes such as anxiety, depression, and antisocial behaviour in older age (Walker et al. 2006). Studies like this do not only indicate the crucial role of parenting and the family in order to build resilience. They also point out that supportive community structures can largely influence these family characteristics and confirm the statement that *"the key to giving young people a good start in life is to help their parents."* (Bartley 2006; p. 5).

In the BELLA study family climate was enquired by items such as "in our family everybody cares about each other's worries" or "we often go to the cinema, visit sport events or go on excursions" (Family Climate Scale, Schneewind et al. 1985). Parental support was measured by means of a scale including items such as "my parents are loving" or "my parents understand my problems and worries" (Currie et al. 2001). However, it also has to be noticed that properties of parents and families that are principally protective may also result in additional problems. Parental overprotection can also hamper a positive development or even result in adverse effects such as antisocial behaviour (Neher and Short 1998). Thus, parental support and supervision are only to a certain degree helpful.

Social resources describe availability of social support outside the nuclear family such as by friends or teachers, relationships in sports clubs or church. Social support has been described as an important psychosocial buffer when confronted with adversity (e.g. Cohen and Wills 1985; Rutter 1987; Werner 1993). It covers not only the objective quantity and function of social relationships, i.e. the degree to which individuals are attached to others. Beyond, the individual's perception of the support being offered and its interaction with the environment are important since social support is not only a characteristic of the social environment but also a function of the person's behaviour. Social support systems relieve the child or adolescent, encourage coping and contribute to the development of individual competences. The protective effects of social support regarding mental health have been shown in a variety of studies (Ezzel et al. 2000; van Aken et al. 1996; Werner 1995; Cederblad et al. 1994) and several measurement devices were developed up to date.

In the BELLA study the level of support received by the child (e.g. by being listened to, being shown affection or being given information) was measured by means of a child-friendly adapted Social Support Scale (Donald and Ware 1984). Peer competence was measured by means of a scale including items such as "it is hard for me to find friends" (Currie et al. 2001). Regarding the broader social context some items referring the school climate were administered. However, it was not possible to measure each factor of interest. Thus, one major limitation of our study is the lack of data regarding structure and function of communities such as neighbourhoods, churches, and further groups that proved to be important to children's mental health (Earls 2001).

7.4 Assets in Socioeconomically Disadvantaged Children: An Example from the BELLA Study

In order to give an example of the benefits of large population-based studies enquiring risks and resources, we will shortly introduce some findings from the BELLA study on mental health in socioeconomically disadvantaged children and the assets they have at their disposal. In order to distinguish a risk group from the rest of our population sample we focused children whose family's socioeconomic status belongs to the most disadvantaged 10% in our sample (according to the Winkler-Index described above). In these children considerably increased rates of mental health problems can be observed (according to the Strengths and Difficulties Questionnaire; Goodman 1997). In the disadvantaged children 18% show seriously high problem scores and 17% of them show at least signs of mental health problems adding up to 35% of the disadvantaged children being affected by mental health problems. The corresponding prevalence rates in the remaining 90% of the children are 9% with seriously high scores and 12% displaying signs of mental health problems, adding up to a considerably smaller number of affected children (21%).

In a second step, we looked at the distribution of assets in these groups. Figure 7.3 displays the distribution of parental support scale scores in the socioeconomically disadvantaged children compared to children with more fortunate backgrounds. It is clearly visible that the "poorer" children report less parental support compared to their peers. This difference corresponds to a small effect (d=0.25) and proves to be important since results from logistic regression (stratified according to the socioeconomic group) show that parental support is a significant predictor of the mental health status. The Odds Ratio of 0.67 (0.58–0.84) in the disadvantaged children and of 0.84 (0.79–0.90) in the remaining population indicate that parental support may be even of higher importance to the disadvantaged group, reducing the chance to suffer from mental health problems by 33% with each additional point on the parental support scale.

A univariate analysis of variance with the mental health total problem score as dependent variable indicates not only significant influences of the factors status group and parental support. It also shows a p-value of 0.054 for the interaction between status group and parental support, indicating a potential buffering effect.

To sum up, it can be concluded that parental support – as an important asset with respect to mental health – is less available in socioeconomically disadvantaged families. Thus, when it comes to promoting mental health in disadvantaged children, it might be reasonable to address their families and to enhance their potential to provide support.

In order to estimate the availability of social resources within this risk group of socioeconomically disadvantaged children, indicators of school climate as reported

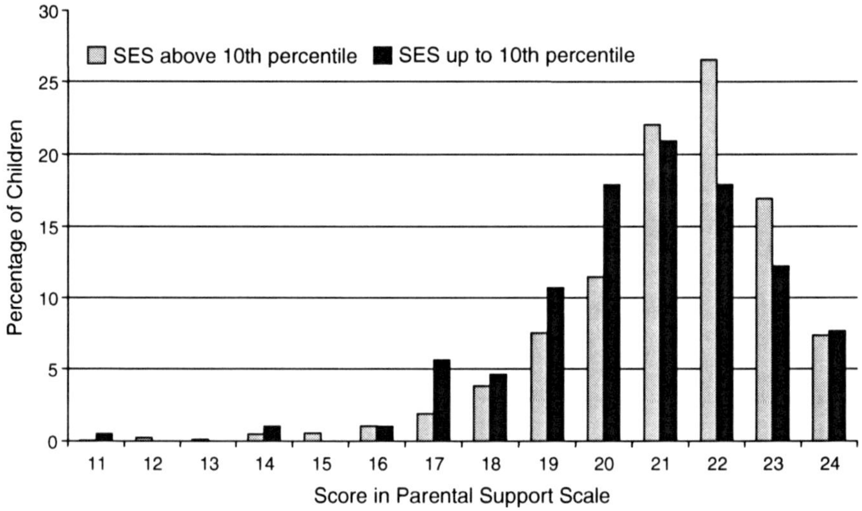

Fig. 7.3 Parental support in different socioeconomicstatus (SES) groups

by the children were compared between the social status groups (10% disadvantaged vs. the remaining population). As Figs. 7.4a–c illustrate children from both groups (dis)agree in similar proportions to statements such as "Most of the students in my class are kind and helpful". However, it has to be mentioned that a χ^2-test indicated significant differences between the groups in 7.4a and 7.4c. These differences obviously result from the "strongly disagree" answers (1% vs. 6% in 7.4a and 0% vs. 2% in 7.4c). In total however, the patterns seem comparable.

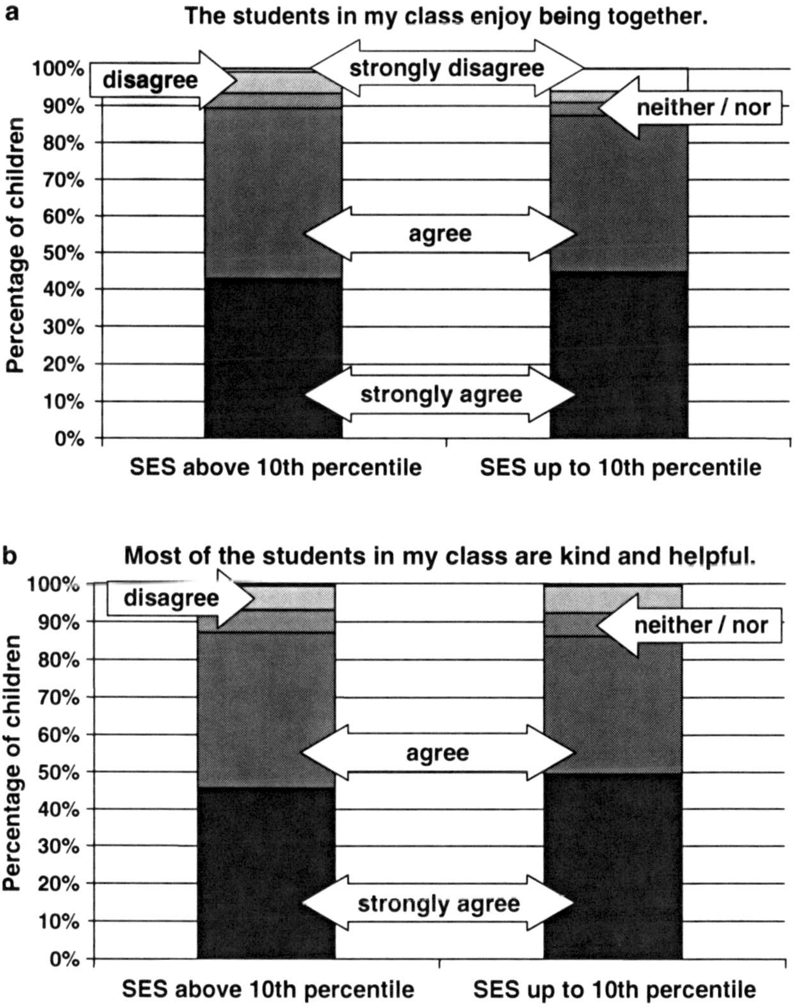

Fig. 7.4 (**a**–**c**) School climate in different socioeconomic status (SES) groups

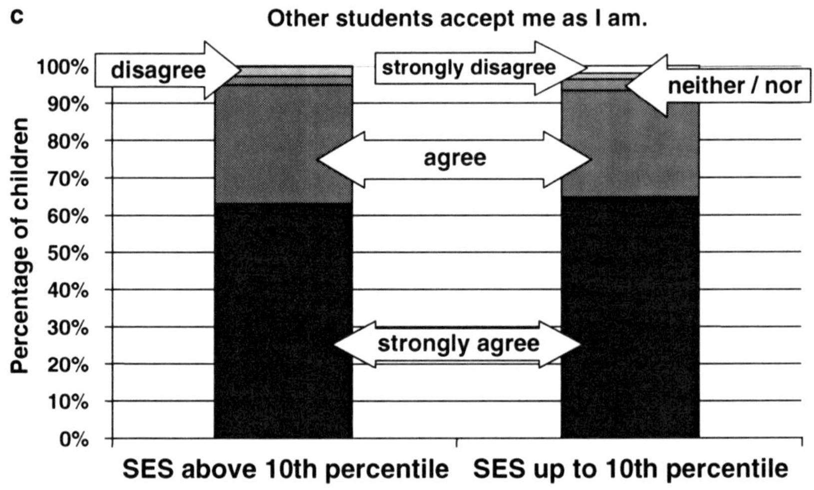

Fig. 7.4 (continued)

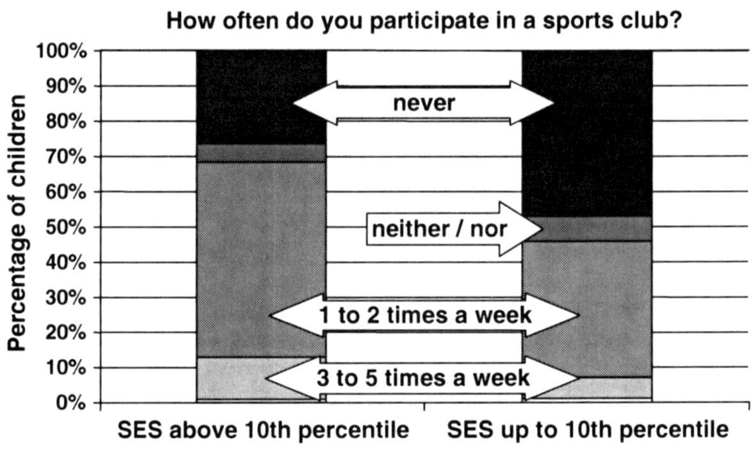

Fig. 7.5 Sport club participation in different socioeconomic status (SES) groups

In order to examine a further source of social support the participation in sports clubs was compared between the groups. Results indicate that about half of the disadvantaged children never participate in organised sport, while this is the case in only a quarter of the children from more fortunate social backgrounds. Thus, a potentially important source of social support is not available in the high risk group (Fig. 7.5).

These results briefly illustrate how large population-based studies can provide crucial information regarding potential approaches to promote the young populations mental health. They do not only enable the identification of particular risk groups. Furthermore the role of resources regarding mental health and differences in the distributions of these assets can be displayed. The results presented here indicate, that in Germany school-based programs focusing peer support may be ineffective regarding a reduction of mental health inequities.

However, it might be a reasonable approach to target the disadvantaged parents' potential to provide support. Furthermore, the participation of their children in sport clubs (or comparable structured leisure time activities) could be enhanced by, e.g. providing easily accessible and inexpensive offers in the community and encouraging participation particularly in groups at risk.

7.5 Conclusions

Findings from epidemiological research on prevalence rates, persistence and negative consequences of mental health problems demonstrate clearly the high public health significance of the topic and the need of action. Supporting resilience in children and adolescents by enhancing key resources is important not only in order to reduce individual suffering and economic costs of treatment and connected burden. In the first instance effective prevention can avoid a huge loss of potential for the individual as well as for society (Belfer 2008). But despite of the large burden on the individuals and on society caused by mental health problems and despite of their growing importance, this topic has been neglected in most countries. A WHO study revealed that 40% of countries do not have a mental health policy (WHO 2001c). Furthermore, in 2002 only 7% of countries worldwide had a specific child and adolescent mental health policy (Belfer 2008).

One reason for the lack of political initiative might be that research often focused on very proximal health determinants that do not necessarily imply political responsibility. Since research on resilience stems from developmental psychology it traditionally focused characteristics of the individual and close relationships. However, the multitude of mental health determinants on different levels shows that an individual's mental health state is also affected by a broad range of factors deriving from, e.g. the economic, environmental, and social sector. Thus, interventions to strengthen mental health by promoting health assets need to address both, proximal and distal determinants. However, this task cannot be solely connected to the health sector but requires socio-political activities as well as intersectoral policies. Since action in settings such as child care, educational institutions, public infrastructure, labour, welfare, justice, housing and environment (WHO 2005) may positively impact on determinants of mental health, all these sectors should be involved in efforts of prevention and mental health promotion. To sum up, available – mainly psychological – expertise regarding individual strengths and family-level assets needs to be integrated within a broader interdisciplinary public health framework in order to identify community-based actions that support resilience.

Besides the fact, that a multi-sectoral approach might reach the most optimal outcome, the broad positive or negative consequences of good or poor mental health should provide a good rationale for many sectors to take responsibility for this major health challenge. E.g. sectors such as education, labour, welfare, and the legal system should be interested in effective mental health promotion since they bear high costs connected to youth mental health problems (Patel et al. 2007). Only approximately 10% of these costs are subjected to the health sector (Belfer 2008).

However, mental health promoting policies require evidence regarding relevant assets that need to be promoted and sustained. As it was pointed out above, public health research has the potential to provide such evidence as a basis for the decisions of policymakers. The measurement of resources besides the assessment of risks in population based studies thus is an important starting point for establishing and improving mental health-related policies. In this regard, the theoretical framework of resilience provides a useful research paradigm. Although research in resilience has been conducted for several decades now, there is still a need for investigating risk and protective factors and their interaction over time as a basis for preventive efforts and early interventions. Beyond, due to ongoing changes in society and consequently changes in living conditions of children and adolescents, future research will be constantly confronted with new questions. The example from our study showed that children with a higher risk burden have at the same time fewer resources at their disposal. However, this primarily applied to parental support and sport clubs as a source of social support but less to reported school climate. Even though more detailed analysis is needed, this suggests that well directed investment in assets of high-risk groups might help to reduce the health gap between disadvantaged children and those who are more fortunate. In this regard our findings correspond to the assumption that *"strengthening of the fundamental nurturing qualities of the family system and community networks"* is essential in youth mental health promotion (Patel et al. 2007; p. 1310).

This contribution primarily dealt with the identification of important assets on a population level to provide an evidence base for policy making, intervention planning and implementation. However, in a second step the availability of psychometrically sound scales further enables the evaluation of such interventions by facilitating pre–post measurements of the protective factors to be enhanced. Future research should increasingly focus the evaluation of programs targeting critical mental health determinants by monitoring changes in these determinants and further documenting the benefits of possible intervention-related improvements (WHO 2005). A further issue, which deserves attention in upcoming research, is the imprecise terminology that was pointed out above. A consensus on the central terms would be helpful not only with respect to ongoing research efforts but also in order to facilitate unambiguous communication of results (Luthar et al. 2000).

Last but not least the meaning of strengthening assets with respect to secondary prevention needs to be addressed. Epidemiological studies have shown that even in high-income countries many children affected by mental health problems do not receive adequate treatment (Kim and The American Academy of Child and Adolescent Psychiatry Task Force on Workforce Needs 2003; Ravens-Sieberer et al. 2008b). Mental health problems in children and adolescents, in particular at an early stage, are likely to be overseen by their everyday environment. The opportunity to provide adequate help by simple measures, such as increased psychosocial support is then missed (Patel et al. 2007). In this regard the assets that were discussed regarding primary prevention might also impact the course of mental health problems and the extent of their negative consequences. Thus, strengthening assets may comprise an even larger potential to reduce the mental health-related burden in the young population that should be further examined by future research.

References

Albee, G.W. (2006). Historical overview of primary prevention of psychopathology: address to the 3rd World Conference on the promotion of mental health and prevention of mental and behavioral disorders, September 15–17, 2004, Auckland, New Zealand. *The Journal of Primary Prevention* 27(5):449–456.

Antonovsky, A. (1987). *Unraveling the mystery of health. How people manage stress and stay well.* San Francisco: Jossey Bass.

Amato, P.R. (2001). Children of divorce in the 1990s: an update of the Amato and Keith (1991) meta-analysis. *Journal of Family Psychology* 15(3):355–370.

American Academy of Pediatrics, Committee on Psychosocial Aspects of Child and Family Health (2001). The new morbidity revisited: a renewed commitment to the psychosocial aspects of pediatric care. *Pediatrics* 108:1227–1230.

American Psychiatric Association (2000). *Diagnostic and statistical manual of mental disorders – DSM-IV-TR, 4th ed., text revision.* Washington, DC:American Psychiatric .

Asendorpf, J.B., van Aken, M.A.G. (1993). Deutsche Versionen der Selbstkonzeptskalen von Harter. *Zeitschrift für Entwicklungspsychologie und Pädagogische Psychologie* 25:64–86.

Bartley, M. (2006). Capability and resilience: beating the odds. London: University College London.

Barbarin, O.A., Richter, L., deWet, T. (2001). Exposure to violence, coping resources, and psychological adjustment. *American Journal of Orthopsychiatry* 71(1):16–25.

Barkmann, C., Romer, G., Watson, M., Schulte-Markwort, M. (2007). Parental physical illness as a risk for psychosocial maladjustment in children and adolescents: epidemiological findings from a National Survey in Germany. *Psychosomatics* 48:476–481,

Belfer, M.L. (2008). Child and adolescent mental disorders: the magnitude of the problem across the globe. *The Journal of Child Psychology and Psychiatry* 49(3):226–236.

Benson, P.L. (1997). All kids are our kids. Minneapolis: Search Institute.

Block, J., Kremen, A. (1996). IQ and ego resiliency: conceptual and empirical connections and separatedness. *Journal of Personality and Social Psychology* 70:349–361.

Bradley, R.H., Corwyn, R.F. (2002). Socioeconomic status and child development. *Annual Review of Psychology* 53:371–399.

Brähler, E., Klaghofer, R. (2001). Konstruktion und teststatistische Prüfung einer Kurzform der SCL-90-R. *Zeitschrift für klinische Psychologie, Psychiatrie und Psychotherapie* 49: 115–124.

Briere, J.N., Elliott, D.M. (1994). Immediate and long-term impacts of child sexual abuse. *The Future of Children* 4(2):54–69.

Bronfenbrenner, U. (1979). The ecology of human development. Experiments by nature and design. Cambridge, MA/London: Harvard University Press.

Caspi, A., McClay, J., Moffitt, T.E., et al. (2002). Role of genotype in the cycle of violence in maltreated children. *Science* 297:851–854.

Caspi, A., Sugden, K., Moffitt, T.E., et al. (2003). Influence of life stress on depression: moderation by a polymorphism in the 5-HTT gene. *Science* 301:386–389.

Cederblad, M., Dahlin, L., Hagnell, O., Hansson, K. (1994). Salutogenic childhood factors reported by middle-aged individuals. Follow-up of the children from the Lundby study grown up in families experiencing three or more childhood psychiatric risk factors. *European Archives of Psychiatry and Clinical Neuroscience* 244:1–11.

Cohen, S., Wills, T.A. (1985). Stress, social support, and the buffering hypothesis. *Psychology Bulletin* 98:310–357.

Costello, E.J., Mustillo, S., Erkanli, A., Keeler, G., Angold, A. (2003). Prevalence and development of psychiatric disorders in childhood and adolescence. *Archives of General Psychiatry* 60:837–844.

Costello, E.J., Egger, H., Angold, A. (2005). 10-year research update review: the epidemiology of child and adolescent psychiatric disorders: I. Methods and Public Health Burden. *Journal of the American Academy of Child and Adolescent Psychiatry* 44:972–986.

Costello, E.J., Foley, D.L., Angold, A. (2006). 10-year research update review: the epidemiology of child and adolescent psychiatric disorders: II. Developmental epidemiology. *Journal of the American Academy of Child and Adolescent Psychiatry* 45: 8–25.

Currie, C., Samdal, O., Boyce, W., Smith, R. (eds) (2001). *Health Behaviour in School-aged Children: a WHO Cross-National Study (HBSC), Research Protocol for the 2001/2002 Survey.* Child and Adolescent Health Research Unit (CAHRU), University of Edinburgh.

Dahlgren, G., Whitehead, M. (1991). Policies and strategies to promote social equity in health. Stockholm: Institute for Future Studies.

Darling, N. (1999). Parenting style and its correlates. ERIC Digest EDO-PS-99-3, clearing house on elementary and early childhood education. Chicago, IL: University of Illinois.

Díaz, R., Gual, A., García, M., Arnau, J., Pascual, F., Cañuelo, B., et al. (2008). Children of alcoholics in Spain: from risk to pathology: Results from the ALFIL program. *Social Psychiatry and Psychiatric Epidemiology* 43(1):1–10.

Donald, C.A., Ware, J.E. (1984). The measurement of social support. *Research in Community and Mental Health* 4:325–370.

Earls, F. (2001). Community factors supporting child mental health. *Child and Adolescent Psychiatric Clinics of North America* 10:693–709.

Evans, G.W. (2004). The environment of childhood poverty. *American Psychologist,* 59(2): 77–92.

Ezzel, C.E., Cupit Swenson, C., Brondino, M.J. (2000). The relationship of social support to physical abused children's adjustment. *Child Abuse & Neglect* 24:641–651.

Fergus, S., Zimmerman, M.A. (2005). Adolescent resilience: a framework for understanding healthy development in the face of risk. *Annual Review of Public Health* 26:399–419.

Fergusson, D.M., Woodward, L.J., Horwood, L.J. (1998). Maternal smoking during pregnancy and psychiatric adjustment in late adolescence. *Archives of General Psychiatry* 55(8):721–727.

Fombonne, E. (1998). Increased rates of psychosocial disorders in youth. *European Archives of Psychiatry and Clinical Neuroscience* 248:14–21.

Ford, T., Goodman, R., Meltzer, H. (2003). The British Child and Adolescent Mental Health Survey 1999: The prevalence of DSM-IV disorders. *Journal of the American Academy of Child and Adolescent Psychiatry* 42(10):1203–1211.

Forehand, R., Wierson, M., Thomas, A., Armstead, L., Kempton, T., Neighbors, B. (1991). The role of family stressors and parent relationships on adolescent functioning. *Journal of the American Academy of Child & Adolescent Psychiatry* 30(2):316–322.

Gardner, F., Johnson, A., Yudkin, P., Bowler, U., Hockley, C., Mutch, L., Wariyar, U., Extremely Low Gestational Age Steering Group (2004). Behavioral and emotional adjustment of teenagers in mainstream school who were born before 29 weeks' gestation. *Pediatrics* 114(3):676–682.

Garmezy, N. (1991). Resiliency and vulnerability to adverse developmental outcomes associated with poverty. *American Behavioral Scientist* 34:416–430.

Garmezy, N., Masten, A., Tellegen, A. (1984). The study of stress and competence in children: a building block for developmental psychology. *Child Development* 55:97–111.

Goodman, R. (1997). The strengths and difficulties questionnaire: a research note. *Journal of Child Psychology and Psychiatry* 38(5):581–586.

Graham, P. (2004). The end of adolescence. Oxford: Oxford University Press.

Grob, A., Lüthi, R., Kaiser, FG., Flammer, A., Mackinnon, A., Wearing, A.J. (1991). Berner Fragebogen zum Wohlbefinden Jugendlicher (BFW). [Bernese questionnaire of subjective well-being]. *Diagnostica* 37:66–75.

Hammen, C., Burge, D., Burney, E., Adrian, C. (1990). Longitudinal study of diagnoses in children of women with unipolar and bipolar affective disorder. *Archives of General Psychiatry* 47(12): 1112–1117.

Hysing, M., Elgen, I., Gillberg, C., Lie, SA., Lundervold, A.J. (2007). Chronic physical illness and mental health in children. Results from a large-scale population study. *Journal of Child Psychology and Psychiatry* 48(8):785–792.

Ihle, W., Esser, G. (2002). Epidemiologie psychischer Störungen im Kindes- und Jugendalter. Prävalenz, Verlauf, Komorbidität und Geschlechtsunterschiede. *Psychologische Rundschau* 53:159–169.

Jenkins, J.M., Smith, M.A. (1991). Marital disharmony and children's behaviour problems: aspects of a poor marriage that affect children adversely. *Journal of Child Psychology and Psychiatry* 32(5):793–810.

Jessor, R., Turbin, M., Costa, F.M. (2003). Adolescent problem behaviour in China and the United States: a cross-national study of psychosocial protective factors. *Journal of Research on Adolescence* 13:329–360.

Jessor, R. (1998). *New prespectives on adolescent risk behaviour.* Cambridge: Cambridge University Press.

Juang, L.P., Silbereisen, R.K. (1999). Supportive parenting and adolescent adjustment across time in former East and West Germany. *Journal of Adolescent* 22:719–736.

Kim, W.J., The American Academy of Child and Adolescent Psychiatry Task Force on Workforce Needs (2003). Child and adolescent psychiatry workforce: a critical shortage and national challenge. *Academic Psychiatry* 27(4):277–282.

Kinard, E.M. (1998). Methodological issues in assessing resilience in maltreated children. *Child Abuse & Neglect* 22(7):669–680.

Klocke, A., Lampert, T. (2005).*Armut bei Kindern und Jugendlichen. Gesundheitsberichterstattung des Bundes (GBE).* Berlin: Robert Koch-Institut.

Lamborn, S.D., Mounts, N.S., Steinberg, L., Dornbusch, S.M. (1991). Pattern of competence and adjustment among adolescent from authoritative, authoritarian, indulgent and neglectful families. *Child Development* 62:1049–1065.

Luthar, S.S. (1993). Annotation: methodological and conceptual issues in research on childhood resilience. *Journal of Child Psychology and Psychiatry* 34(4):441–453.

Luthar, S.S., Cicchetti, D., Becker, B. (2000). The construct of resilience: a critical evaluation and guidelines for future work. *Child Development* 71(3):543–562.

Markel, H., Golden, J. (2005). Successes and missed opportunities in protecting our children's health: critical junctures in the history of children's health policy in the United States. *Pediatrics* 115(4 pt 2):1129–1133.

Masten, A.S. (2001). Ordinary magic. Resilience processes in development. American Psychologist 56(3):227–238.

Masten, A.S., Coatsworth, J.D. (1998). The development of competence in favorable and unfavorable environments. Lessons from research on successful children. *American Psychologist* 53(2):205–220.

Masten, A.S., Reed, M-G.J. (2002). Resilience in development. In: C.R. Snyder, S.J. Lopez (eds.) *The handbook of positive psychology* (pp. 74–88). Oxford: University Press.

McLeod, J.D., Kaiser, K. (2004). Childhood emotional and behavioral problems and educational attainment. *American Sociological Review* 69:636–658.

Murray, C.J.L., Lopez, A.D. (1996). Evidence-based health policy-lessons from the global burden of disease study. *Science* 274:740–743.

Murray, C.J.L., Lopez, A.D. (1997). Alternative projections of mortality and disability by cause 1990–2020: Global Burden of Disease Study. *Lancet* 349:1498–1504.

Neher, L., Short, J. (1998). Risk and protective factors for children's substance abuse and antisocial behavior following parental divorce. *American Journal of Orthopsychiatry* 68(1):154–161.

Palfrey, J.S., Tonniges, T.F., Green, M., Richmond, J. (2005). Introduction: addressing the millennial morbidity – the context of community. *Pediatrics* 115:1121–1123.

Patel, V., Flisher, A.J., Hetrick, S., McGorry, P. (2007). Mental health of young people: a global public-health challenge. *Lancet* 369:1302–1313.

Prosser, J., McArdle, P. (1996). The changing mental health of children and adolescents: evidence for deterioration? *Psychological Medicine* 26:715–725.

Ravens-Sieberer, U., Kurth, B.M. BELLA study group, KiGGS study group (2008a). The mental health module (BELLA study) within the German Health Interview and Examination Survey of Children and Adolescents (KiGGS): study design and methods. *Eur Child Adolesc Psychiatry* 17(Suppl 1):10–21.

Ravens-Sieberer, U., Wille, N., Erhart, M., et al. (2008b). Prevalence of mental health problems among children and adolescents in Germany: results of the BELLA study within the National Health Interview and Examination Survey. *European Child & Adolescent Psychiatry* 17(Suppl 1):22–33.

Razum, O., Breckemkamp, J. (2007). Kindersterblichkeit und soziale Situation: Ein internationaler Vergleich. [Mortality in children under 5 years and social situation: international comparison] *Deutsches Ärzteblatt* 104(43) A2950–A2956.

Richardson, G.E. (2002). The metatheory of resilience and resiliency. *Journal of Clinical Psychology* 58(3):307–321.

Roberts, R.E., Attkisson, C.C., Rosenblatt, A. (1998). Prevalence of psychopathology among children and adolescents. *American Journal of Psychiatry* 155:715–725.

Rolf, J.E. (1999). Resilience: an interview with Norman Garmezy. In: M.D. Glantz & J.L. Johnson (eds.) *Resilience and development. Positive life adaptations*. New York: Kluwer Academic/Plenum.

Rutter, M. (1971). Parent-child separation: psychological effects on the children. *Journal of Child Psychology and Psychiatry* 12:233–260.

Rutter, M. (1985). Resilience in the face of adversity. Protective factors and resistance to psychiatric disorder. *British Journal of Psychiatry* 147:598–611.

Rutter, M., Smith, D.J. (1995). *Psychosocial disorders in young people: time trends and their causes*. Chicester: Wiley.

Rutter, M., Yule, B., Quinton, D., Rowlands, O., Yule, W., Berger, M. (1975). Attainment and adjustment in two geographical areas: III. Some factors accounting for area differences. *British Journal of Psychiatry* 126:520–533.

Rutter, M. (1987). Psychosocial resilience and protective mechanisms. *American Journal of Orthopsychiatry* 57(3):316–331.

Rutter, M., Quinton, D. (1984). Parental psychiatric disorder: effects on children. *Psychological Medicine* 14:853–880.

Rutter, M., Tizard, J., Yule, W., Graham, P., Whitmore, K. (1976). Isle of Wight studies 1964–1974. *Psychological Medicine* 6:313–332.

Sameroff, A.J., Seifer, R., Bartko, W.T. (1997). Environmental perspectives on adaptation during childhood and adolescence. In: S.S. Luthar, J.A. Burack, D. Cicchetti, J. Weisz (eds.), *Developmental psychopathology: perspectives on adjustment risk and disorder* (pp. 507–526). New York: Cambridge University Press.

Scheier, M.F., Carver, C.S. (1985). Optimism, coping and health: assessment and implications of generalized outcome expectancies. *Health Psychology* 4:219–247.

Scheithauer, H., Petermann, F. (1999). Zur Wirkungsweise von Risiko- und Schutzfaktoren in der Entwicklung von Kindern und Jugendlichen. *Kindheit und Entwicklung* 8:3–14.

Schneewind, K., Beckmann, M., Hecht-Jackl, A. (1985). *Familienklima-Skalen. Bericht 8.1 und 8.2. Institut für Psychologie – Persönlichkeitspsychologie und Psychodiagnostik*. München: Ludwig Maximilians Universität.

Schwarzer, R. (1994). Optimistische Kompetenzerwartung: Zur Erfassung einer personalen Bewältigungsressource. *Diagnostica* 40:105–123.

Schwarzer, R., Jerusalem, M. (1999). *Skalen zur Erfassung von Lehrer- und Schülermerkmalen. Dokumentation der psychometrischen Verfahren im Rahmen der Wissenschaftlichen Begleitung des Modellversuchs Selbstwirksame Schulen*. Berlin: Institut für Psychologie, Freie Universität Berlin.

Starfield, B., Riley, A., Ensminger, M., Green, B., Ryan, S., Kim-Harris, S. (1994/1997/2000). *Manual for the Child Health and Illness Profile-Adolescent Edition (CHIP-AETM)* Baltimore: The Johns Hopkins University.

Steinhausen, H.C., Winkler Metzge, C. (2001). Risk, compensatory, vulnerability, and protective factors influencing mental health in adolescence. *Journal of Youth and Adolescence* 30(3):259–280.
van Aken, M.A.G., Asendorpf, J.B., Wilpers, S. (1996). Das soziale Unterstützungsnetzwerk von Kindern: Strukturelle Merkmale, Grad der Unterstützung, Konflikte und Beziehung zum Selbstwertgefühl. *Psychologie Erziehung Unterricht* 43:114–126.
von Rueden, U., Gosch, A., Rajmil, L., Bisegger, C., Ravens-Sieberer, U., the European KIDSCREEN group (2006). Socioeconomic determinants of health related quality of life in childhood and adolescence: results from a European study. *Journal of Epidemiology and Community Health* 60:130–135.
Walker, S.P., Chang, S.M., Powell, C.A., Simonoff, E., Grantham-McGregor, S.M. (2006). Effects of psychosocial stimulation and dietary supplementation in early childhood on psychosocial functioning in late adolescence: follow-up of randomised controlled trial. *BMJ* 333:472–476.
Ward, C.L., Flisher, A.J., Zissis, C., Muller, M., Lombard, C. (2001). Exposure to violence and its relationship to psychopathology in adolescents. *Inj Prev* 7:297–301.
Ware, J.E., Kosinski, M., Keller, S.D. (1996). A 12-Item Short-Form Health Survey (SF-12): construction of scales and preliminary tests of reliability and validity. *Medical Care* 32:220–233.
Werner, E., Smith, R.S. (1982). *Vulnerable but invincible: a study of resilient children.* New York: McGraw-Hill.
Werner, E., Smith, R.S. (1992). *Overcoming the odds: high risk children from birth to adulthood.* Ithaca: Cornell University Press.
Werner, E. (1993). Risk, resilience, and recovery: perspectives from Kauai. *Development and Psychopathology* 5:503–515.
Werner, E. (1995). Resilience in development. *Current Directions in Psychological Science* 4:81–85.
Williams, J.H., Ross, L. (2007). Consequences of prenatal toxin exposure for mental health in children and adolescents: a systematic review. *European Child & Adolescent Psychiatry* 16(4): 243–253.
Winkler, J., Stolzenberg, H. (1999). Social class index in the Federal Health Survey [Der Sozialschichtindex im Bundes-Gesundheitssurvey]. *Das Gesundheitswesen* 61 (Sonderheft 2):178–183.
WHO. (1992). *The ICD-10 classification of mental and behavioural disorders: clinical descriptions and diagnostic guidelines.* Geneva: World Health Organization.
WHO. (2001a). *The world health report. Mental health: new understanding, new hope.* Geneva: World Health Organization.
WHO. (2001b). *Strengthening mental health promotion.* Geneva: World Health Organization. (Fact sheet, No. 220).
WHO. (2001c). *Mental health policy project. Policy and service guidance package. Executive summary.* Geneva: World Health Organization.
WHO. (2005). *Promoting Mental Health. Concepts, Emerging Evidence, Practice. Summary Report.* World Health Organization, Department of Mental Health and Substance Abuse in collaboration with the Victorian Health Promotion Foundation and the University of Melbourne. Geneva: World Health Organization.
Wolin, S.J., Wolin, S. (1993). *Bound and determined: Growing up resilient in a troubled family.* New York: Villard.

Chapter 8
Measuring Children's Well-Being: Some Problems and Possibilities

Virginia Morrow and Berry Mayall

Keywords Children's well-being • WHO Health Behaviour in School-aged Children (HBSC) • Research with children

8.1 Introduction

This chapter explores the concept of children's well-being and discusses how it has been measured and operationalised in research. We raise some critical questions about the concept of 'well-being' in general, about how children's well-being is researched, and how the United Nations (UN) Convention on the Rights of the Child is invoked in such research. We discuss as an example the United Nations Children's Fund (UNICEF) Innocenti Report Card 7, published in 2007, (UNICEF 2007, henceforth the UNICEF Report) entitled *Child poverty in perspective: An overview of child well-being in rich countries: a comprehensive assessment of the lives and well-being of children and adolescents in the economically advanced nations* which received a great deal of publicity in the British news media. It placed UK's children at the bottom of the league table of rich nations in relation to emotional well-being and 'happiness'. The report seems to have entered the public, or at least news media, consciousness to an unprecedented degree. We have not undertaken a systematic analysis of media reports (this would be an overwhelming task) but to take one recent example as illustration: *Time* magazine, 7th April 2008, had a front page illustration of a young man in a hooded top (hoodie), peering through a Union Jack flag, with the title '*Unhappy, Unloved and Out of Control: An epidemic of violence, crime and drunkenness has made Britain scared of its young. What's causing the crisis?*' This example is worth mentioning because it refuelled the initial furore. Eighteen months on, the unhappiness of UK children is routinely, almost offhandedly, reported as fact. For instance, in an article about rates of mental ill-health, a senior representative of the National Union of Teachers reportedly said: 'As the UNICEF survey last year showed, children in the UK are among the unhappiest in the world. Unhappy children

V. Morrow (✉)
Institute of Education, University of London, London, UK
e-mail: v.morrow@ioe.ac.uk

A. Morgan et al. (eds.), *Health Assets in a Global Context: Theory, Methods, Action*,
DOI 10.1007/978-1-4419-5921-8_8,

are more likely to be stressed, which can lead to emotional and mental health problems.' (Guardian Education, 2nd September 2008, p. 25).

Such approaches to research based on data gathered from children and young people, and the subsequent reporting of the research in news media clearly emphasise negative attributes of young people and their lives (see Mayall 2002; Morrow 2000). A more positive approach is currently being developed by the WHO European Office for Investment in Health Development based on 'health assets'. This approach, described in Chap. 1, involves identifying factors and resources that enhance the capacities of "individuals, groups, communities, populations, social systems and/or institutions to maintain and sustain health and well-being and to help reduce health inequities". In relation to young people, such an approach includes not only exploring individual competencies such as resilience, but also community level attributes such as supportive social networks, strong intergenerational relationships and so on. It would also include a consideration of organisational or institutional structures, such as: "environmental resources necessary for promoting physical, mental and social health, employment security and opportunities for voluntary service, safe and pleasant housing, political democracy and participation opportunities, social justice and enhancing equity".

These important contextual political, economic and structural factors are often missing from individualistic research on health risk behaviours (Morrow 2000). In Chap. 1, Morgan and Ziglio suggest that an assets approach would balance the deficit model approach, not least by relating individuals to their social context in a much more systematic way than has tended to be the case in (dominant) deficit model research on young people's health risk behaviours.

The chapter is structured in three parts: the first part explores the rise of the term 'well-being' and asks some critical questions about its use. The second part looks in some detail at what the UNICEF Report was measuring, and considers the value of the measurements and conclusions drawn. Finally, the third section considers ways in which the UN Convention on the Rights of the Child has been invoked in well-being research. We conclude with a brief discussion of how the assets approach could be useful in future research, and how the problems we have identified in relation to the concept of well-being need to be clarified before this can proceed effectively.

8.1.1 Summary of UNICEF Report

The UNICEF Report claims to 'provide a comprehensive assessment of the lives and well-being of children and young people in 21 nations of the industrialised world. Its purpose is to encourage monitoring, to permit comparison, and to stimulate the discussion and development of policies to improve children's lives' (p. 2).

The report represents a significant advance on previous titles in the UNICEF Report Card series which have used income poverty as a proxy measure for overall child-well being in the Organisation for Economic Co-operation and Development

(OECD) countries. Specifically, it attempts to measure and compare child well-being under six different headings or dimensions: material well-being; health and safety; education; peer and family relationships; behaviours and risks; and young people's own subjective sense of well-being. In all it draws upon 40 separate indictors relevant to children's lives and children's rights (UNICEF 2007; p. 2).

The report points to the fact that the UK government has led the way in providing indicators and measuring how the UK is progressing. This initiative can be seen as positive, but also as simultaneously fuelling social concern about childhood.

The main findings of the UNICEF Report are as follows: The Netherlands heads the table of overall child well-being in the OECD countries studied, ranking in the top ten for all six dimensions. European countries dominate the top half of the overall league table, with northern countries – the Netherlands, Sweden, Denmark and Finland – claiming the top four places, closely followed by Spain, Switzerland and Norway. The UK and USA are in the bottom third of rankings for five of the six dimensions. No single dimension stands as a reliable proxy for child well-being and several OECD countries have widely differing rankings to the dimensions. There is no obvious relationship between child well-being and GDP per capita.

8.1.2 *Why Are We Writing This Chapter?*

We write as two sociologists who, over the past 20 and more years, have been carrying out research with and about children, and exploring the status of childhood in the UK and the positioning of children in research. As noted, children have traditionally been studied through what might be termed a 'deficit-model' lens (Mayall 2002; Morrow 2000).

We welcome the fact that it is now possible to find statistical information about (or from) children that takes children as the unit of analysis, whereas previously they were subsumed under the category of household or family (Qvortrup 1991, 1994). The UNICEF Report moves on from a narrow focus on child poverty as measured by family income. It is also a useful 'start' in trying to compare countries. It is generally very fair – the authors admit that they can use only what is available, they acknowledge problems with what they do use, deficiencies, and gaps and limitations in data from some countries. They also acknowledge that some of the data used are quite old, and that government initiatives may have made a difference, such as staying on at school, provision of resources for childhood (though not, apparently, child poverty rates). However, we think it is important that a report is sound, and that it does what it says it will, and that it is worth looking more closely at than just at its summary findings.

Secondly, we accept that childhood, in some respects, is in a bad way in the UK. Rates of poverty mean disadvantaged childhoods for some. News media and government comments on children tend to accentuate the negative, and in the case of government, children are valued in terms of future human capital (becoming) over the present (being) (though this is changing). A balanced debate can be difficult to achieve because of sensational events and the emotive way in which notions of childhood are discussed in the media (Alexander 2009).

There have been few critiques of the UNICEF Report, but a helpful starting point for us has been a paper by Ansell et al. (2007). They suggest:

> "...given the limitations of the report... it is worrying that its findings have been accepted unproblematically by much of the UK media and many policy makers. With a more critical approach, however, it does have the potential to contribute to many key debates currently surrounding childhood." (Ansell et al. 2007; p. 29)

Thirdly, we emphasise that we are not statisticians, but are looking at the presentation of statistics from the point of view of sociologists. We raise a series of (perhaps naïve) questions about the use of statistics, the meaning of well-being, and the use of rights-talk in relation to children's well-being. We draw on a range of material, and emphasise that this is not a systematic review but a selective one. We suggest that the UNICEF Report makes some dubious assumptions, which to some extent reflect normative ideas about childhood. We question how far it makes sense to compare small, relatively homogeneous, societies with much larger diverse ones. Is competition between governments a good thing? Are league tables like this really helpful? Ansell et al. (2007) note:

> "The report has an unashamedly instrumental purpose. It is intended not simply to document geographical patterns, but to demonstrate what can be achieved at the national level. By encouraging competition between governments, the aim is to shame them into enacting policies that will ultimately improve the well-being of children across the rich world."Ansell et al. 2007; p. 329)

8.2 What Is "Well-Being"?

The concept of 'well-being' has become popular in the past 5 years in UK social policy documentation in general. Dinham (2007), for example, writing in the context of community development, suggests well-being 'has joined 'community', 'participation', and 'empowerment' and a range of other perceived positives in the pantheon of New Labour language for civil society' (p. 3) – it is a 'hurrah' word. However, as Dinham notes:

> "Well-being lacks definition, both as a concept and in practice. Thus there emerges a range of factors identified as inherent in it or against which it is recognizable and/or measurable. Yet, at the same time, there is little or no consensus about what it really means or looks like and therefore to produce and reproduce it, and to know that it is there, proves highly difficult except in the most general of terms." (Dinham 2007; p. 3)

Previously 'well-being' was an appendage to 'health' (one of us has used it in this way, in research based upon another popular policy/academic/lay term: social capital – without defining well-being adequately, see Morrow (1999)). The roots of the connection of well-being to health can be located in the WHO definition of health as:

> "A state of complete physical, mental and social well-being and not merely the absence of disease or infirmity." (WHO 1946)

Subsequently, well-being has increasingly become a feature in the language of public health and health promotion. However, as Cameron et al. (2006) point out (writing in relation to health promotion)

> "Well-being seems to be used in a curiously unconsidered way, involving assumptions and with little systematic attention. A considered (i.e. generous) view might see this notion of 'well-being' as indicating engagement with a broad model of health and a focus on the 'non-medical." (Cameron et al. 2006; p. 349)

They continue: 'it suggests an emphasis on positive health rather than negative health, and also highlights the subjective rather than objective aspects of health. On the face of it... a focus on well-being may appear useful...' (p. 349). However, they (Cameron et al. 2006) suggest that 'well-being':

> "as currently used, contributes to a muddying rather than a clarification of all-important conceptual waters around health. The lack of definition in much health policy and practice typically leaves the term "well-being" as an open-ended, catch-all category." (Cameron et al. 2006; p. 349)

The question is whether adding the term well-being to health enhances our understanding or is redundant. Cameron et al. (2006) carried out qualitative research to explore concepts of health, being well, and well-being with various groups of adults (community and professional groups) and found a range of interpretations of well-being. They conclude that "the often unexplained addition of 'well-being' to health is merely confusing and unhelpful" (p. 353).

Other public health researchers relate the emphasis on well-being to dilemmas in modern western societies: Carlisle and Hanlon (2007), also writing in the context of public health and health promotion, suggest that:

> "although we have seen an unprecedented growth in wealth and comfort over recent decades and many past causes of suffering have now been eliminated or reduced, average levels of well-being have not increased... large numbers remain deeply unhappy..." (Carlisle and Hanlon 2007; p. 262)

Carlisle and Hanlon suggest that 'these are clearly cultural as well as social problems, but that this tends to remain under-recognised: the burgeoning literature on well-being tends to omit any acknowledgement of the importance of 'culture' in influencing well-being at various levels – individual, social and global...' (p. 262). They point to the capitalist system of production and consumption and the rise of consumer culture, and note that the 'problem' for economists is that subjective well-being rose for a decade or two after World War II, but has since remained static, despite rising living standards and increased wealth, and that economists need to explain this. Carlisle and Hanlon (2007) point out that well-being is now "firmly part of popular discourse, ... used interchangeably with notions of 'happiness' and 'positive emotions" (p. 264).

Here we ask what happens when questions about well-being are applied to children. To what extent is it appropriate to ask these questions (that derive from what is essentially a problem for economists in relation to adults) about children, for whom (subjective) well-being may well involve much more than wealth and affluence? The (Western) norm is that children should 'be happy'; children are expected to be smiling, and dominant imagery projects this (Ennew and Milne 1989; Holland 1992). Social historian Hugh Cunningham (2007) points out that "The belief that childhood should be a time of happiness is now deeply embedded, but it had scary any purchase before the later eighteenth century" (p. 19). This is related to powerful cultural constructions of childhood that the sociology of childhood has been exploring and problematizing over the past two decades (James and Prout 1990/1997; Mayall 2002). Spencer (2007) found that young people frequently discussed adult expectation and pressure to always 'be happy', when at times they felt quite miserable. It seems children and young people are not 'allowed' to feel 'unhappy', yet they have increasing pressure on them from school, home, friends and the media.

The policy implications of well-being research for public health (for adults) appear to be therapeutic interventions with individuals (Carlisle and Hanlon 2007):

> "scientific solutions to the problem of static well-being are often cast in individualist and biomedical terms, from drug treatments, psychotherapy and the practice of medication as a way of reducing stress and enhancing well-being for the minority experiencing mental illness to personal psychology modification for the reasonably discontented majority" (p. 265).

In the case of children, there have been suggestions that they should have 'happiness' lessons in school (though journalists also tend to elide 'well-being' and 'happiness' and use the terms interchangeably, see for example Thomas-Bailey (2008) describing a recent UK government initiative entitled Social and Emotional Aspects of Learning, DCSF 2007). Some argue that academic and professional concern has led to the 'medicalisation' of children's problematic behaviour (see Coppock 2001; Ecclestone 2004, 2008) with the concomitant idea that there are (individual) therapeutic solutions that can be bolted on.

Sointu (2005) also points to the individualistic nature of the debates. She undertook a sociological analysis of the changing meaning of well-being based on analysis of newspaper articles 1985–2003 (and in relation to adults not children). She suggests that the idea of personal well-being has emerged in a specific social context, one that 'emphasises proactive agency and self-responsibility as meaningful and normal…' (p. 255). Carlisle and Hanlon also suggest:

> "we need to ask whether the cultivation of individual happiness is an adequate and appropriate goal for health promotion. Focusing simply on personal growth and development can be just another form of consumption and would arguably sell health promotion short." (Carlisle and Hanlon 2007; p. 266)

On the other hand, well-being may be a useful concept in multi-disciplinary research becausee it is understandable to researchers from a range of theoretical backgrounds as well as to policy-makers. This is surely something to be welcomed. Huppert and Baylis (2004) (co-founders of 'The Well-being Institute' at the University of Cambridge) suggest (somewhat evangelically) that well-being is not only a rapidly evolving field of study, but also 'an exquisite example of a truly multidisciplinary endeavour' (p. 1,447; see Hulme and Toye (2006) for international development studies). Huppert and Baylis (2004) draw on an eclectic range of disciplines, including sociobiology, evolutionary theory, positive psychology, neurobiology, and epidemiology, and political science (narrowly derived from Putnam's ideas about social capital, Putnam 2000) and argue that a range of factors, ranging from individual genes, maternal nutrition, brain activity, early childhood development, and 'positive' emotions all determine (individuals') levels of well-being.

However, the use of terms like well-being should be critically considered, because if (like social capital) it is a kind of unit of exchange that works across cultures and nations, this is in itself politically loaded and problematic. Is well-being (simply) a word that economists can work with and understand? In the arguments for inter-disciplinarity, there is no mention made of critical sociology, political or social theory, and no consideration of the risks involved in transferring concepts between disciplines, cultures and languages, which we suggest should be acknowledged when concepts such as 'well-being' are studied.

A final point is that the links between children's well-being and poverty are not well-elaborated or well understood, and it is not straightforward to trace causal pathways – setting aside material well-being, it is not possible to demonstrate that poor children are necessarily the most unhappy and most stressed. There is (developmental psychological) research evidence from the USA that suggests that children of affluent parents are at a greater 'risk' of various non-trivial threats to their psychological well-being than their poorer counterparts: risks such as higher rates of substance use, anxiety and depression, that are linked to two sets of factors: excessive pressure to achieve, and physical and emotional isolation from parents (Luthar 2003; Luthar and Latendresse 2005).

In summary, well-being is conceptually muddy, but has become pervasive. There is some critical thinking about the concept in relation to adults. Would other European countries simply refer to 'children's welfare'? Is the focus on well-being inherently individualistic and thus, is it a way of NOT talking about welfare and responsibilities of governments towards children? Does it replace welfare as a conceptual device, and what are the implications of this?

8.3 Measuring Well-Being

As noted, the UNICEF Report UNICEF 2007 focuses on six dimensions of well-being – these are: material well-being; health and safety; education; peer and family relationships; behaviours and risks; and young people's subjective sense of well-being. The authors of the report argue at the outset that their report represents a significant advance on previous reports in the Innocenti series, which have used income poverty as a proxy for child well-being. They go on to argue that comparing child well-being in differing countries is necessary, for, in order 'to improve something, first measure it' (p. 3). Internationally, these measurements and comparisons show what can be achieved and what each country's strengths and weaknesses are. Above all, such reports show that levels of child well-being are not inevitable, but are policy-susceptible.

However, the authors go on to say, the study could use only what data were available. The only data collected with children themselves comes from the WHO Health Behaviour in School-Aged Children (HBSC) survey, a cross-national survey that has been running since 1982, and repeated every 4 years with 11, 13 and 15-year-olds, which maps trends in children's health risk behaviours (so it has a very specific focus). Some comparisons could not be made because data are not comparable (for instance on levels of violence in the home, on participation rates of children in early childhood services; and on children's mental health and emotional well-being). Furthermore, as the authors note during the course of their presentation of the data, much of it is old – and so, we may add, may be unrepresentative of progress made in countries which have introduced policies to improve childhood (such as the UK since 1997). The problem of dealing with necessarily dated data is discussed by Jonathan Bradshaw elsewhere (Bradshaw 2007). We also identify some problems with the uses that have been made of the HBSC data. Some of the claims made seem to be based on unreflective developmental assumptions and on cultural assumptions, as we shall demonstrate. Further, some indicators are rather oddly selected.

We now proceed to consider each of the six dimensions of well-being, and the indicators used to arrive at them. We note that averaging the indicators means that each is given equal weight (UNICEF 2007; p. 5) and we are not sure this works well for the data in all cases. We also note that for most dimensions 18–21 countries are being compared. We cannot present here findings for all the countries, but concentrate on the UK, since findings have been so widely reported, as facts, in the news media.

8.3.1 Dimension 1: Material Well-Being

Indicators used here are: relative income poverty; percentages of children in households without jobs; and reported deprivation (averages of children's reports on low family affluence, numbers of educational resources and fewer than ten books in the home). It is no surprise that the UK is second from the bottom on income poverty and near the bottom on workless households (see UNICEF (2007); Figs. 1.1 and 1.2; henceforth all figures refer to UNICEF (2007)). But as the authors point out, differences in national wealth need to be taken into account – a poor child in the UK and the USA may be less disadvantaged relatively than a poor child in Hungary or Poland. And it is also necessary to take account of the point that some countries have more equal distribution of income (so fewer children will fall below the 50% of the national median). In other words we are talking about social exclusion rather than poverty. These points become relevant when we consider 11, 13 and 15 year-old children's reports on three topics: on household ownership (of cars, own bedroom, holiday with family, and computers) (UK comes eighth in the ranking); on ownership of education-related possessions (UK seventh); and on household ownership of ten or more books (UK 17th) (Fig. 1.3a–c).

But the averaging of these three sets of reports by children into one component of the dimension, which is then averaged with income poverty and households without jobs, means that the UK's overall score on this dimension is near the bottom, along with the USA, Ireland, Hungary, and Poland. The authors argue that 'children appear to be most deprived of educational and cultural resources in some of the world's most economically developed countries (UNICEF 2007; p. 11). Perhaps we should note, however, that a wider encompassing of social factors might provide a (somewhat) differing picture; thus, for instance, in more affluent nations, books and computers and space to work are freely available in schools and libraries. We suggest that there is a need to combine quantitative and qualitative data in order to interpret findings more systematically and accurately when attempting to make international comparisons.

8.3.2 Dimension 2: Health and Safety

Indicators used here are: health at age 0–1 (averages of infant mortality rates and low birth-weight rates); percentage of children aged 12–23 months immunised against measles, DPT and polio; and deaths from accident and injury, age 0–19. The authors regret that there was no comparable indicator of children's mental and emotional health; or of child abuse and neglect.

Overall, the UK is ranked at 12th place on the average of these (Fig. 2.0). Again there is variation in the UK ranking on each indicator, for whilst the UK ranks some way down on the first two (Figs. 2.1a, b and 2.2), the UK is second from the top (after Sweden) on preventing death from accident and injury (Fig. 2.3).

It is difficult to know what to make of these findings, apart from the point that it seems unhelpful to average the indicators. One point, however, is that as with many of the indicators, it is the more socialist countries that do best on infants' health and immunisation rates. More neo-liberal societies (Esping Andersen 1996), and possibly countries with more diverse populations, do less well on prevention in early childhood and on persuading people to take up immunisation. The authors also note that the indicators do not include children's own views on their health – yet these are included under the dimension subjective well-being; so it is not clear how choices were made about what to include where.

8.3.3 Dimension 3: Educational Well-Being

The indicators used here are: school achievement at age 15 (including averages of achievement in literacy, numeracy and science); percentage of young people aged 15–19 in full- or part-time education; and the transition to employment (including averages of percentage not in education, training or employment, and percentage of 15-year-olds expecting to find low-skilled work). Again, the authors deplore that adequate, comparable data were not available on the quantity and quality of early years provision (UNICEF 2007; p. 21).

This dimension (Fig. 3.0) includes indicators that perhaps are so disparate as to defy averaging; and this may account for the unusual group of those who top the ranking: Belgium, Canada, Poland and Finland; and those at the bottom: France, Austria, Italy and Portugal. Overall the UK ranks at 17th place on this dimension; but does better on the first one: achievement at age 15 (ranked ninth) (Fig. 3.1). We have some difficulties with these indicators. Whilst it is the case, as the authors argue, that we need to know how well the education system serves our children, it does not follow, we submit, that a long time (after compulsory school-leaving age) in that system has to be regarded as a good; there seem to be some cultural pre-conceptions here: that more education in school is necessarily a good thing. And/or it may be that the economic welfare of the country, rather than children's 'educational well-being', determined the choice of these indicators. Many people, including children, would argue that we learn more out of school than in school; and an indicator under material well-being – possession of educational resources at home (Fig. 1.3b), puts the UK near the top (in seventh place). Possession of computers at home is among the highest in the world. The indicator covering full-time or part-time engagement with education, may encompass a very wide range in rates of participation – from 100% down to perhaps 10% and is maybe not a very useful indicator. The indicator about 15-year-olds' expectations of doing low skilled work by the time they are 30 finds the USA, for once, in top ranking – that is with lower percentages than any other country saying yes, they had such low expectations; perhaps this means the answers given to the question reflect less the realities of their futures, than the log-cabin-to-White-House optimism we are told US citizens enjoy.

8.3.4 Dimension 4: Family and Peer Relationships

This is the dimension which aroused most of the media hype about children in the UK. The indicators used here are: family structure (including averages of percentage of children living in single-parent families and percentage of children living in stepfamilies); family relationships (including averages of percentage of children who report eating the main meal of the day with parents several times a week and percentage of children who report that parents spend time 'just talking' to them); and peer relationships (percentage of 11, 13 and 15-year-olds who report finding their peers kind and helpful). We note that there is a developmental assumption in this dimension, since it is relationships with parents that are prioritised: eating meals with parents and parents talking with children; of course measuring relationships is difficult, as the authors note (UNICEF 2007; p. 22), but limiting relations in this way omits other people in the family with whom children have important relations – notably siblings and grandparents (see, for example, Dunn and Deater-Deckard 2001; Edwards et al. 2005; Mayall 2002; Morrow 1998; Smart et al. 2001; Punch 2008; Mason and Tipper 2008).

Overall the UK ranks at the bottom of the table on this dimension (Fig. 4.0), along with the USA. On the first indicator, the authors note that it may be thought unfair or insensitive to use it – children may be happy or unhappy in a range of family types. But they justify the choice on the grounds that statistics show children growing up in single-parent and stepfamilies have greater risk to well-being in the future (leaving school early, poor health, leaving home early, low skills, poor pay); and that these risks persist even when poverty levels are taken into account; however they also note that the research has been conducted mainly in the UK and USA. So it can be argued that the authors are prioritising the future of these children and that the indicator does not seem to capture well child–adult relations in the present. It is notable that the Nordic countries (Finland, Sweden, Denmark and Norway) have high rates of lone-parenting and stepfamilies (Fig. 4.1a, b), which drags down their overall rating on this dimension. Southern European countries (Italy, Portugal, Spain and Greece) scored in the top group for this indicator; and this pushed their overall score upon the dimension as a whole.

The first component of the second indicator – children and parents eating the main meal together – points to one of the starkest cultural assumptions; as is borne out by the relevant table (Fig. 4.2a). Finland, for once, comes bottom of the ranking; and this must be because by tradition, bolstered by social policy, the main meal of the day is eaten at midday – children get a free school meal, and adults a subsidised meal at their workplaces. The UK, USA and New Zealand occupy the next lowest rankings. However, the authors also note that even in the lowest ranking countries, almost two-thirds of children report eating a meal several times a week with their parents. There is much greater variation on the question do 15-year-olds think their parents spend time 'just talking to them' several times a week, with a range of 90–40% (Fig. 4.2b). The authors also note that this finding does not square with other UK studies, which have found high proportions of children reporting good relations with their parents; and they say findings on this dimension should be treated with caution for they are only a 'first step' towards monitoring children's relationships.

Finally on the third indicator – percentage of 11, 13 and 15-year-olds who find their peers 'kind and helpful' – the UK was ranked at the bottom of the table (Fig. 4.3). And this has been re-phrased by the UK news media as a clear factual finding that children do not have good friendships. But we have to note that the question was part of a series on life at school, and relates not to 'peers' nor to friends, but to 'class-mates'. Given the individualistic and competitive character of the current English education system, it is not surprising that children do not all regard all class-mates as friends. However, the media seized on this finding, for instance:

> "The report presents a sad picture of relationships with friends, which are so important to children. Not much more than 40% of the UK's 11, 13 and 15 year-olds find their peers 'kind and helpful', which is the worst score of all the developed countries" (Guardian 14.02.07).

Oddly, other sections of the HBSC survey referred to here did have questions specifically about friends; perhaps these could have been used in this dimension.

8.3.5 Dimension 5: Behaviours and Risks

The three indicators here are: health behaviours (including averages of percentage of children who eat breakfast, who eat fruit daily, are physically active and are overweight); risk behaviours (including averages of 15-year-olds who smoke, have been drunk more than twice, use cannabis, have sex by age 15, use condoms, and teenage fertility rate); experience of violence (including percentages of 11, 13 and 15-year-olds involved in fighting in last year, and reporting being bullied in last 2 months).

The UK is ranked by some considerable margin worst on this dimension (Fig. 5.0). On health behaviours the UK is fifth from the bottom, although on physical exercise near the top (Fig. 5.1c). On risk behaviours the UK is ranked at the bottom by a large margin (Fig. 5.2). And on experience of violence third from the bottom (Fig. 5.3). As the authors note, on this last indicator perception and definition play a large part, and more adequate measures, especially on exposure to violence in the home, are needed.

8.3.6 Dimension 6: Subjective Well-Being

In some ways this is the most puzzling dimension, since as far as the UK is concerned it seems to work against earlier dimensions. The indicators used are: self-appraisal of health (percentage of young people aged 11, 13 and 15 rating their health no more than 'fair' or 'poor'); school life (percentage of young people 'liking school a lot'); personal well-being (average of percentage of children rating themselves above the mid-point of a life satisfaction scale, and percentage of children reporting negatively about personal well-being).

The UK scores at the bottom of the ranking on children's self-appraisal of health (Fig. 6.1); and the Nordic countries, which do so well on the health dimension, are distributed through the table, with Norway fourth from the bottom and Finland fourth from the top, after Spain, Switzerland and Greece. We wonder if the word 'fair' was confusing; it can mean 'good' in English! Presumably national messages to children affect their self-appraisal. Across the board, girls were unhappier than boys about their health status. On liking school a lot, in all countries no more than 38% of children agreed, with most, including the UK, bunched at around 20% (Fig. 6.2). Yet when young people were asked to rate their current satisfaction with themselves and their lives on a scale of 1–10, in most countries, including the UK, 80% or more reached a score of 6 or more (Fig. 6.3a), with 15-year-old boys, across the board, more satisfied than girls (p. 37). Similarly, a question designed to explore feelings of awkwardness, loneliness and being an outsider led to most 15-year-olds – about 90% rejecting these perceptions of themselves. Indeed only one country (Japan) stood out – for 30% of the young people there agreed with the statement 'I feel lonely', almost three times higher than the next highest-scoring country.

These findings seem to suggest that overall UK children are as 'happy' as others in OECD countries, except on their own assessment of their health – and this may be a function of the question (or possibly related to high poverty rates?). It is this self-assessment score which presumably accounts for the UK having the worst overall score on this dimension (Fig. 6.0). Again, we suggest that averaging the indicators does a disservice to the data; and that discussion of the separate indicators would be more useful.

8.3.7 Discussion of These Dimensions

We agree with the authors that a start has been made towards using a range of indicators on children's well-being. And we agree that child poverty may underlie many of the findings, and may account for the UK's poor showing on some dimensions, although the precise relationships are not clear. Rather than average all the dimensions, it was useful to maintain a focus on children's well-being as a multi-dimensional issue, requiring a range of policy responses. Somehow a balance had to be struck between retaining each facet of the problem in separate tables and combining them through averaging. In some cases we think averaging did a disservice to the data, as we have indicated.

One feature of the data used is that much of it is negative – especially as regards risky behaviours. It would be good to explore ways of tapping into children's everyday lives and experiences in the neighbourhood, and their involvement in decisions which affect their lives (Ansell et al. 2007; p. 326).

One message we should like to emphasise is to commentators, who have a duty to read such reports carefully before referring to them. Our consideration is motivated more by our concerns about the relatively low status of children in the UK and the deplorable way that the report has been so misrepresented in the media. And we know that these misrepresentations affect adults' perceptions. In the Primary Review (an independent review of primary education in England being conducted at the University of Cambridge, funded by Esmée Fairbairn Foundation see www.primaryreview.org.uk), parents, teachers, local authority staff and children's organisations presented a gloomy vision of today's childhood; and this too long established vision was bolstered by the media representation of the UNICEF Report (Alexander and Hargreaves 2007).

8.3.8 Overall Comments

The UNICEF Report focused, in many of the indicators, on deficits – what children do not have, negatives, rather than positives, particularly in relation to 'risky health behaviours'. We already know from our own research (Mayall 2002; Morrow 2002) (not specifically about well-being) that children feel subordinated to adults, not able to make their own decisions (not often consulted), not having to take major responsibility for decisions (and they accept these points); they regard good personal relations as key to their happiness (but it doesn't have to be two parents, and friends are crucial as defence and company at school). For example, in middle childhood (say 8–12 years), playing out is their preferred activity, but often circumscribed by anxious parents. So what matters to children differs from what concerns adults (Mayall 2002; Morrow 1998, and many other examples could be cited here). Research specifically on well-being has explored what children's understandings of well-being are see Fattore et al. (2007); Heady and Oliveira (2008); Ben-Arieh and Frones (2007); OFSTED (2007); 11 Million (2008).

In Australia, Fattore et al. (2007) undertook qualitative research with 8–15-year olds and found that:

> "Well-being is defined through feelings, in particular happiness, but integrating sadness is also relevant. Well-being is about feeling secure, particularly in social relations... also as being a moral actor in relation to oneself (when making decisions in one's best interest) and when one behaves well towards others. ... well-being is the capacity to act freely and to make choices and exert influence in everyday situations. This was not necessarily being independent from others. Children articulated the social relations upon which autonomy was premised, including stable, secure relationships with adults. ... Children told us fear and insecurity affects their well-being and that feeling and being safe is an important part of well-being. This included fears about personal safety, particularly feeling alone and fear of being a victim of crime. Children also expressed more global fears about war and terrorism, particularly feeling helpless to do anything about world events. Children... identified factors that make them feel afraid and place restrictions on their ability to participate in social life, including design of the built environment and parental concerns about children's safety." (Fattore et al. 2007; p. 18)

They also found that children articulated clear ideas about the importance of having a positive sense of themselves, material resources, physical environment and home. Sixsmith et al. (2007) in Ireland undertook research with 8–12 year olds, using qualitative methods (photography) to explore children's, parents' and teachers' views of child well-being. They found marked differences between these three groups about what constitutes children's well-being, with different emphasis being placed on aspects of well-being by children. These qualitative studies show great potential for complementing, or expanding upon, larger scale survey research by providing deeper insights into children's everyday lives and what matters to them from their point of view (an important factor to consider when developing health promotion policies) (Morrow 2000).

In the specific case of the UK, adults construct children and childhood as a social problem. This is linked to social class divides. It is entirely possible that media, teachers and even parental concern about childhood affects children's self-image and accounts for any low scores on that. If the UNICEF Report is correct, and UK childhood is (objectively) bad and children think so too, could this be because children have internalised their risky and at risk status? What is the impact on children's views of societal denigration of children and childhood?

8.4 Rights: The UN Convention on the Rights of the Child

The UNICEF Report claims to be grounded in the UN Convention on the Rights of the Child (CRC) 1989 (UNHCHR 1989). The CRC is an international treaty to be used to assess laws and policies relating to children. It was ratified by the UK Government in 1991. Its articles are deliberately vague and open to interpretation by countries. It is not intended to be a means of interpreting or analysing children's lives, though the linkages between research evidence and implications for children's rights can usefully be made. The UNICEF Report selects various articles and mentions them in isolation, for example, Article 29 relating to children's development (p. 19); Article 24 (the right to the highest attainable standard of health care) and Article 27, relating to 'an adequate standard of living'. In doing so, the Report seems to be focusing on provision rights. However, rights – to provision, protection and participation – are indivisible. The CRC does use the term 'well-being', but it does not define it. For example, the preamble to the UN CRC states:

> "Convinced that the family, as the fundamental group of society and the natural environment for the growth and well-being of all its members and particularly children, should be afforded the necessary protection and assistance so that it can fully assume its responsibilities within the community." (UN CRC Preamble)

The term 'well-being' is also used Articles 3, 9, 17, 40 (UNHCHR 1989). Nor does the CRC define 'poverty' explicitly, and work is currently underway to elaborate connections between child poverty, social exclusion, capabilities and children's rights (see Redmond 2008).

The UNICEF Report cites Article 12 of the UN CRC – text of which is as follows:

> "States parties shall assure to the child who is capable of forming his or her own views the right to express those views freely in all matters affecting the child, the views of the child being given due weight in accordance with the age and maturity of the child... For this purpose, the child shall, in particular, be provided with the opportunity to be heard in any judicial and administrative procedures affecting the child."

The UNICEF Report claims that "the report takes note of the child's right to be heard and, to this end, incorporates a dimension that is based solely on children' own subjective sense of their own well-being [sic]" (p. 40). However, these claims need to be balanced with a consideration of whether and/or how children can freely 'express their views' in a necessarily circumscribed questionnaire. Ennew (2008); see also Beazley et al. (2006) has been arguing for some time that children have 'the right to be properly researched' Article 12: opinion, Article 13, modes of expression, Article 3a standards, and Article 36, other forms of exploitation – these are basic principles of dignity and respect.

Additionally, there is the vexed question of the relationship between mass news media and representations of children in respect of children's rights in the UK. Article 17 of the UN Convention on the Rights of the Child explicitly connects the media and children's well-being:

> "States Parties recognize the important function performed by the mass media and shall ensure that the child has access to information and material from a diversity of national and international sources, especially those aimed at the promotion of his or her social, spiritual and moral well-being and physical and mental health. To this end, States Parties shall:
>
> (a) Encourage the mass media to disseminate information and material of social and cultural benefit to the child…"

The Oslo Challenge (MAGIC 1999), which marked the tenth anniversary of UN CRC, was a collaboration between the Norwegian Government and UNICEF, and included the following challenge to media professionals at all levels and in all media:

> "to work ethically and professionally to sound media practices and to develop and promote media codes of ethics in order to avoid sensationalism, stereotyping (including by gender) or undervaluing of children and their rights." (MAGIC 1999)

The publicity surrounding the publication of the UNICEF Report can hardly be said to have 'avoided sensationalism'. The CRC represents a framework for action, but has yet to be taken seriously as an instrument of social change. A holistic approach to children's human rights, that holds governments accountable to every article of the convention, rather than a selected few, is vital as a way forward (CRAE 2008).

8.5 Conclusions

We have suggested that a close reading of the data upon which some very bold claims were made suggests that continued caution is needed in attempts to measure and interpret findings about children's well-being. Firstly, the UNICEF Report presents a de-contextualised childhood, childhood as a separate space, utterly disconnected from adulthood. It is technically a report that focuses mainly on people aged 11–15 and, thus, is not 'comprehensive'. Indeed, this idea of childhood/youth as disconnected from wider society has been constantly emphasised in news media reports – for example, Lord Layard, is quoted as saying "Young people live in a world with very little meaningful contact or engagement with adults" (Mayer 2008; p. 39). However, there have been few attempts to explore whether and if so why this may be the case, and why this matters; and this vision in itself leads to the 'tribal' child idea, and reinforces stereotypical views of children and young people. The intention of the UNICEF Report appears to have been overtly political – it certainly grabbed headlines. However, there are important questions to be raised about the ethics of research dissemination (Alderson and Morrow 2004).

From our own research studies, we learn that children have very clear ideas about how they are represented, and how adults view them (Mayall 2002; Morrow 2000). A recent survey of children's views on what makes them 'happy and healthy' by the Office of the Children's Commissioner for England found:

> "The dominant negative portrayal of young people as 'thugs' and 'yobs' and a group to be feared directly impacts on children and young people, and contributes to making them feel unhappy and unhealthy. They told us that they feel their lives as teenagers are pre-determined by stereotypes such as risk-taking binge drinkers with no positive alternatives." (11 Million 2008; p. 7)

A conference entitled Health in Schools: Participation and Partnerships held at the Institute of Education, University of London in 2008 included a presentation from a group of school children/young people. They showed the image from the front cover of *Time* Magazine described at the start of this chapter, and posed a question to the audience: 'Is it time for a different view?' They did not use the word 'well-being'. In response to a question about what health in schools meant to them, they said:

> "... we'd like you to know that we feel happy and healthy when our good points and our achievements are recognised, respected and celebrated. ... We'd also like you to know that how we feel about ourselves at school is affected by the way adults and society see young people and we ask you to help us change the negative views and stereotypes of young people that exist in today's society. Let us show you how much we can do, instead of focusing on how bad we are, or what we can't do." (Institute of Education 2008).

The emphasis placed by young people about the importance of adults recognising their achievements and capabilities clearly reflects the assets-based approach to health described in Chap. 1.

Secondly, children's well-being is rarely analysed in the context of adults' well-being, or population well-being in general. It is important to remember that the roots of research exploring levels of happiness and well-being relate to specific historical and economic circumstances, and above all to a particular question about *adults'* levels of life satisfaction in rich countries. The interconnections and interdependencies of childhood with adulthood have yet to be fully elaborated, and we suggest that we need to hold a mirror up to adult worlds and see how they reflect back to children, particularly in relation to how research findings are reported in the news media. After all, in relation to research findings and media representations based on such research findings, children have little power or status to answer back, or challenge, or redress the balance, (nor indeed do many adults, especially disadvantaged people). In relation to their health, they may exercise their agency through resistance to top-down health and education messages, and this resistance is then defined by adults as evidence of their wilful, risky, problematic behaviour (Spencer 2007). Children also positively take on important aspects of their own health care from early ages (Mayall 1996). Research that focuses on problems and deficits tends to overlook reasonably healthy behaviours by the majority.

Thirdly, discussions about children's well-being are rarely contextualised in understandings of structural, political and economic pressures and constraints on children's lives. As Ansell et al. (2007) note:

> "Without addressing broader political considerations regarding what shapes well-being (for example, access to resources and an ability to participate in decisions within society) it may not have any meaningful impact on children's 'well-being" (p. 330).

The extent to which well-being (emphasising responsibilities of individuals to be happy and to seek therapy if they are not) has replaced welfare (emphasising responsibilities of states to their citizens) could usefully be explored.

In conclusion, well-being may be a useful umbrella concept for exploring important aspects of children's lives, and the focus on the here-and-now and the present tense of childhood (Mayall 2002) is welcome because it moves on from the focus on outcomes and what children become. However, we suggest that greater clarity is required when claims are made about 'children's well-being'. We suggest that existing indicators (while needed to 'measure' change over time) could usefully be complemented by (and perhaps ultimately replaced by) research that attempts to incorporate children's experiences from their viewpoints, and that emphasises what they value. Children's positive 'assets' (as outlined in Chap. 1) could be the focus, rather than their deficiencies. This concurs with what children themselves seem to demand, and would be one way to respect their rights in research terms – not to be stigmatised and demonised.

Many definitions of well-being exist, but variations in understanding of this term have not been sufficiently recognised in the analysis, nor have the complications of measurement that arise from different interpretations. The extraordinarily negative image of children and youth in the UK has been compounded by news media reporting of the UNICEF Report, and young people seem to be aware of this (though thorough research on the relationships between news media representations of children and their 'well-being' has yet to be undertaken). Current attempts to measure children's well-being are problematic because they fail to incorporate an analysis of broader contextual structural and political factors; if we are to retain the use of the term 'well-being', then children's well-being could usefully be considered in the context of 'well-being' of people in general. Five suggestions emerge from this discussion. Firstly, care needs to be taken with conceptualisation of complex concepts such as 'well-being'. There remains a danger that a focus on well-being is ultimately an individualistic, subjective approach that risks depoliticising children's lives. Secondly, there needs to be great caution exercised when reporting research relating to children, not least because of the danger of over-simplification through international comparisons. We have suggested that cultural factors may play an important and hitherto under-researched part in what is conducive to children's 'well-being'. Thirdly, we suggest that involving children and young people in the conceptualisation of well-being could enhance the potential usefulness of the concept. Fourthly, qualitative and quantitative approaches could be usefully combined to improve understanding and measurement. Finally, we have suggested that greater understanding of UN Convention on the Rights of the Child is needed in working towards a genuinely rights-based approach to monitoring children's everyday lives that emphasises the low social status of children in western societies.

Acknowledgements The authors would like to thank Grace Spencer, Priscilla Alderson, Maggie Black, Tom Burke, Georgia Towers, Helen Roberts and Ian Warwick for very helpful comments on an earlier draft, as well as members of the seminar audience at the Social Science Research Unit, Institute of Education, University of London, where this chapter was first presented.

References

11 Million (2008). *Happy + Healthy. Summary of children and young people's views on what makes them happy and healthy*. London: 11 Million. www.11million.org.uk cited 4 June 2008.

Alderson, P., & Morrow, V. (2004). *Ethics, social research and consulting with children and young people*. Barkingside: Barnardo's.
Alexander, R., & Hargreaves, L. (2007). *Community soundings. Primary review briefings*. Cambridge: Faculty of Education, University of Cambridge.
Alexander, R. (ed) (2009) Children, their World, their Education: final report and recommendations of the *Cambridge Primary Review*. London: Routledge
Ansell, N., Barker, J., & Smith, F. (2007). UNICEF 'child poverty in perspective' report: a view from the UK. Viewpoint. *Children's Geographies*, 5, 3, 325–330.
Beazley H., Bessell, S., Ennew, J., & Waterson, R. (2006). *What children say. Results of comparative research on the physical and emotional punishment of children in Southeast Asia and the Pacific, 2005*. Bangkok, Thailand: Save the Children Sweden.
Ben-Arieh, A., & Frones, I. (2007). Indicators of children's well-being – concepts, indices and usage. Guest editorial. *Social Indicators Research*, 80, 1–4.
Bradshaw, J. (2007). Some problems in the international comparison of child income poverty, In H. Wintersberger, et al. (eds.) *Childhood, generational order and the welfare state: exploring children's social and economic welfare*. (pp. 93–107) Odense: University Press of Southern Denmark.
Cameron, E., Mathers, J., & Parry, J. (2006). 'Health and well-being': questioning the use of health concepts in public health policy and practice. *Critical Public Health*, 16, 4, 347–354.
Carlisle, S., & Hanlon, P. (2007). Well-being and consumer culture: a different kind of public health problem? *Health Promotion International*, 22, 3, 261–268.
Coppock, V. (2001). Medicalising children's behaviour. In B. Franklin (ed.) (Second edition) *The new handbook of children's rights. Comparative policy and practice*. (pp. 139–154) London: Routledge.
CRAE (Children's Rights Alliance for England) (2008). Alternative NGO report to the Committee on the Rights of the Child. London: CRAE.
Cunningham, H. (2007). Childhood and happiness in Britain. *GRAAT*, 36, 19–30.
DCSF (Department for Children, Families and Schools) (2007). Social and emotional aspects of learning. www.dcsf.gov.uk.
Dinham, A. (2007) Raising expectations or dashing hopes? Well-being and participation in disadvantages areas. *Community Development Journal*, 42, 2, 181–193.
Dunn, J., & Deater-Deckard, K. (2001). *Children's views of their changing families*. New York: Joseph Rowntree Foundation/YPS.
Ecclestone, K. (2004). Learning or therapy? The demoralisation of education. *British Journal of Educational Studies*, 52, 2, 112–127.
Ecclestone, K. (2008). *The rise of the fragile learner: why assessing emotional well-being undermines education*. Inaugural lecture. Oxford: Oxford Brookes University.
Edwards, R., Mauthner, M., Hadfield, L. (2005) Children's sibling relationships and gendered practices: talk, activity and dealing with change. *Gender and Education*, 17, 5, 499–513.
Ennew, J., & Milne, B. (1989). *The next generation. Lives of third world children*. London: Zed Press.
Ennew, J. (2008). Children's rights in the driving seat? Muddles in the interface between policy, programme and information about children since 1989. Plenary address, Child and Youth Research Network Conference: *Child and youth research in the 21st century: a critical appraisal*. European University, Cyprus, 28–29 May 2008.
Esping Andersen, G. (1996). *Welfare states in transition*. London: Sage.
Fattore, T., Mason, J., & Watson, E. (2007). Children's conceptualisation(s) of their well-being. *Social Indicators Research*, 80, 5–29.
Heady, L., & Oliveira, A. (2008). *On the bright side. Measuring the impact of charities on children's well-being*. London: New Philanthropy Capital.
Holland, P. (1992). *What is a child? Popular images of childhood*. London: Virago.
Hulme, D., & Toye, J. (2006). The case for cross-disciplinary social science research on poverty, inequality and well-being. *Journal of Development Studies*, 42, 7, 1085–1107.

Huppert, F., & Baylis, N. (2004). Well-being: towards an integration of psychology, neurobiology and social science. *Philosophical Transactions of the Royal Society of London*, 359, 1447–1451.

Institute of Education (2008). Conference participants. *Health in schools: participation and partnerships*, Day conference, Institute of Education, University of London, March 2008.

James, A., & Prout, A. (eds.) (1990/1997). *Constructing and reconstructing childhood*. London: Falmer Press.

Luthar, S. (2003). The culture of affluence: psychological costs of material wealth. *Child Development*, 74, 6, 1581–1593.

Luthar, S., & Latendresse, S. (2005). Children of the affluent. Challenges to well-being. *Current Directions in Psychological Science*, 14, 1, 49–52.

MAGIC (1999). Briefing on the Oslo challenge. Available online: http://www.unicef.org/magic/briefing/ cited 2 September 2008.

Mason, J., and Tipper, B. (2008). Being related: how children define and create kinship. *Childhood: A Journal of Global Child Research*, 15, 4, 441–460.

Mayall, B. (1996). *Children, health and the social order*. Buckingham: Open University Press.

Mayall, B. (2002). *Towards a sociology for childhood. Thinking from children's lives*. London: Open University Press.

Mayer, C. (2008). Unhappy, unloved and out of control. *Time Magazine*, 7 April 2008.

Morrow, V. (1998). *Understanding families: children's perspective*. London: National Children's Bureau/Joseph Rowntree Foundation.

Morrow, V. (1999). Conceptualising social capital in relation to the well-being of children and young people: a critical review. *The Sociological Review*, 47, 4, 744–765.

Morrow, V. (2000). 'Dirty looks' and 'trampy places' in young people's accounts of community and neighbourhood: implications for health inequalities. *Critical Public Health*, 10, 2, 141–152.

Morrow, V. (2002). Children's rights to public space: environment and curfews. In Bob Franklin (ed.) (Second edition) *The new handbook of children's rights. Comparative policy and practice*. London: Routledge.

OFSTED (2007). Tell us 2 survey results, press release. www.ofsted.gov.uk cited 4 June 2008.

Punch, S. (2008). You can do nasty things to your brothers and sisters without a reason: siblings' backstage behaviour. *Children & Society*, 22, 333–344.

Putnam, R.D. (2000). *Bowling alone: the collapse and revival of American community*. New York: Simon & Schuster.

Qvortrup, J. (1991). Childhood as a social phenomenon: introduction to a series of national reports. *Eurosocial Report 36*. Vienna: European Centre.

Qvortrup, J. (1994). Introduction. In J. Qvortrup, et al. (eds.) *Childhood matters: social theory, practice and politics*. (pp. 1–23) Aldershot: Avebury Press.

Redmond, G. (2008). Child poverty and child rights: edging towards a definition. *Journal of Children and Poverty*, 14, 1, 63–82.

Sixsmith, J., Nic Gabhainn, S., Fleming, C., O'Higgins, S. (2007). Children's, parents' and teachers' perceptions of child wellbeing. *Health Education*, 107, 6, 511–523.

Smart, C., Neale, B., & Wade, A. (2001). *The changing experience of childhood: families and divorce*. Cambridge: Polity.

Sointu, E. (2005). The rise of an ideal: tracing changing discourses of wellbeing. *The Sociological Review*, 53, 2, 255–274.

Spencer, G. (2007). *Young people's perspectives on health related risks*. MRes Dissertation, Faculty of Children and Health, Institute of Education, University of London.

Thomas-Bailey, C. (2008). Call for happiness lessons as teenage depression increases. *The Guardian*, 10 September 2008.

UNHCHR (1989) (Office of the UN High Commissioner for Human Rights). *UN Convention on the Rights of the Child 1989*.

UNICEF (2007). Child poverty in perspective: an overview of child well-being in rich countries. *Innocenti Report Card No.* 7, UNICEF Innocenti Research Centre, Florence, Italy.

WHO (1946). Preamble to the Constitution of the World Health Organization as adopted by the International Health Conference, New York, 19–22 June, 1946; signed on 22 July 1946 by the representatives of 61 States (Official Records of the World Health Organization, no. 2, p. 100) and entered into force on 7 April 1948.

Chapter 9
The Relationship Between Health Assets, Social Capital and Cohesive Communities

Ichiro Kawachi

Keywords Community • Role models • Neighbourhood • Earthquake (Kobe) • Machizukuri • Social cohesion • Social capital

9.1 Social Cohesion and Health: Theoretical Links to Health

The determinants of community health can be described from a deficits perspective or an assets perspective. *Deficit models* draw attention to the presence of pathology – for example, the level of "social disorganization" within communities. According to Shaw and McKay (1942) original description of this concept, certain structural characteristics of urban neighborhoods – such as persistent poverty and high population turnover – impede the development of secure social attachment to a community, and hinder the ability of residents to realize common goals.

Such conditions, Shaw and McKay argued, result in the lowered ability of communities to control problems such as delinquency and crime. Within public health, the presence of social disorganization in communities has been measured through indicators such as the presence of social and physical disorder (e.g. "broken windows"), and a growing number of studies have linked such deficits to outcomes such as sexually-transmitted infection (Cohen et al. 2000), asthma (Wright and Fisher 2003), and the unwillingness of community residents to engage in outdoor physical activity (King et al. 2000).

By contrast, an *assets based model* of health emphasizes the *positive capacity* of communities to promote the health of its members, and is thus linked to the concept of salutogenesis championed by Antonovsky (Lindström and Eriksson 2005). By enhancing the capacity of communities to preserve and maintain health, social cohesion sits squarely in the assets based model of health.

I. Kawachi (✉)
Department of Society, Human Development and Health, Harvard School of Public Health, 677 Huntington Ave, Boston, MA 02115, USA
e-mail: ikawachi@hsph.harvard.edu

A. Morgan et al. (eds.), *Health Assets in a Global Context: Theory, Methods, Action*,
DOI 10.1007/978-1-4419-5921-8_9,

It is important at the outset to stress two crucial caveats: First, community assets are not simply the absence of community deficits, and vice versa. The tendency to equate social capital with the absence of community "bads" (such as crime) has prompted critics to (reasonably) argue that the measurement of social capital often constitutes a tautology – if the community does not exhibit deficits, then it must be because it is endowed with high stocks of social capital. In reality, assets based models and deficits based models of health production are not mutually exclusive. Most communities are characterized by the presence of both assets *and* deficits. For example, significant variations have been found in the levels of social cohesion across communities that looked similar with respect to their level of deficits (e.g. level of poverty and deprivation). The "orthogonality" of community assets and deficits provides a cogent rationale for a deeper exploration of the concept of salutogenesis.

A second important caveat to note is that community assets are not unqualified "goods". As we shall describe in greater detail in this chapter, it is now widely acknowledged that there are important "downsides" of social cohesion that may harm, rather than protect, the health of certain community members. Any policy or intervention to boost social cohesion must therefore anticipate these side effects and attempt to minimize them.

Examples of "assets" that residents of cohesive communities can access and mobilize to protect their health consist of norms, trust, and the exercise of sanctions. In turn, examples of social *processes* through which these assets become translated into improved health status include collective socialization, informal social control, and collective efficacy. These are discussed in turn.

9.1.1 Collective Socialization

In the urban sociology literature, collective socialization refers to the role of community adults – not just a child's own parents – in enhancing child developmental outcomes. For example, the presence of adult role models helps to transmit important environmental cues to youth concerning expected norms of behaviour within the community. According to the ethnographer Elijah Anderson (1990), who conducted extensive fieldwork between 1975 and 1989 in an urban, low-income, and predominantly black community in the US, male role models – dubbed "old heads" – were *"traditionally [men] of stable means who believed in hard work, family life, and the church. He was an aggressive agent of the wider society whose acknowledged role was to teach, support, encourage, and in effect socialize young men to meet their responsibilities regarding work, family, the law, and common decency"* (Anderson 1990, p. 3). Anderson's qualitative insights have been corroborated by quantitative analyses suggesting the importance of adult role models within the community in protecting against outcomes such as teen pregnancy rates and high school dropouts (Crane 1989).

The loss of adult role models is an often overlooked consequence of structural deficits afflicting deprived communities, such as high unemployment rates. Unemployment is undoubtedly damaging to the families that are affected, but it also produces collateral effects on the rest of the community. When work disappears, the adverse impacts of unemployment become amplified throughout the community via the loss of adult role models. As youth begin to perceive that adults around them are not getting up in the mornings to report to work, or only doing so to work in low-paying insecure jobs, their expectations for the future become diminished, and dropping out of school may begin to seem like a rational response to their circumstances.

9.1.2 Informal Social Control

A related concept to collective socialization is informal social control, which refers to the capacity of a community to regulate the behaviour of its members according to collectively desired (as opposed to forced) goals. In contrast to legal sanctions (such as police crackdowns), informal social control represents *"the effectiveness of informal mechanisms by which residents themselves achieve public order"* (Sampson et al. 1997). In urban sociology, informal social control has been studied as a mechanism through which communities prevent the onset and occurrence of juvenile delinquency – for example, when adults step in to intervene in situations such as suspected truancy, vandalism, public fights, and so forth. However, informal social control is of equal potential relevance to public health outcomes. In Japanese society, for example, informal control used to be the traditional mechanism which communities relied upon to regulate cigarette smoking among school-aged children, despite very high prevalence rates among adults (at least among adult males) and the nearly ubiquitous presence of cigarette vending machines. In more recent years, however, as the authority of community adults and teachers has become eroded, smoking among Japanese youth has soared, prompting calls to ban vending machines or to restrict the hours during which cigarettes can be purchased.

9.1.3 Collective Efficacy

Collective efficacy, which can be thought of as the community-level counterpart to individual self-efficacy, refers to the ability of community members to undertake collective action for mutual benefit. In turn, the willingness of local residents to intervene for the common good depends critically on the presence of mutual trust and solidarity among neighbors (Sampson et al. 1997). The ability of residents to organize and engage in collective action turns out to be relevant for health promotion in several ways. For example, coordinated action enables residents of communities to lobby for the passage of local ordinances (e.g. restrictions on smoking in public places), or to rally against the threatened closure of local services (e.g. health clinics), or to manage physical hazards (e.g. the location of toxic waste sites) (Kawachi and Berkman 2000; Browning and Cagney 2002). In each instance, coordinated action is facilitated by the presence of local organizations, measured by proxy indicators such as the density of neighborhood based organizations and self-reports of social participation. In other words, the presence of locally based organizations represents the *capacity* of a community to respond to external threats and trauma.

Community variations in collective efficacy are strikingly illustrated by differential rates of recovery following natural disasters, such as earthquakes, hurricanes, floods, and tsunamis. Nakagawa and Shaw (2004) found that variations in recovery following major earthquakes in Kobe, Japan (1995) and Gujarat, India (2001) were in part explained by the presence of locally based organizations that pre-dated the disasters.

In Kobe, official rescue teams were quickly overwhelmed in the immediate aftermath of the January 17, 1995 earthquake. Once this realization dawned, some neighborhoods within Kobe began to organize their own rescue and relief efforts. Nakagawa and Shaw argue that the presence of community based assets – in the form of town development associations (called *machizukuri*) – accounted for the neighborhood differences in the immediate response phase as well as subsequent recovery. These associations originated in the 1960s when residents launched protest movements to curb polluting factories nearby. Subsequently, the same organizations changed their mission to focus on issues such as community development, health care of the aged, and the provision of voluntary services (Nakagawa and Shaw 2004).

In the aftermath of the earthquake, the presence of *machizukuri* associations sped up rescue operations, evacuation to nearby schools, the establishment of community kitchens, and organization of night watchmen to guard abandoned property. During the post-relief phase, the same associations facilitated building inspection surveys, publication of weekly community newsletters, as well as the management of shelters and retrofitting of damaged houses.

9.2 The Measurement of Social Cohesion

As alluded to above, the social capital literature describes two distinct definitions and approaches to measurement, based respectively, on the "network" concept of social capital, and the "social cohesion" concept. In the network approach, social capital has often been conceptualized as an individual-level asset, and the corresponding measurement techniques involve the methods of sociometric analysis. Examples of measurement techniques for network based social capital include Lin's Position Generator (Lin 2001), which asks individuals (egos) to nominate others in their network (alters) who provide them with access to valued resources, e.g. prestige, political connections. Alternatively, van der Gaag (2005) has developed the Resource Generator, which is a multidimensional index that taps an individual's access to resources across several domains of life (e.g. at home and in the work place), and spans across a range of goods from the material (e.g. borrowing money) to the symbolic (e.g. prestige, influence).

A network based definition of social capital is not exclusively based upon the assessment of ego-centred network resources, however. Whole network analysis involves saturation surveys of all existing social connections within a defined collective (e.g. a school or a workplace), and the resulting data can then be manipulated to derive different structural properties of the network (Hawe et al. 2004).

As pointed out by Moore et al. (2004), however, the public health literature – including much of the empirical evidence published to date – has focused heavily on the social cohesion definition of social capital. The social cohesion approach emphasizes social capital as an asset of communities (or other collectives), not of individuals. Measurement approaches therefore typically *aggregate* individual cognitive perceptions (such as perceptions of trust and reciprocity) up to the community level, or they aggregate other proxy indicators (such as density of community organizations, frequency of social participation) up to the community level (Harpham et al. 2002). Validated scales to assess concepts such as informal social control have also been developed – for example, from the Community Survey of the Project on Human Development in Chicago Neighborhoods (Sampson et al. 1997). However, the more commonly practiced approach to measure social cohesion has been to develop multi-item scales to tap domains such as interpersonal trust, reciprocal exchanges of support, social participation, and informal patterns of socializing.

One criticism of the social cohesion literature has been that, in the absence of primary data, investigators have resorted to a diverse – and many say increasingly tenuous – set of proxy indicators ranging from voting behaviour, volunteering, local crime rates, and perceptions of corruption (Paldam 2000). Some of these indicators may be precursors or consequences of social cohesion, but they should not be conflated with the community based assets that we are interested in.

An important refinement that has emerged in the measurement of social capital is the bonding/bridging distinction. Bonding social capital refers to trusting and cooperative relations between members of a group who are similar in terms of social identity (e.g., race/ethnicity), whereas bridging social capital refers to connections between individuals who are dissimilar with respect to their social identity (e.g. race, ethnicity, social class) (Szreter and Woolcock 2004). The relevance of making this distinction lies in the fact that each type may have different effects on health outcomes.

Although few studies so far have examined the difference between bonding and bridging social capital, Mitchell and La Gory (2002) carried out a small cross-sectional study among residents of a disadvantaged, predominantly minority community in Birmingham, Alabama, in which they found that that while bridging social capital (measured by the strength of trust and associational ties with others of a different race and educational background as the respondent) was associated with lower levels of mental distress, bonding social capital was related to health in the opposite direction, i.e. greater distress. Additional studies from Baltimore, Maryland (Caughy et al. 2003), and Adelaide, Australia (Ziersch et al. 2005), suggest that stronger bonding ties within disadvantaged communities may turn out to be a detriment to the health of residents.

In the Baltimore study, lower community attachment among mothers was associated with fewer behavioural and mental health problems among children living in low-income areas (Caughy et al. 2003). In a cross-sectional survey of a working class suburb in Adelaide, Ziersch et al. (2005) reported that involvement in community groups was associated with worse physical health as measured by the SF-12. Qualitative interviews with residents in the same study found that respondents were more apt to link their participation in community groups with negative mental and physical health outcomes.

9.3 Social Cohesion and Health: Empirical Findings

Empirical studies of social capital and health have been conducted at four distinct levels of aggregation: (1) at the macro-social level, linking social cohesion at the national or state level to population health; (2) at the meso level such as cities, neighborhoods, schools, and workplaces; (3) at the micro level, involving the mapping of social networks; and (4) at the individual level, in which perceptions of trust or individual reports of social participation have been linked to individual health status (Macinko and Starfield 2001).

From an assets perspective, the concept of social capital is potentially relevant to health at all four levels of analysis. At the broadest level of social organization, Wilkinson (1996, 2005) has argued that egalitarian societies – characterized by a more equal distribution of incomes – tend to be more cohesive, and that in turn social cohesion promotes better health by mitigating the adverse psychosocial consequences of social stratification such as feelings of shame, inferiority, social exclusion, envy, and frustration. Social cohesion at the macrosocial level has also been hypothesized to influence population health through political mechanisms. For instance, at the country level, markers of social cohesion have been linked to lower levels of corruption (Easterly et al. 2005) as well as to the smoother functioning of democracy (Putnam 1993). Kawachi and Kennedy (2002) argue that social cohesion at the state level within the US federal system is associated with more generous provision of welfare services, e.g. income support for the poor, health care access for the indigent, and a fairer distribution of social resources. These macro-level processes are possibly distinct from the community-level mechanisms (discussed above) which are believed to link community cohesion to health outcomes, i.e. collective socialization, informal control, and collective efficacy.

From a methodological perspective, empirical studies of community cohesion and health can be categorized into three types: (1) ecological studies, which attempt to link aggregated community characteristics (e.g. average rates of social participation) with aggregated health outcomes (e.g. the community rate of mortality); (2) multilevel studies, which examine the variation in individual health outcomes nested within different communities; and (3) individual-level studies, which link individual perceptions of neighborhood characteristics (e.g. perceptions of the trustworthiness of neighbors) to individual health outcomes.

Within the community assets framework, the most illuminating study design is arguably the multilevel study design. The reason is because individual *perceptions* of community assets (such as the perception of the trustworthiness of neighbors) is likely to be confounded by other unobserved individual attributes such as temperament and personality. Ecological studies are similarly limited in their ability to distinguish between the influence that the social context exerts on people's health versus the compositional influence of individual characteristics on the aggregated health status of a given locality. If the investigator's interest is focused on demonstrating the influence of community contexts on individual health status, then the multilevel analytical framework is the most appropriate study design (Subramanian et al. 2003).

By incorporating attributes at both the individual *and* the community level, multilevel study designs permit the investigator to examine the independent contextual influence of community assets on health, in addition to exploring cross-level interactions between community and individual-level characteristics.

This unique advantage is illustrated by a multilevel study of community trust (as a measure of social cohesion) and individual self-rated health carried out by Subramanian et al. (2002). The authors analyzed the Social Capital Community Benchmark Survey involving 21,456 individuals nested within 40 US communities. The analysis found no main effect of community levels of social trust on the self-rated health of individuals, once individual perceptions of trust were taken into account. However, a significant cross-level interaction was found between community levels of trust and individual trust perceptions. Among individuals who reported higher levels of trust, self-rated health was higher among those who resided in communities where others also shared the same perceptions. By contrast, a trend was found in the opposite direction for individuals expressing mistrust of others: the more trusting the community in which they lived, the lower was their rating of health.

The two opposing trends cancelled each other out in the main effects model. However, the complexity and heterogeneity of the effects of community trust on health – suggesting a benefit for some groups, but also harm for other groups – is possibly relevant for forecasting the effects of boosting community cohesion on health.

A summary of the empirical evidence linking community cohesion to health outcomes has been provided in extensive recent reviews by Kawachi et al. (2004) and Islam et al. (2006a) for physical health outcomes and health behaviours, as well as by Almedom (2005) and De Silva (2006) for mental health outcomes. Islam et al. (2006a) identified 42 studies of social capital and health published between 1995 and 2005, including 30 single level studies (either individual-level or ecological studies) as well as 12 multi-level studies from different countries.

Regardless of study design, the review found a fairly consistent association between social capital and a range of health outcomes. However, in the multilevel studies, the between-area variance (random effect) in health tended to be substantially lower in egalitarian countries compared to unequal countries. That is, the intra-class correlations (ICCs) for health outcomes were considerably lower in studies carried out in more egalitarian countries (e.g. Sweden) compared to countries with greater levels of inequalities, such as the United States. For example, ICCs from studies of neighborhood influences on health typically range from 5–10% in US studies, but they tend to range between 1–2% for studies in Sweden. One implication is that in egalitarian societies with strong safety nets and adequate provision of public goods, neighborhood contexts (including the level of social cohesion) may be less salient for the health of residents in contrast to segregated and unequal societies such as the United States. Consistent with this interpretation, a recent panel-data multilevel study of 275 Swedish municipalities found a modest fixed effect association between voting participation (as a marker of social cohesion) and health-related quality of life (Islam et al. 2006b). However, 98% of variation in health was attributed to the individual level, and only 2% to the municipality level.

For social capital and mental health outcomes, De Silva et al. (2005) identified 21 studies that met the criteria for inclusion in their review. Taken together, these studies indicated a fairly consistent inverse relationship between individual perceptions of social cohesion and mental illness; however, there were far fewer studies of social cohesion assessed as a community attribute, and these studies were more mixed with respect to their findings. Two of the papers included in the review measured social cohesion at both the individual and the community level.

Cutrona et al. (2000) found no significant association between markers of social capital (measured at either the community or individual level), once individual characteristics were controlled for. By contrast, a Canadian study (Veenstra 2005) found that while indicators of community cohesion were not associated with common mental disorders, individual perceptions of social capital was associated with reduced depression scores.

To summarize the state of the empirical evidence, the preponderance of studies indicates a link between community cohesion and physical health outcomes (including self-rated health) and health-related behaviours, whereas the evidence for mental health so far has remained more sparse and mixed. The overwhelming majority of studies have been carried out in developed countries (North America in particular), and more evidence is needed from other societal contexts – for example, in Asia and in less developed countries. Community cohesion (as a health asset) appears to be more salient in societies characterized by the deficient provision of material infrastructure (i.e. services and amenities provided to assist the poor).

A common weakness across all existing studies, uniformly noted by the systematic reviews, has been the heterogeneity in the measurement approaches used to assess social capital and social cohesion. Studies have used remote proxies (obtained from secondary data sources) to assess social cohesion, or included measures that do not reflect common definitions of social capital. Other studies have concatenated different aspects of social capital into a single index or score. Very few studies have sought to examine the distinction between bonding and bridging forms of social capital (De Silva 2006).

9.4 Is Investing in Social Cohesion a Practical Strategy for Health Promotion?

Social capital remains a contested concept in public health not just on account of the comparative infancy or mixed nature of the empirical knowledge base. A number of criticisms have been directed at the concept on more theoretical grounds. For example, critics have expressed scepticism about the utility of "investing" in social cohesion as a public health improvement strategy (Pearce and Davey Smith 2003).

"Social capitalists" have been accused of downplaying the health liabilities associated with living in more cohesive communities. Social cohesion is clearly not a panacea for population health, and can sometimes facilitate negative or perverse consequences (Kawachi and Berkman 2001). Portes (1998) acknowledges four instances of the negative consequences of socially cohesive communities. They include: exclusion of outsiders from resources controlled by network members; excess claims made on "conscientious citizens" by free-riding fellow members; demands for conformity (including intolerance of diversity) and restrictions on individual freedoms; and the downward levelling of norms, which may block members of historically oppressed groups from participation in mainstream society.

For instance, Japan is frequently cited as an example of a socially cohesive (and high longevity) society (Wilkinson 1996). Yet the flip side of cohesion is conformity, which is expressed in the popular proverb that "The nail that sticks out gets hammered down." The price of conformity is particularly steep for marginalized groups such as gay men. Japanese society has long maintained a duality in social relationships characterized by the concepts of *honne* (one's true nature) and *tatemae* (a person's outward appearance which he/she presents to society). Homosexuality is tacitly acknowledged in Japanese society, so long as proper *tatemae* is preserved (e.g. gay men who marry and have families). Strengthening social cohesion in such circumstances may therefore result in the further marginalization of particular groups, unless the form of capital that is being built is of the bridging kind.

Meanwhile, mapping the strength of social cohesion across diverse communities runs the risk of labelling some communities as being deficient in certain assets (often defined according to some bourgeois notion of "what a community ought to be like"), which is tantamount to "blaming the community" for its problems (Muntaner et al. 2001). This critique is particularly cogent when asset mapping is carried out in the absence of an analysis of broader structural problems and power differentials that confront socially-excluded communities, such as the lack of employment opportunities, policies that perpetuate residential segregation, and the deliberate starving of services and amenities by municipal authorities. In other words, investing in social capital should be thought of as a complement to broader structural interventions (e.g. improving access to job markets), not as a replacement for them (Szreter and Woolcock 2004). Building social cohesion cannot be sold as a "cheap" way to solve the problems of poverty and health inequalities.

The third and final criticism levelled at the concept of social capital pertains to the lack of clarity about how to go about building social cohesion. Social capitalists have been frequently (and perhaps unfairly) portrayed as advocating a return to more "traditional" forms of social organization, where neighbors help one another, people are nice to each other, and busy housewives volunteer in schools and local block groups to provide the social "glue" that binds communities together. In reality, it is clear that in a globalised economy where dual earner couples are spending increasing hours of their day at work or commuting to and from work, there is no practical way to turn the clock back to such a nostalgic vision of the past (nor would it be necessarily desirable). Although demonstrations of interventions to build community cohesion are still scarce, a few principles seem worth mentioning.

Firstly, there is unlikely to be a single magic bullet to build community cohesion. What we know about the topic suggests that success in shoring up social cohesion is likely to be accomplished by making a series of "smart bets" (Sander and Lowney 2005). Several examples of such smart bets – involving the principles of community organizing (e.g. establishing neighborhood based associations to solve collective problems) – have been described in the Social Capital Building Toolkit, developed by the Saguaro Seminar of the Harvard University Kennedy School of Government (Sander and Lowney 2005). As the Social Capital Building Toolkit cautions, it is important at the outset to emphasize that besides community organizing, one should not overlook the importance of broader *structural* interventions aimed at boosting the capacity of individuals and communities to organize. Broader structural interventions include job creation as well as private sector reform to improve the work/family balance of employees.

A second principle of social capital building is to pay attention not just to the *level* of social capital but also to the *type* of social capital. For example, theory would suggest that it is not sufficient (or may be even harmful) to build bonding social capital among unemployed youth. It would be more helpful instead to build bridging capital between unemployed youth and employed adults to provide access to role models and mentoring (Sander and Lowney 2005).

Thirdly, any strategy to build social capital needs to pay close attention to the *distribution* of costs and benefits, including the possibilities of unintended consequences (or the "downsides" of social capital mentioned above). A gendered analysis of social capital would suggest that the mobilization and provision of support to others in the community tends to fall disproportionately on the shoulders of women. A health promotion strategy that supports one group in the community (e.g. men) at the expense of burdening another group (women) would only lead to a zero-sum outcome.

Lastly, in order to be sustainable, a social capital investment strategy requires more than the donated voluntary efforts of "do-gooders" in a community. Investing in social capital is likely to require real money, and hence a government (as well as private sector) that is committed to such a strategy. Historically, the sustenance of social cohesion has depended on state support and stewardship, not just on voluntarism and the energy of communities (Szreter and Woolcock 2004). Perhaps the most compelling economic rationale for governments to be involved in building social capital is that community cohesion – as a collective asset – produces externalities, i.e. collateral benefits to the rest of society that reach beyond the immediate members of networks. Often these externalities are invisible, and the benefits may not become apparent except during a community crisis (such as an earthquake or other natural disaster). When left in the hands of private initiatives, economic theory suggests that communities tend to under-invest in the production of such collective assets.

By applying these principles, public health practitioners may begin to harness the potential of social cohesion as a community asset. We conclude this section by describing a recent demonstration project to build social capital carried out within the city of Baltimore, Maryland (Glass et al. 2004). Called the Experience Corps, the program places older volunteers (mean age 69 years, 93% African-American, 90% women, 84% with annual incomes below the poverty threshold) in public elementary schools for 15 or more hours per week in roles designed to improve the academic outcomes of children. The randomized demonstration program placed 113 older volunteers within six urban elementary schools. After 4–8 months of follow-up, participation in the program led to health benefits for the senior volunteers, including higher physical activity, increases in cognitive activity, and more people that they could turn to for help (Fried et al. 2004). Among the 1,194 schoolchildren enrolled in grades K-3, the program also resulted in significantly higher reading scores on standardized tests, as well as fewer referrals for disruptive classroom behaviour (Rebok et al. 2004).

Beyond these win-win outcomes for the individuals involved, there are also likely to be broader benefits to society. They include: the building of inter-generational bridging social capital (harnessing the productive capacity of older individuals and enhancing inter-generational communication); maintaining the functional independence of community-dwelling seniors, and thereby enhancing their capacity for civic engagement in other spheres; and – from a life course perspective – fostering optimal child development for a new generation of kids through mentoring and the transmission of wisdom.

9.5 Conclusions

Social cohesion, if approached through a careful delineation of theory and the weighing of costs and benefits, represents an example of a community asset. Improvements in research practices and further demonstrations of interventions offer the prospect of harnessing this community asset for health promotion.

References

Almedom, A. (2005). Social capital and mental health: an interdisciplinary review of primary evidence. *Soc Sci Med,* 61(5):943–964.

Anderson, E. (1990). Streetwise. Race, class and change in an urban community. Chicago: The University of Chicago Press

Browning, C. R., & Cagney, K. A. (2002). Collective efficacy and health: neighbourhood social capital and self-rated physical functioning in an Urban Setting. *J Health Soc, Behav* 43:383–399.

Caughy, M. O., O'Campo, P. J., & Muntaner, C. (2003). When being alone might be better: neighbourhood poverty, social capital, and child mental health. *Soc Sci Med*, 57:227–237.

Cohen, D., Spear, S., Scribner, R., Kissinger, P., Mason, K., & Wildgen, J. (2000). Broken windows and the risk of gonorrhoea. *Am J Public Health*, 90(2):230–236.

Crane, J. (1989). The epidemic theory of ghettos and neighborhood effects on dropping out and teenage childbearing. *Am J Sociol*, 95:1226–59.

Cutrona, C. E., Russell, D.W., Hessling, R. M., Brown, P. A., & Murry, V. (2000). Direct and moderating effects of community context on the psychological well-being of African American women. *J Personal Soc Psychol*, 79(6):1088–1101.

De Silva, M. J., McKenzie, K., Huttly, S. R., & Harpham, T. (2005). Social capital and mental illness: a systematic review. *J Epidemiol Comm Health*, 59(8):619–627.

De Silva, M. J. (2006). A systematic review of the methods used in studies of social capital and mental health. In: McKenzie, K., & Harpham, T., eds. *Social capital and mental health.* London: Kingsley.

Easterly, W., Ritzen, J., & Woolcock, M. (2005). *Social cohesion, institutions, and growth. World Bank working paper.* Washington DC: The World Bank. www.worldbank.org/wbi/governance/pdf/wps2448.pdf cited May 2009.

Fried, L. P., Carlson, M. C., Freedman, M., Frick, K. D., Glass, T. A., Hill, J., et al. (2004). A social model for health promotion for an aging population: initial evidence on the Experience Corps model. *J Urban Health*, 81(1):64–78.

Glass, T. A., Friedman, M., Carlson, M. C., Hill, J., Frick, K. D., Ialongo, N., et al. (2004). Experience corps: design of an intergenerational program to boost social capital and promote the health of an aging society. *J Urban Health*, 81(1):94–105.

Harpham, T., Grant, E., & Thomas, E. (2002). Measuring social capital within health surveys: key issues. *Health Policy and Plan*, 17(1):106–111.

Hawe, P., Webster, C., Shiell, A. (2004). A glossary of terms for navigating the field of social network analysis. *J Epidemiol Comm Health*, 58:971–975.

Islam, M. K., Merlo, J., Kawachi, I., Lindstrom, M., Gerdtham, U.-G. (2006a). Social capital and health: does egalitarianism matter? A literature review. *Int J Equity in Health*, 5(1):3.

Islam, M. K., Merlo, J., Kawachi, I., Lindstrom, M., Burstrom, K., Gerdtham, U.-G. (2006b). Does it really matter where you live? A panel data multilevel analysis of Swedish municipality level social capital on individual health-related quality of life. *Health Econ, Policy and Law*, 1(3):209–235.

Kawachi, I., & Berkman, L. F. (2000). Social cohesion, social capital, and health. In: Berkman, L. F., & Kawachi, I., eds. *Social epidemiology*. New York: Oxford University Press, pp. 174–190.

Kawachi, I., & Berkman, L. F. (2001). Social ties and mental health. *J Urban Health*, 78(3):458–467.

Kawachi, I., & Kennedy, B. P. (2002). *The health of nations: why inequality is harmful to your health.* New York: The New Press.

Kawachi, I., Kim, D. J., Coutts, A., & Subramanian, S. V. (2004). Reconciling the three accounts of social capital (commentary). *Int J Epidemiol*, 33(4):682–690.

King, A. C., Castro, C., Wilcox, S., Eyler, A. A., Sallis, J. F., & Brownson, R. C. (2000). Personal and environmental factors associated with physical inactivity among different racial-ethnic groups of U.S. middle-aged and older-aged women. *Health Psych*, 19(4):354–364

Lin, N. (2001). *Social capital. Theory and research.* New York, NY: Aldine de Gruyter.

Lindström, B., & Eriksson, M. (2005). Salutogenesis. *J Epidemiol Comm Health*, 59(6):440–442.

Macinko, J., & Starfield, B. (2001). The utility of social capital in research on health determinants. *Milbank Q* 79(3):387–427.

Mitchell, C., & La Gory, M. (2002). Social capital and mental distress in an impoverished community. *City Community*, 1(2):199–222.

Moore, S., Shiell, A., Hawe, P., Haines, V. A. (2004). The privileging of communitarian ideas: citation practices and the translation of social capital into public health research. *Am J Public Health*, 95:1330–1337.

Muntaner, C., Lynch, J., Davey Smith, G. D. (2001). Social capital, disorganized communities, and the third way: understanding the retreat from structural inequalities in epidemiology and public health. *Int J Health Serv*, 31(2):213–237.

Nakagawa, Y., & Shaw, R. (2004). Social capital: a missing link to disaster recovery. *Int J Mass Emerg Disasters* 22(1):5–34.

Paldam, M. (2000). Social capital: one or many? Definition and measurement. *J Econ Surveys* 14(5):629–653.

Pearce, N., & Davey Smith, G. (2003). Is social capital the key to inequalities in health? *Am J Public Health* 93(1):122–129.

Putnam, R. D. (1993). *Making democracy work. Civic traditions in modern Italy.* Princeton, NJ: The Princeton University Press.

Portes, A. (1998). Social capital: its origins and applications in modern sociology. *Annu Rev Sociol*, 24:1–24.

Rebok, G. W., Carlson, M. C., Glass, T. A., McGill, S., Hill, J., Wasik, B. A., et al. (2004). Short-term impact of Experience Corps participation on children and schools: results from a pilot randomized trial. *J Urban Health,* 81(1):79–93.

Sampson, R. J., Raudenbush, S. W., & Earls, F. (1997). Neighbourhoods and violent crime: a multilevel study of collective efficacy. *Science,* 277:918–924.

Sander, T. H., & Lowney, K. (2005). *Social capital building toolkit, version 1.1.* Cambridge, MA: Harvard University John F. Kennedy School of Government. www.ksg.harvard.edu/saguaro/pdfs/skbuildingtoolkitversion1.1.pdf cited May 2009.

Shaw, C., & McKay, H. (1942). *Juvenile delinquency in urban areas.* Chicago: University of Chicago Press.

Subramanian, S. V., Kim, D. J., & Kawachi, I. (2002). Social trust and self-rated health in US communities: a multilevel analysis. *J Urban Health,* 79(4) Suppl 1: S21–S34.

Subramanian, S. V., Jones, K., & Duncan, C. (2003). Multilevel methods for public health research. In: Kawachi, I., & Berkman, L. F., eds. *Neighbourhoods and health.* New York: Oxford University Press, pp. 65–111.

Szreter, S., & Woolcock, M. (2004). Health by association? Social capital, social theory, and the political economy of public health. *Int J Epidemiol,* 33:1–18.

van der Gaag, M. (2005). *Measurement of individual social capital.* Amsterdam: F&N Boekservices.

Veenstra, G. (2005). Location, location, location: contextual and compositional health effects of social capital in British Columbia, Canada. *Soc Sci Med,* 60(9):2059–2071.

Wilkinson, R. G. (1996). *Unhealthy societies. The afflictions of inequality.* London: Routledge.

Wilkinson, R. G. (2005). *The impact of inequality. How to make sick societies healthier.* New York: The New Press.

Wright, R. J., & Fisher, E. B. (2003). Putting asthma into context: community influences on risk, behaviour, and intervention. In: Kawachi, I., Berkman, L. F., eds. *Neighbourhoods and health.* New York: Oxford University Press, pp. 233–262.

Ziersch, A. M., Baum, F. E., MacDougall, C., & Putland, C. (2005). Neighbourhood life and social capital: the implications for health. *Soc Sci Med,* 60(1):71–86.

Part III
Health Assets in Action

Chapter 10
Community Empowerment and Health Improvement: The English Experience

Jennie Popay

Keywords Community development • Community empowerment • Community participation • Community engagement • Choosing health

10.1 Introduction

Involving communities of place and/or interest in all aspects of the development, implementation and evaluation of health development and social regeneration programmes has become common place and is now an explicit requirement of many government strategies promoting social models for action to tackle health inequalities (DH 1999; CSDH 2008). The primary purpose of engaging communities from a policy perspective is to promote more responsive public services, to help improve quality and to support civic renewal (Hamer 2005). However, despite the commitment to community level action in policy terms – at least at the rhetorical level–the practice of how to do it effectively has proved highly complex. Morgan and Ziglio (2007) also highlight that asset based approaches can only be effective if we avoid "community involvement activities becoming tokenistic and separated from the main decision making processes of professionals". One way that this can be achieved is to have a clear definition of community involvement and its associated vocabulary and to make explicit how its different forms can help achieve different objectives. This chapter starts that process by unravelling the multitude of terms and definitions used to encapsulate the involvement of communities in the health development process. It also offers a framework for clarifying how we might build an evidence base that identifies the most effective approaches to community involvement for different purposes and in different contexts.

J. Popay (✉)
Division of Health Research, School of Health and Medicine, Lancaster University, Lancaster, LA 1 4YT UK
e-mail: j.popay@lancaster.ac.uk

A. Morgan et al. (eds.), *Health Assets in a Global Context: Theory, Methods, Action*, DOI 10.1007/978-1-4419-5921-8_10, © Springer Science+Business Media, LLC 2010

10.2 Community Empowerment, Development and Involvement

There are many different ways of describing activities that broadly speaking are focused on enabling communities (defined in terms of place of residence or shared interest) to have greater control over decisions that affect their lives. These activities are elements of policies and actions aiming to improve population health and/or reduce health inequalities in many countries. A number of different terms are used to describe these activities notably: *community engagement, community empowerment, community participation and community involvement.* Although there is considerable overlap between the meanings attached to these phrases there are also important distinctions to be drawn between them.

Community development refers to a form of *professional practice* whose practitioners typically have formal qualifications and there are extensive international networks of community development workers. The World Health Organization (WHO) has defined community development as:

> ...a way of working underpinned by a commitment to equity, social justice and participation that enables people to strengthen networks and identify common concerns and supports them in taking action related to them. It respects community-defined priorities, recognizes community assets as well as problems, prioritises capacity-building and is a key mechanism for enabling effective community participation and empowerment (WHO 2002).

As the WHO definition highlights, *community empowerment* is both central to the process of community development and an outcome of this process. According to WHO, empowerment at both individual and community level is a pre-requisite for health improvements and the reduction of health inequalities (WHO 1997).

The World Bank also highlights both process and outcomes when it argues that empowerment in the context of poverty reduction is concerned with:

> ...the expansion of assets and capabilities of poor people to participate in, negotiate with, influence, control and hold accountable institutions that affect their lives (Narayan 2002).

The practice of community development and community empowerment is extremely diverse but it is possible to identity common characteristics of these participative strategies including: group dialogue; collective action; advocacy and leadership training; organisational development; and activities aimed at giving more power to community members (Wallerstein 2006). The literature points to three key indicators of successful community development and empowerment: the enhanced agency of communities; the transformation of power relationships between communities, institutions and government; and the removal of formal and informal barriers to effective community action.

Community development activities aimed at increasing individual and community empowerment may be implemented as interventions in their own right – as is the case with many community development and health projects. Alternatively, community development methods may be used as a way of delivering interventions focusing on a specific health issue (e.g. interventions aimed at reducing coronary heart diseases or injury prevention interventions) or interventions aiming to address the wider social determinants of population health and health inequalities (e.g. neighbourhood regeneration initiatives).

Community engagement or *involvement* is more commonly used in the UK than community empowerment. This is a more eclectic arena of activity that lacks the defining value base underpinning community development and community empowerment. There are no specific formal qualifications for practitioners of "engagement" or "involvement" and many different types of professionals are involved. As Rogers and Robinson (2004) have argued, community engagement involves community members being engaged in different ways and to differing degrees. They may:

- Be given and/or take different degrees of power and responsibility from one off consultations, which have no impact on power relationships, to initiatives involving power being fully devolved to communities.
- Have more or less formal roles in shaping, governing and/or running services taking elected posts for example or attending public meetings.
- Govern and scrutinise public services, operate as "co-producers" in the running of a service or own and deliver the service themselves.
- Be enabled to lead activities from the bottom up or be expected to react to top down initiatives from public sector organisations.

Goodlad (2002) taking a different approach to Rogers and Robinson (2004) distinguishes between three broad types of community engagement: (1) the engagement of community members or voluntary organisations in partnership with formal organisations in deciding what is to be done and then implementing it; (2) membership of voluntary and community organisations getting things done, fostering community links and building skills, self-esteem and networks; and (3) informal community engagement involving social support mechanisms based on kinship, friendship and neighbourhood networks.

Given this diversity it is clear that community engagement activities do not rest on a readily identifiable body of knowledge. They may adopt a community development approach and explicitly encompass the aim of community empowerment or their objectives may be more modest than this. A wide array of specific methods are used including, for example: citizens panels and juries; rapid appraisal techniques; neighbourhood committees; community forums; participatory evaluation and research and community champions. The latter are people chosen in some way from a local community (of place or interest) to provide leadership in support of action in a particular area such as health improvement. Unlike community development, community engagement activities are not undertaken in their own right but rather are mechanisms for delivering specific policies/actions/interventions or may be linked to audit or research such as health equity audits and/or health impact assessment.

The aims of community empowerment, community development and/or community engagement initiative are diverse and can be more or less explicit. They may include:

- Increasing the appropriateness, responsiveness and ultimately the effectiveness of services.
- Promoting community governance and delivery of services.
- Fostering the development of stronger community "social capital" (networks of mutual support and reciprocity based on trust and common interest).
- Empowering communities to define their own needs and solutions and supporting them to meet these needs across a wide policy landscape (e.g. housing, employment, leisure, transport, health and social care etc.).
- Contributing to democratic renewal.

10.3 Community Empowerment and Health Improvements

In theory there are a number of possible interlinked pathways between activities aimed at increasing community engagement and/or empowerment and health outcomes including both improved population health and reduced health inequalities. Most of these pathways suggest that the relationship is indirect mediated by: (1) changes in the effectiveness of services/interventions; (2) improvements in social and material circumstances (including social relationships/capital); and (3) greater control and self efficacy (at individual and community levels). A theoretical framework for thinking about the relationship between different levels of community engagement and/or empowerment and different types of outcomes are shown in Fig. 10.1. Four possible pathways are highlighted.

Pathway 1. Health outcomes resulting from improved *Information flows*: Identifying population needs more accurately and obtaining better quality information from communities on factors operating as barriers to service uptake will contribute to the design of more appropriate and accessible services/interventions. In theory this can lead to health improvements and reduce health inequalities through an increased uptake of more effective services and/or more effective interventions.

Pathway 2. Governance and guardianship: Promoting and supporting community engagement in or control of a service and/or interventions can increase the appropriateness and accessibility of services/interventions, increase uptake and effectiveness and hence have positive health outcomes.

Pathway 3. Social capital development: Enhanced community empowerment and/or engagement may also contribute to the development of relationships of trust, reciprocity and exchange within communities, strengthening social capital, which has been shown to be linked to improved health.

Pathway 4. Control and empowerment: Community empowerment and/or engagement can also result in communities acting to change their social, material and political environments. This pathway requires the transformation of power relationships between communities, institutions and government increasing the capacity and competence of individuals and their communities to exercise choice and to act

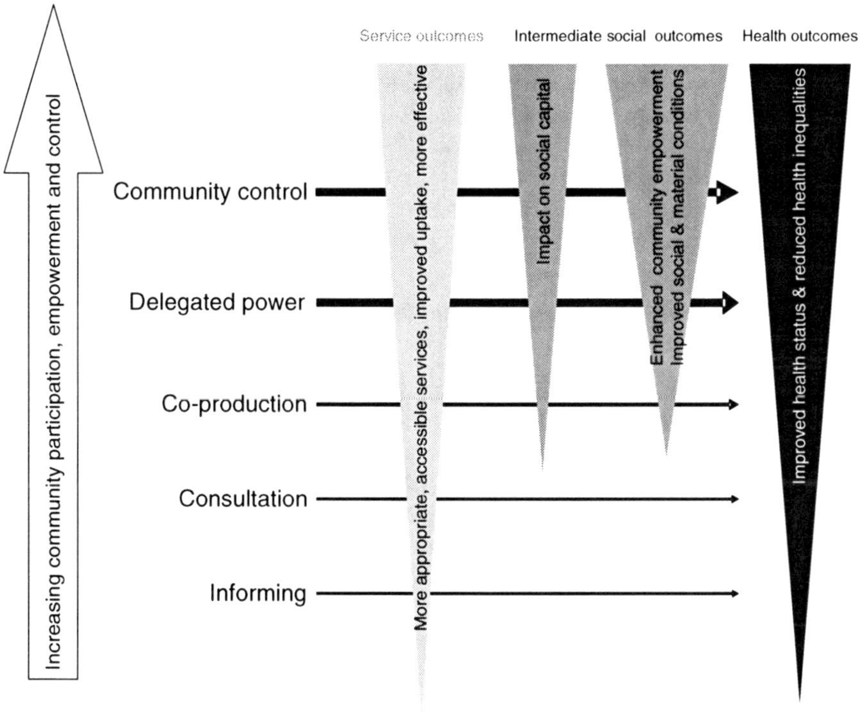

Fig. 10.1 Pathways from community empowerment and engagement to health improvement

on these choices. Health improvement and inequality reduction may therefore result from improvements in individual self-efficacy and control; from collective community action resulting in improved community relationships and material conditions (e.g. increased employment opportunities or improved housing); and from improved effectiveness of services/interventions.

In theory, different pathways to health outcomes will be operating at different "levels" of empowerment and/or engagement. The diagram suggests that at one end of an empowerment/engagement spectrum approach that involves the more or less passive transfer of information from communities to professionals and/or organisations may impact on the appropriateness, accessibility, uptake and ultimately the effectiveness of services but will not impact on dimensions of social capital or result in significant empowerment of a community. Hence the impact on health at population or individual level will be modest. In contrast, the greater the emphasis on giving communities more power and control over decisions that affect their lives, the more likely there are to be positive impacts on service quality, social capital, socioeconomic circumstances, community empowerment and ultimately on population health and health inequalities.

Conversely, it is also important to recognise that whilst the diagram highlights the possible contribution of community engagement/development to health improvement it is also theoretically possible that community engagement and/or community development initiatives may have negative impacts on service use, social capital and individual and population health. This may result, for example, if "engaged" individuals are not appropriately supported and at the population level if, for example, community expectations of involvement, influence and/or control are not met (Popay and Finegan 2005).

10.4 Community Engagement in Public Health Policy and Practice

Whilst the language of policy is always changing, attempts to promote and support the empowerment or engagement of communities through the development and implementation of public policy have a long history in the United Kingdom and internationally. One of oldest initiatives in the UK was the Community Development Project (CDP) that ran from 1969 to 1978. This was a Home Office initiative that aimed to tackle poverty and deprivation in 12 of the most disadvantaged neighbourhoods at a cost of £5 million which Loney (1983) argued was Britain's largest ever government funded social-action experiment.

Internationally the concept of empowerment is now enshrined in the Ottawa Charter (WHO 1986) and the Jakarta health promotion declaration (WHO 1997) extending the focus on community participation in the 1978 WHO's Alma Ata Declaration (WHO 1978). It is a central plank of international development efforts embedded in the United Nation's Millennium Development Goals (UN 2000), the World Bank's Strategic Framework (Narayan 2002) and the work of the WHO (Sachs 2004).

In the UK, whilst policies focusing on democratic and neighbourhood renewal tend to use the phrase community empowerment, it is community engagement and involvement that are central to national strategies for health promotion and the reduction of health inequalities. An increasing number of public health interventions utilise community engagement as a mechanism for delivering change to achieve population health improvements. The English Public Health White Paper "Choosing Health" (DH 2004) placed great emphasis on the role of communities of place and interest working in partnership with health agencies and local government to address the wider determinants of population health and health inequalities. Key elements of this strategy include:

- An increased role for voluntary and community organisations in the provision of services seeking to engage with the most disadvantaged groups and/or to increase opportunities for people to make healthy lifestyle choices. Specific proposals in the White Paper included funding for community food initiatives in deprived communities, and the Safer and Stronger Communities Fund which was intended to support improvement in parks and public spaces. There was also to be a roll-out of initiatives arising from Local Exercise Action Pilots

including, for example, a Physical Activity Promotion Fund and the appointment of regional physical activity coordinators.
- The development of new forms of community leadership with:
  - "Communities for health" pilots being established in 12 localities, with the aim of promoting action across organisations on a locally chosen health priority.
  - A network of health champions being developed drawn from communities as well as from public, private and voluntary sector organisations to help share good practice.
- Wide consultation with and involvement of communities in health related decision making at a local level.

Similar initiatives are evident across the wider UK policy landscape and the political spectrum including local government reform, urban regeneration, policing, education, housing and devolution where the engagement and/or empowerment of communities in identifying needs, and developing and implementing solutions is now seen to be a pre-requisite for success and sustainability.

10.5 The Challenge of Community Empowerment and Engagement for Health Development

Successful community empowerment and engagement requires communities that are willing and able to engage and public organisations and workers willing and able to share power and influence with communities. Whilst recent reviews of research evidence have identified examples of good practice in community empowerment and engagement they have also identified many significant barriers to more effective practice (see for example, Popay et al. 2007). For example, research on barriers to community involvement in the health sector funded by the Department of Health (Pickin et al. 2002) identified five types of barriers to more effective practice:

- The capacity and willingness of communities to "engage".
- The skills and competencies of health professionals staff.
- The dominance of professional cultures and ideologies.
- The organisational ethos and culture; and
- The dynamics of the local and national political system.

Formal evaluations in England of a number of recent high profile health related initiatives with a commitment to engage with communities at all levels have also pointed to difficulties in the implementation of this policy aspiration (Popay and Finegan 2006; Bridge Consortium 2005; Barnes et al. 2003; Woods et al. 2003; Sullivan et al. 2004; Lloyd 2003; Crawshaw et al. 2003; CRESR 2004; Ball 2002; Myers et al. 2004; Cropper and Ong 2003). There is little evidence, for example, that the strategic directions of Health Action Zones, New Deal for Communities (urban renewal) initiatives or Sure Start schemes focusing on child health were shaped by local communities although these initiatives did appear to succeed in fostering active community participation in specific health improvement initiatives and in the delivery of services. Attempts to share power and influence with communities in all these initiatives were severely constrained. In particular, the later neglect of the principles of common purpose espoused during the opening stages of these national initiatives. Community participants experienced this as a lack of respect, undermining their motivation to maintain relationships and in so doing undermining any social capital built in the early stages. National evaluations of these initiatives point to deficits in the skills and competencies required for effective working with active communities within public sector organisations at a local, regional and national level including government departments. Whilst those Healthy Living Centres with a stronger community development orientation may have avoided some of these difficulties, the evaluation suggests that they have become marginalised from mainstream policy developments and that learning from their experiences has been limited.

If activities aimed at community empowerment and engagement are to be effective they require both community and organisational capacity. Capacity as used here refers to the values, knowledge, skills, competencies and motivation required by community members, community and public sector organisations and individual professionals to engage effectively in joint discussions, decision making, governance and intervention/programme delivery and evaluation. Whilst methods for engaging and/or empowering communities have received significant critical attention there has been far less attention given to ways of building the capacity for community engagement within public sector organisations. This will require structural and cultural changes at the organisational level as well as improvements in appropriate knowledge, skills and competencies amongst public sector employees.

As always, there is a need for more research into the methods needed to develop appropriate capacities in communities and organisations (whether public or private) to support more collaborative action to promote health and reduce health inequalities. However, there is also a great deal of existing research evidence that can inform the development of good practice in community empowerment and engagement.

10.6 Reviewing Evidence on Good Practice in Community Empowerment, Community Engagement and Community Development and the Impact on Health and Health Inequalities

Community engagement, empowerment and development are not separate, clearly defined, consistently applied activities or interventions. As already noted, the objectives of initiatives can range from relatively passive information provision and/or exchange to community empowerment and control. Practice is typically characterised by an eclectic assortment of techniques although more formalised methods such as the "community collaborative approach" and "community development approaches" are used. Community development initiatives will always aim to promote and support community empowerment although in practice empowerment is defined in more or less radical ways. The constituent elements of community development practice are also diverse.

Evidence based recommendations to improve practice need to span this diverse field in a meaningful and manageable way. In theory, an evidence review would aim to provide:

- Clear and succinct descriptions of:
- The values and theories of change (Weiss 1998)[1] underpinning different approaches to community empowerment and engagement.
- The key characteristics of these different approaches and the specific methods they use
- An assessment of the impact of different approaches to, and specific methods for, community empowerment and engagement in different communities of interest and/or place on a range of outcomes including:
  - Type, levels and sustainability of empowerment and engagement and the characteristics of people engaged
  - Service appropriateness, accessibility and uptake
  - Social capital/social relationships
  - Community empowerment
  - Individual and community health status including where available impact on health gradients
- Detailed descriptions of the factors and/or processes (operating within the public sector and/or private sector and/or communities) that have been shown to inhibit the effectiveness of approaches to community empowerment and engagement
- An assessment of the effectiveness of approaches that aim to reduce these barriers
- An assessment of the cost-effectiveness of community empowerment and engagement initiatives and if feasible an assessment of cost-effectiveness

In practice, however, the available evidence is still very limited and few of these issues can be addressed in any detail.

---

[1] The notion of a "theory of change" was developed by Weiss, and refers to "the chain of causal assumption that link programme resources, activities, intermediate outcomes and ultimate goals". It is concerned with how an intervention is expected to work, why, and for whom. A clear understanding of the theory that is intended to underpin a particular approach to or method for community engagement/development can help in the design of the approach/methods and help implementers to ensure that the initiative remains on course as it is implemented.

10.7 Evaluative Evidence on Community Engagement/Development

Evaluating the impact of community engagement and/or development initiatives as interventions with the potential to improve population health and/or reduce health inequalities is challenging. Key documents (Wallerstein 2006; Connell 2004; PAHO 2005; Rootman 2001; Alsop and Heinsohn, 2005; Narayan 2005) in this field suggest that the following factors are crucial in considering the evaluation of community engagement/development and empowerment initiatives.

- The simpler the engagement initiative (focusing for example on the provision and/or exchange of information or on community engagement in the (re) design of services) the more easily it can be evaluated but the less likely it is to have discernable impacts on intermediate social capital and/or community empowerment outcomes or on population health or health inequalities.
- The stronger the focus on community empowerment then the more action will be needed at local, regional and even national levels to support the changes required and the more difficult it will be to clearly delineate a project or programme for evaluation.
- The greater the emphasis on community empowerment then the more dynamic the intervention processes can be expected to be. Genuine community empowerment requires a continual cycle of evaluation and reformulation of the objectives sought and the methods employed. Because the goals and methods can change over time to meet the priorities of those involved, in particular the community, it is difficult to evaluate these initiatives using traditional research designs.
- Community involvement in participative evaluative research is becoming increasing common as a method for engagement and empowerment. This may have implication for the type of methods to be adopted in the evaluation and for the outcomes to be measured.
- With any community empowerment and/or engagement initiative the local context will be a powerful force shaping implementation and impact. The scope for generalising from evaluative research is therefore dependent on the quality of the implementation evaluation undertaken and must depend in part on theoretical reasoning rather than statistical probability.
- Where community engagement is used as one aspect of the delivery mechanisms of a project or programme it will be difficult to link specific outcomes to engagement per se.
- Initiatives aiming to promote community empowerment and/or engagement can be expected to generate positive and/or negative outcomes in different domains (individual, organisational and community), at different levels in a system (local, regional and national), and beyond the specific system, or service area itself. Community representatives may wish to measure different outcomes than those required by the public or private sector participants. The outcomes to be measured may therefore need to be negotiated between all stakeholders and compromises may be needed. Additionally, the inclusion of the communities "voice" in

the assessment of the success of any initiative is now widely recognised to be vital. This will require more qualitative methods aimed at describing experiences of evaluation alongside methods concerned to provide quantitative estimates of effects and "thick" descriptions of context and implementation processes.
- Impacts on health outcomes are unlikely to be seen in the short and perhaps medium terms so long term evaluation is required but this is often beyond the funding available.
- Outcomes on a community's capacity to act for change will not be static. Impacts on intermediate and end health outcomes may be identified for a particular initiative. However, it cannot be assumed that the conditions that enabled these impacts to be achieved will remain in place, or that the capacity acquired by a particular community will be readily transferred to another situation or another time.

Limitations in the evidence base relevant to community empowerment and engagement can be addressed by future research. There is a need for more comparative research and for more research addressing questions of cost and cost-effectiveness. Methodological research is also needed on whether, and how, traditional experimental methods can be adapted for the evaluation of these initiatives, including, for example, new approaches to the construction of controls or place based approaches to allocation (Popay et al. 2005). However, as the WHO has argued the use of randomised controlled trials for the evaluation of complex social intervention is *"in most cases inappropriate, misleading and unnecessarily expensive"* (WHO 1999).

It is inevitable therefore that the evidence to inform recommendations to improve practice in community empowerment and engagement will, of necessity, be very diverse. There is an extensive evidence base available, as recent reviews demonstrate, but this includes a wide range of different evaluative methods including: case study research utilising both qualitative and quantitative methods; ethnographic research; survey research; participative research; the analysis of routine data sources and other approaches including a limited body of experimental research. Many studies are focused exclusively on the process of empowerment and engagement with fewer providing empirical data on outcomes, however defined.

Given this diversity in the evidence base there is a strong case for synthesising it in such a way that the process is able to both populate and test theoretical models of the pathways between different approaches to, and specific methods for, community empowerment and engagement and the various types and levels of outcomes that have been identified some of which have been discussed in this paper. There are a number of such models available in the literature (Wallerstein 2006; Rifkin 2003), in addition to the one developed in Fig. 10.1.

References

Alsop, R., Heinsohn, N. (2005). Measuring empowerment in practice: structuring analysis and framing indicators. In *Policy Research Working Paper Series, 3510.* Washington DC: World Bank

Ball, M. (2002). *Sure Start national evaluation. Getting Sure Start Started.* Nottingham: Department for Education and Science Publications

Barnes, M., Sullivan, H., Matka, E. (2003) *National Evaluation of HAZs. The Development of Collaborative Capacity in Health Action Zones. A final report from the national evaluation.* Birmingham: University of Birmingham

Bridge Consortium. (2005). *The evaluation of the Big Lottery Fund Healthy Living Centres. Third Annual Report of the Bridge Consortium.* London: Big Lottery Fund

Commission on the Social Determinants of Health (CSDH). (2008). *Closing the gap in a generation – health equity through action on the social determinants of health. Final report of the Commission on the Social Determinants of Health.* Geneva: World Health Organisation

Connell, J.P. (2004). Eds. *New Approaches to evaluating community initiatives: concepts, methods and contexts.* New York: Aspen Institute

Crawshaw, P., Bunton R., Gillen K. (2003). Health Action Zones and the problem of community. *Health and Social Care in the Community*, 11(1), 36–44

CRESR. (2004). *New Deal for Communities: The National Evaluation. The Programme Wide Annual Report 2003/04.* Sheffield: Centre for Regional Economic and Social Research, Sheffield Hallam University

Cropper, S., Ong, P. (2003). Salford SARP: Final Year Report of the Process Evaluation – lessons and evidence

DH (1999). *Saving lives: our healthier nation.* London: The Stationery Office

DH. (2004). *Choosing health: making healthy choices easier.* London: Department of Health

Goodlad, R. (2002) "Neighbourhood regeneration policy: rebuilding community?" in: Reclaiming Community, editor V. Nash, London: Institute for Public Policy Research, pp. 65–84 Lloyd, N., O'Brien, M., Lewis, C. (2003). *Sure Start national evaluation summary. Fathers in Sure Start local programmes*

Hamer, R.B. (2005). *Community engagement for health: a preliminary review of training and development needs and existing provision for public sector organisations and their workers.* London: NICE

Lloyd, N., O'Brien, M., Lewis, C. (2003) *Fathers in Sure Start local programmes. Sure Start national evaluation summary.* The National Evaluation of Sure Start (NESS) Institute for the Study of Children, Families and Social Issues, Birkbeck, University of London, UK

Loney, M. (1983). *Community against government: the British community development programme, 1968–78: a study of government incompetence.* London: Heinemann

Morgan, A., Ziglio, E. (2007). *Revitalising the evidence base for public health: an assets model.* IUHPE – Promotion and Education Supplement 2. pp. 17–22

Myers, P., Barnes, J., Brodie, I. (2004). *Sure Start national evaluation. Partnership working in Sure Start Local Programmes. A synthesis of early findings from local programme evaluations*

Narayan, D. (2002). *Empowerment and poverty reduction: a sourcebook.* Washington DC: World Bank

Narayan, D. (Ed.) (2005). *Measuring empowerment: cross disciplinary perspectives.* Washington DC: World Bank

PAHO. (2005). *Participatory evaluation of healthy municipalities.* Washington DC: Pan American Health Organisation

Pickin, C., Popay, J., Staley, K., Bruce, N., Jones, C., Gowman, N. (2002). Promoting organisational capacity to engage with active lay communities: developing a model to support organizational change for health, *Health Service Research and Policy*, 7 (1), 34–46

Popay, J., Finegan, H. (2006). *Learning about effective community engagement from selected national initiatives. National Collaborating Centre for Community Engagement Working Paper 5.* Lancaster: Lancaster University

Popay, J., Finegan, H. (2005). *Learning about effective community engagement from selected national initiatives: NCCCE working paper 5.* Report prepared for National Institute for Health and Clinical Excellence

Popay, J., Attree, P., Hornby, D., Milton, B., Whitehead, M., French, B., et al. (2007). *Community engagement to address the wider social determinants of health: A review of evidence on impact, experience & process,* National Institute for Health & Clinical Excellence, London. Available http://www.nice.org.uk/guidance/index.jsp?action=folder&o=34709. cited November 2009

Popay, J., McLeod, A., Kearns, A., Nazroo, J., Whitehead, M. (2005). *New Deal for Communities and health inequalities: A report on work exploring the feasibility of undertaking secondary analysis of the relationship between health inequalities and the NDC policy initiative. Final Report.* Submitted to the Department of Health, May 2005

Rifkin, S.B. (2003). A framework for linking community empowerment and health equity: it is a matter of choice. *Journal of Health, Population and Nutrition*, 21 (3), 168–180

Rogers, B., Robinson, E. (2004). *Active Citizenship Centre Report – The benefits of community engagement. A review of the evidence*. London: Home Office

Rootman, E. (2001). *Evaluation in health promotion: principles and perspectives.* Geneva: World Health Organisation, European Regional Publications

Sachs, J.D. (2004). Health in the developing world: achieving the millennium development goals. *Bulletin of the World Health Organization*, 82 (12), 947–949

Sullivan, H., Judge, K., Sewel, K. (2004). In the eye of the beholder: perceptions of local impact in English Health Action Zones. *Social Science and Medicine*, 59, 1603–1612

UN. (2000). *United Nations Millennium Declaration.* New York: United Nations General Assembly. http://www.un.org/millennium/declaration/ares552e.htm cited May 2009

Wallerstein, N. (2006). *What is the evidence on effectiveness of empowerment to improve health? Copenhagen, WHO Regional Office for Europe (Health Evidence Network report);* http://www.euro.who.int/Document/E88086.pdf cited May 2009

Weiss, C.H. (1998). *Evaluation: methods for studying programs and policies.* New Jersey: Prentice-Hall

Woods, S., Lake, J., Springett, J. (2003). Tackling health inequalities and the HAZ smoking cessation programme: the perfect match? *Critical Public Health*, 13 (1), pp. 61–76

WHO. (1978). Declaration of Alma-Ata. *International Conference on Primary Health Care, Alma-Ata, USSR, 6–12 September 1978.* World Health Organization

WHO. (1986). Ottawa Charter for Health Promotion. *The Move Toward A New Public Health, Ottawa 17-21 November 1986.* World Health Organization

WHO. (1997). The Jakarta Declaration on Leading Health Promotion into the 21st Century. *Fourth International Conference on Health Promotion. Jakarta, 1997* http://www.who.int/hpr/NPH/docs/jakara_declaration_en.pdf cited May 2009

WHO. (1999). *Report on recommendations for health promotion effectiveness.* Geneva: World Health Organization

WHO. (2002). *Community participation in local health and sustainable development: approaches and techniques.* World Health Organization Regional Office for Europe, Copenhagen. Available http://www.euro.who.int/healthy-cities/UHT/20050201_11 cited November 2009

Chapter 11
Strengthening the Assets of Women Living in Disadvantaged Situations: The German Experience

Alfred Rütten, Karim Abu-Omar, Sabine Seidenstücker, and Sabine Mayer

Keywords Physical activity • Movement • Inequality

11.1 Introduction

The promotion of physical activity has become a top public health priority over the last decade. Stirred by alarming rates of obesity and the dominance of chronic diseases in the industrialised world, efforts to combat sedentary lifestyles have surged on national and supranational levels (US Department of Health and Human Services 1996). Due to the documented benefits of physical activity for a variety of health conditions and its potential for cost savings in medical expenditures, increasing rates of population level physical activity has been labelled as a "magic bullet" and as a "best buy" (Munro et al. 1997) for public health. Responding to calls for more successful strategies to promote physical activity at the population level, public health has refined its tools for combating sedentary lifestyles and has shifted from prescribing exercise regimes to recommending "health-enhancing physical activities" as a part of daily life. Furthermore, emerging evidence for the impact of environmental and policy factors on physical activity levels have stimulated the debate for designing interventions that result in physical activity friendly environments and policies (Sallis et al. 2005). In the meantime, meta-analysis and reviews on successful interventions to promote physical activity have been conducted, and have resulted in detailed recommendations (Zaza et al. 2005; Hillsdon et al. 2005).

Despite such progress, public health has still to resolve two important issues in order to increase physical activity at the population level: (1) reaching most vulnerable population subgroups such as ethnic minorities and low-income groups (Taylor

---

A. Rütten (✉)
Institute of Sport Science and Sport, University of Erlangen-Nuremberg, Germany
e-mail: alfred.ruetten@sport.uni-erlangen.de

A. Morgan et al. (eds.), *Health Assets in a Global Context: Theory, Methods, Action*,
DOI 10.1007/978-1-4419-5921-8_11, © Springer Science+Business Media, LLC 2010

et al. 1998), and (2) producing and documenting sustained effects (King et al. 2002). Current deficits in these areas might be partially caused by the concept of "physical activity" that has been utilised in public health. This concept does, from our point of view, not lend much room for an integration of physical activity promotion in the broader context of health promotion. This chapter will therefore try to suggest an alternative approach, i.e. the concept of "movement", as being more appropriate for promoting active lifestyles in the context of health promotion (Rütten 2006).

The concept of "movement" was developed and tested in a multi-centre study with a particular focus on women from a lower social class background. The purpose of the study was to develop, implement, and evaluate innovative intervention strategies for this group in three different settings (e.g. neighbourhood, company, sports club). A participatory approach was used to plan and implement interventions in the three settings, and combined the "investment for health" model with the newly designed "health assets" approach, as discussed in Chap. 1, to health promotion. This chapter focuses on the experience of using the asset approach in the neighbourhood setting. In the first part, the theoretical foundation of the concept of movement and its differences to the concept of physical activity are described. In the second part, the methodology that was used to collect and use "assets for movement" in the planning phase of the intervention is described. The third part demonstrates how assets were adopted in the later stages of the project and discusses the usefulness of the methodology.

11.2 The Concept of Movement in a Health Promotion/ Health Assets Framework

The purpose of this section is to introduce "movement" as a core concept of healthy living. From our point of view, the concept of "movement" goes far beyond the concepts of sport/exercise and physical activity and is closely related to generic health promotion categories such as empowerment, social connectedness, social capital and community capacity. In this section, assets for movement are conceptualised as a particularly fruitful set of assets for health.

11.2.1 Beyond Sport and Physical Activity

Present public health literature is full of evidence regarding the various health effects of physical activity. High levels of physical activity have been associated with lower risks of developing type II diabetes, cardiovascular diseases, and several cancers, and an overall prolonged life expectancy. Furthermore, physical activity has been associated with increased quality of life, and some studies have suggested that physical activity may improve mental conditions such as anxiety and depression (US Department of Health and Human Services 1996; Sallis and Owen 1998; Bauman 2004). Although data from longitudinal studies suggest that it may not be sufficient to exercise regularly in order to reduce weight (Bensinhom et al. 2006), physical activity may assist in controlling body weight. The World Health Organization (WHO) has estimated that annually about 1.9 million people die prematurely due to insufficient levels of physical activity and a sedentary lifestyle (WHO 2002a).

As a consequence of the mounting evidence for the health benefits and its potential for counteracting obesity, increasing population levels of physical activity has become a key focus for public health and health promotion in recent years. Supranational organisations such as the WHO (Global Strategy on Diet, Physical Activity and Health, WHA 2004), and the European Union (EU Platform on Diet, Physical Activity and Health; EU Physical Activity Guidelines (EU 2006, 2008)) as well as many nations (e.g. "Healthy People 2010" and Physical Activity Guidelines Advisory Committee Report 2008 (US Department of Health and Human Services 2000, 2008)) have responded by developing strategies to promote physical activity in populations. However, these strategies tend to follow a predominantly traditional public health concept of sport and exercise (or the more recently established concept of health-enhancing physical activity) and are, for several reasons, of very limited use within the context of health promotion (see Fig. 11.1).

The concept of sport and exercise, which dominated public health research until the 1990s, mainly focused on health benefits through processes of training and physiological adaptation of the human body. This concept attributes health benefits

concept	main processes	main outcomes
sport / exercise	training → physiological adaptation: endurance, strength etc	fitness, physical health
Broaden the context of processes (active lifestyle) within traditional public health		
physical activity	work, transportation, training → physiological adaptation: calorie expenditure	fitness, physical health
From traditional public health to a new public health (health promotion) context		
movement	work, transportation, training social action → individual & social development: empowerment	physical, mental & social health community connectedness & engagement supportive environments

Fig. 11.1 Comparison of concepts: sport/exercise – physical activity – movement

of regular exercise to increased muscle strength and aerobic capacity. Within this concept, 3–5 exercise bouts per week of 15–60 min and 60–90% of the maximum heart rate were recommended for adults by the American College of Sports Medicine (1978, 1990). In line with this concept, the goal of public health efforts was to convince populations to take part in regular exercise programmes.

Triggered by the discouraging results of large scale trials, that failed to demonstrate that populations would adopt exercise regimens, and by increasing evidence of the health benefits of moderate intensities of physical activity, public health concepts shifted in the 1990s (Blair et al. 1992). The concept of "health-enhancing physical activity" (HEPA) was introduced and has dominated public health ever since. The HEPA concept attributes health benefits of physical activity to increased caloric expenditures. Based on study results that demonstrated health benefits of moderate intensities of physical activity outside the context of exercise (e.g. physical activity at work or for transportation) recommendations were reframed and shifted towards accumulating a minimum of 30 min of (almost) all types of physical activity of moderate intensity on most, or preferably all days of the week (Pate et al. 1995; US Department of Health and Human Services 1996). In 2007, these recommendations were adjusted by adding that 20 min of vigorous aerobic physical activity on 3 days per week would provide comparable health benefits as 5 days of 30 min of moderate physical activity per week (Haskell et al. 2007). Within the concept of HEPA, domestic work (e.g. vacuum cleaning, car washing), physical activity for transportation (e.g. riding a bicycle for running errands), and physical activity at work can yield important health benefits that are comparable to those of traditional forms of exercise. Following the HEPA concept, current public health efforts focus on convincing people to take every opportunity to be physically active (e.g. use stairs instead of elevator), and to integrate physical activity into their daily life (Sallis et al. 2005).

The shift from a traditional concept of exercise to HEPA has resulted in some efforts that are in line with general health promotion ideas. For example, efforts to encourage populations to walk or ride a bicycle in everyday life have stirred discussions about safety of pedestrians and cyclists in traffic and resulted in calls for pedestrian/cyclists friendly environments (WHO 2002b, 2006). On the other hand, research on the health benefits of physical activity remains focused on processes of physiological adaptation/caloric expenditures and seeks to demonstrate effects of short activity bouts with low levels of intensity. Moreover, "calories counting", i.e. measuring calories expenditure, has become a major topic of research and public health discussion.

From our point of view, such research interests neglect the profound effects that certain types of physical activity can have beyond processes of physiological adaptation of the human body. We would like to argue that getting together with friends at the bowling lane, walking with a neighbour through the community, or cycling through a nearby park effect health and well being through pathways other than physiological body adaptation and caloric expenditures. In the view of the current concepts, such pathways are rarely considered. We would like to suggest concentrating on such pathways from physical activity to health and well being, and thus employ the social potential and social impact of physical activity for health promotion. Doing this might require a new understanding of physical activity. We have, thus developed the concept of "movement" that follows a different (new public health) paradigm to define relevant pathways and outcomes in regard to physical activity and might therefore have more relevance for health promotion as the current concept of physical activity (see Fig. 11.1). We would like to suggest that possible pathways affected by "movement" may include the following dimensions: the regulatory, educational, social, environmental, and political:

- First of all, unlike the current concept of physical activity the concept of movement has a fundamental regulatory dimension which closely relates to individual physical capacity, independency, and health: From the first steps in our life, where we learn to explore und cope with our environment until the oldest age, where fragility may limit our activities of daily living and our potential to control the determinants of our life, we very much rely on our physical capacity to move. The ability to move and "exercise" control over our physical environment is closely related to psychological parameters such as self-esteem and self-efficacy (Fuchs 1997). As such, movement can be seen as an asset for an independent and self-determined life.
- Secondly, the concept of movement has a fundamental educational dimension which relates to the ability to learn, concentrate and increase cognitive function. Moving can reduce the decline in cognition associated with aging among adults (Dishman et al. 2006), and study results suggest that moving might enhance the ability of children to learn (Weuve et al. 2004; Singh-Manoux et al. 2005; Dishman et al. 2006). Programmes that use movement to enhance learning and personal development have been developed, particularly in the context of older people and children. As such, movement can be seen as an asset for education.
- Thirdly, movement has a fundamental social dimension. We have to "move ourselves" – in a physical and sometimes also in a mental way – to get together with others. Moreover, moving creates specific opportunities for social contacts and social networking. Someone may become a better friend with her/his neighbour by joining her/him regularly for walking. In addition, people who come together to exercise in a sport club may broaden their social networks, develop closer social relationships, and receive social support. The social context of movement may even relate to community connectedness. For example, in Germany, members of sports clubs show a higher degree of belonging to the community than the rest of the population (Wieland and Rütten 1991). Studies have also shown that lower levels of physical activity are associated with lower levels of social participation (Lindström et al. 2001), and that social participation and perceptions of political efficacy might affect individual's health (Rütten et al. 2000). As such, movement can be seen as an asset for social contacts.
- Fourthly, movement has a fundamental environmental dimension. Movement is not only a prerequisite for coping with or changing the environment. Movement may directly be related to the creation of better environmental conditions and support

healthy living. For example, studies have shown relationships between neighbourhood safety and physical activity. Neighbourhoods with higher crime rates, local people are less likely to walk to get public transport or, reversing causality, neighbourhoods where residents walk for transport feature lower crime rates (CDC 1999). Movement can therefore be seen as an asset for healthy living.

- Fifthly, on a policy level, movement has a fundamental political dimension. For example, promoting safe walking and cycling has led to discussions about the reduction of inner city car traffic and has thus supported policy efforts for a healthier environment. In the meantime, urban planning has identified and called for community designs that are attractive for movement (Frank and Engelke 2001). Encouraging movement has served as a catalyst for cross-sector working in health, environment, transportation and urban planning. Movement can therefore be seen as an asset for intersectoral health promotion efforts.

Following these examples where movement might have beneficial effects, different outcomes of movement in comparison to physical activity should be considered. The outcomes of increased movement could have an impact at both the individual and community level:

- At an individual level, our model predicts movement has the potential to have a positive impact on all three dimensions of the original WHO definition of health (WHO 1948): i.e. physical health, mental health and social health. Movement could increase an individual's physical capacity to live an independent and self-determined life (physical health). While, movement may increase an individual's capacity to cope with life events and life stressors (mental health). Finally, movement could also help to enlarge an individual's social network and increase resources of social support (social health). The Ottawa Charter (WHO 1986) defined health as a resource for everyday life. Our concept shares the Ottawa Charter's emphasis on personal skills and social resources, as well as physical capacities (WHO 1986).
- Regarding community level indicators, we would predict that movement could strengthen social, environmental, and political outcomes relevant for public health. Movement may increase the connectedness of neighbourhoods and communities, and strengthen the social capital of communities (social outcome). Higher levels of movement could increase social contacts among community members, and reduce crime rates in communities. Additionally, movement may aid the creation of better environmental conditions and thereby support healthy living (environmental outcome). For example, promoting inner city walking and cycling might reduce car traffic and air pollution. Finally, movement may increase the community capacity for intersectoral work and health promotion (political outcome). For example, engaging political parties in a discussion about inner city walking and cycling, might lead policy sectors who have been previously withdrawn from health promotion efforts (e.g. transportation, urban planning) to recognise and consider health promotion issues in their daily work.

Considering the described pathways and outcomes, the concept of movement, might have higher applicability for health promotion than the concept of physical activity. Movement, as proposed by us, might very well serve as an asset for health promotion in itself. The described community level outcomes that efforts to promote movement might yield a unique return of investment, comparable to efforts in the areas of smoking cessation or healthy nutrition.

11.2.2 Movement and Social Inequality

Within the present study, the concept of movement was applied to promote the health of women in difficult life situations. Federal interest for the study stemmed from national health data which indicated that women from lower social class background report highest levels of sedentary lifestyles and obesity (Rütten et al. 2005). These data are confirmed by European studies, indicating that adults in the lowest national quartile of gross household income report lower rates of days with vigorous and moderate physical activity per week compared to other income quartiles (Rütten and Abu-Omar 2004). Also, Margetts et al. (1999) identified associations between educational level and physical activity. The study found that adults with primary education had lower rates of physical activity compared to adults with secondary or tertiary education.

Within the traditional view of the concept of physical activity, higher prevalence of sedentary lifestyles among disadvantaged population groups is linked to individual determinants of physical activity such as attitudes and health beliefs. From our point of view, the concept of movement provides clues to (re)consider the role of social support, community connectedness and the built environment as determinants and outcomes of a physically active lifestyle. In this section we will explore, the degree to which such dimensions can be linked to physical activity, and touch on the issue of social inequality.

11.2.2.1 Movement: Social Support and Inequality

Influences of social networks and social support on health have been described since the 1970s and 1980s (e.g. Berkman and Syme 1979; Cohen and Syme 1985). Today, it is widely accepted that low resources of social support and social isolation result in a variety of adverse health outcomes and effect overall mortality rates. Some studies suggest that the risk of receiving low levels of social support is greater among members of lower social classes than for members of the middle and upper class (Matthews et al. 1999).

The significance of adequate social support for physical activity has been demonstrated by a number of studies. Stahl et al. (2001) identified perceived motivation from family and friends to engage in physical activity as an important determinant of physical activity. Also, having friends to exercise with has been associated with a physically active lifestyle (Giles-Corti and Donovan 2002). Eyler et al. (2001) found that among minority women, high levels of social support are related to an active lifestyle but not to exercising regularly.

11.2.2.2 Movement: Community Connectedness and Inequality

Beyond social networks and social support, community connectedness and social capital have been linked to health outcomes (Kawachi and Berkman 2000). Studies suggest that, after controlling for individual level factors such as low socioeconomic status, living in communities that features higher levels of social capital might lead to important health benefits (Kawachi et al. 1999a). Social capital has also been linked to social inequality. Kawachi et al. (1999b) identified relationships between poverty and social capital on the state level as potential causes for mortality differences.

To our knowledge, very few studies have explored associations between measures of community connectedness and physical activity. Lindström et al. (2001) demonstrated that low social participation might result in lower levels of physical activity.

11.2.2.3 Movement: The Built Environment and Inequality

Studies have shown that neighbourhood characteristics such as availability of amenities (e.g. shops, public parks, and public sport facilities), cleanliness, or crime and traffic are related to health outcomes (Sooman and Macintyre 1995; Balfour and Kaplan 2002). Frumkin et al. (2004) found that relationships between the socioeconomic status of neighbourhoods, air quality, injury rates and health outcomes were especially strong in the US.

Recent reviews suggest an influence of the built environment on physical activity (Frank and Engelke 2001; Humpel et al. 2002), and also suggest influences of environmental perceptions on health (Rütten et al. 2001). Studies have shown that living close to exercise facilities (Sallis et al. 1990) or in coastal proximity (Bauman et al. 1999) might increase participation rates in leisure-time physical activity. Also, aspects of safety and aesthetics of neighbourhoods have been associated with physical activity (Booth et al. 2000; Ball et al. 2001). In general, such results might suggest that living in a poor neighbourhood could be associated with fewer opportunities for, and consequentially lower levels, of physical activity. For one US community it has been demonstrated, that neighbourhoods with lower socioeconomic status feature significantly fewer recreational facilities that can be used free of charge than neighbourhoods with higher socioeconomic status (Estabrooks et al. 2003). While some studies have provided evidence that living in a poor neighbourhood results in decreased physical activity levels (Yen and Kaplan 1998), other studies could not find such an association (Ross 2000).

11.3 Assets for Movement

The present study applied the WHO "Assets for health and development programme" concept to the promotion of healthy behaviour (movement) among women in difficult life situations. To create sustainable and effective interventions for this group, the "Assets for health and development" concept was adapted towards an "asset for movement" concept.

As outlined in Chap. 1, a health asset can be defined as "*...any factor (or resource), which enhances the ability of individuals, communities and populations to maintain and sustain health and well-being. These assets can operate at the level of the individual, family or community as protective (and/or promoting) factors to buffer against life's stresses*". This definition was adapted to the specific health behaviour of movement. An asset for movement was defined as any factor (or resource), which enhances the ability of individuals, communities and populations to begin, maintain and sustain movement. As with the broader concept of health assets, assets for movement can operate on the individual, family, or community level. Within our theoretical framework, we operationalised assets for movement on the individual, organisational, and infrastructural level.

11.3.1 Individuals as an Asset for Movement

Studies have demonstrated that supportive social environments are an important predictor of a physically active lifestyle (Stahl et al. 2001). Individuals who report supportive social environments (e.g. friends or family members who support being physically active) are more likely to be physically active compared to individuals who lack such social contacts. Following these research results, individuals could function as an asset for movement, if they provide others with a supportive social environment for movement. For example, a person could be seen as an asset for movement if she/he would be available to assist in organising exercise classes, or is willing to assist in recruiting participants to exercise classes.

11.3.2 Organisations as an Asset for Movement

Within the German sport system, organisations (e.g. sport clubs) play a key role in providing opportunities for leisure-time physical activity. German sport clubs traditionally support competitive and also recreational sport. As such, sport clubs represent one type of organisation that could be seen as an asset for movement. On the other hand, about 80% of leisure-time physical activity takes place outside the realm of sport clubs. Fitness gyms, companies, or sickness funds are organisations that, within the German system, offer opportunities to exercise and thus could support movement. As such, organisations could be seen as an asset for movement if they already offer opportunities for leisure-time physical activity or would consider offering new opportunities for leisure-time physical activity. Additionally, an organisation could represent an asset for movement. For example, if women of the target group developed a relationship with an organisation and were then receptive to health promotion messages from the organisation. In this case, organisations as well as individuals could function as a supportive social environment for movement.

11.3.3 Infrastructures as an Asset for Movement

In recent years, studies have provided evidence that infrastructural opportunities for physical activity are important predictors of a physically active lifestyle (e.g. Humpel et al. 2002). Such infrastructural opportunities could include walking trails, parks, sidewalks, bicycle lanes, or exercise and recreational facilities. In the context of the present study, infrastructures were seen as an asset for movement if they could provide a place, where women of the target group felt safe and comfortable to meet and exercise. This could be parks or recreational facilities, but also buildings/grounds that could host new opportunities for movement (e.g. gym in elementary school, community room in a local village).

11.4 Assessing Assets for Movement

11.4.1 Methodology of Asset Assessment

In order to collect information on potential assets for movement, the following methodology was applied: In the first phase, two focus group meetings took place in the setting neighbourhood. One focus group meeting was organised for women of the target group who lived in the neighbourhood, and one for local experts of the neighbourhood and the municipality. The goal of the focus group meetings was the identification of assets for movement in the setting neighbourhood at the level of "individual assets", "organisational assets", and "infrastructural assets". Initially information on assets for movement was collected separately for women of the target group, in order to avoid a bias towards perceived assets of experts. Secondly, participants of the two focus group meetings were invited to a workshop. In the workshop, representatives of the two focus groups reported on identified assets in the focus groups and participants discussed assets that both groups had identified (overlapping assets for movement). Thirdly, at the end of the workshop, all participants visualized overlapping assets for movement and brainstormed about potential interventions to promote movement among women of the target group.

11.4.2 Implementation of Asset Assessment

In the first phase of the project, five women of the neighbourhood were interviewed about assets and barriers to movement by the project staff. These women had been identified and initially contacted by local experts (e.g. Reverend of local church, Pharmacist). After qualitative interviews about assets and barriers to movement, these women were asked for referral of friends/women they knew who were in similar life situations and would be willing to participate in an interview. All of these women were invited to the focus group meeting. Some other women were identified through visits of the project staff at organisations of the neighbourhood (e.g. Turkish cultural club, local kindergarten), and then invited to take the interview and participate in the focus group meeting.

The focus group meeting was attended by 21 women, seven of whom were of German nationality, and 14 belonged to different ethnic minorities (most of them of Turkish nationality). The meeting started with some introductory remarks from the project staff about the project, the purpose of the meeting and the concept of assets for movement. Project staff adapted language and contents to ensure that it was appropriate and accessible to the target group and non-native speakers. After the introductory remarks, women were asked to identify assets for movement at the individual, organisational and infrastructural level. To help women to identify assets that they perceived as important for promoting movement, the group was divided into subgroups of 3–5 women. Most subgroups were accompanied by one member of the research staff who recorded assets on each of the three levels. At the end, groups gathered to exchange information on the collated assets for movement.

Experts were contacted by the project staff, informed about the project, and invited to attend an expert focus group meeting. Experts were contacted, if it was perceived that their institution could support the goals of the project. The organisational sectors of the municipality that were contacted were health (e.g. local health authority), religion (e.g. different religious communities), women (e.g. equal opportunity office of municipality), social inequality (organisation to support single mothers of municipality), migrants (e.g. migrants council of municipality), urban affairs (e.g. office of city planning and exercise facility management of municipality), sociocultural work (office for cultural activities of municipality), education (e.g. kindergarten and public schools of municipality), and sport (e.g. neighbourhood sport club). A total of 14 experts formed the second focus group, which followed the same general procedure as the women's focus group.

A workshop was held about 6 weeks after the focus group meetings, the purpose of which was the identification of overlapping assets between both focus groups. All participants and invitees of the two focus groups were invited to take part in the workshop. Additionally, some people who were named as individual assets in the focus groups were also invited to the workshop. After some introductory remarks from the project staff, clipboard cards were used to map identified assets for movement of the two focus groups separately on the walls of the conference rooms (organised by level of assets). Participants were then asked to review clipboards, and place overlapping assets (assets that had been recorded by women and experts) in a separate space. During this process participants continued to discuss the assets. At the end of the information-sharing session, one woman from the target group and one expert jointly presented the overlapping assets for movement to the project staff.

In the second part of the workshop, participants brainstormed about potential interventions to promote movement among the target group. Project staff encouraged participants to consider the identified overlapping assets for movement in the brainstorming process.

11.4.3 Results of Assets Assessment

On the organisational level, focus groups and the workshop generated a number of potential assets for movement. Organisations referred to as potential assets for movement included clubs, volunteer organisations, branches of municipality, and commercial organisations. In the focus group of experts 43 potential assets on the organisational level were identified, women of the target group named 27 organisations as an asset for movement. The workshop identified 12 overlapping assets for movement between both focus groups (Fig. 11.2).

On the individual level, focus groups identified 40 (experts) and 23 (women) people as an asset for movement. Among the people mentioned were, staff of the municipality, exercise instructors, reverends of several churches, citizens, and owners of small businesses in the community. The workshop resulted in nine people being contacted, who were referred to by both focus groups (Fig. 11.3). These people were invited to join the cooperative planning process.

On the infrastructural level, focus groups identified 27 (experts) and 53 (women) assets for movement. Infrastructural assets identified ranged from parks and recreational facilities to community rooms, unused grounds in the neighbourhood, and exercise facilities of schools and sport clubs. The workshop identified 14 overlapping assets (Fig. 11.4).

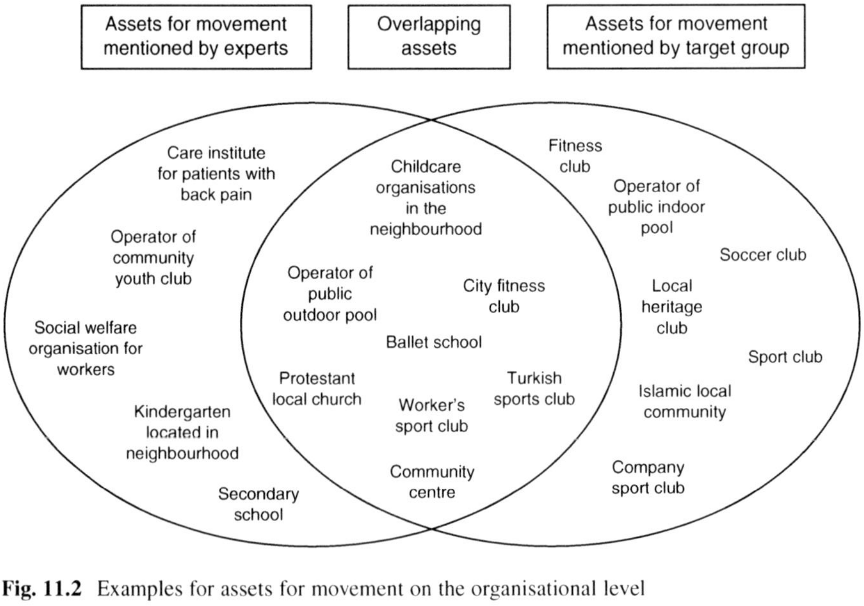

Fig. 11.2 Examples for assets for movement on the organisational level

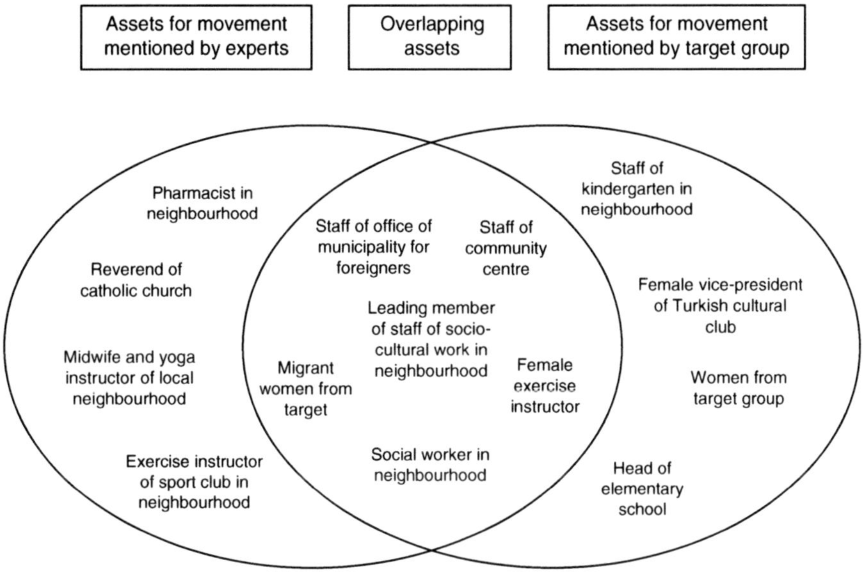

Fig. 11.3 Examples for assets for movement on the individual level

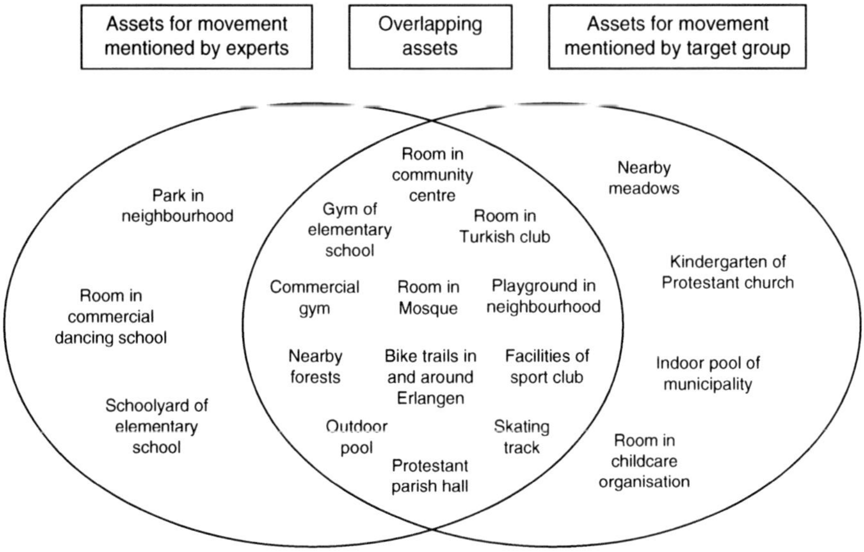

Fig. 11.4 Examples of assets for movement on the infrastructural level

11.5 Applying Assets for Movement in the Planning Process

11.5.1 Methodology of Asset Application

In the next step, identified overlapping assets for movement were utilised in the development of interventions for the promotion of movement among women of the target group. In order to empower women of the target group to take part in the planning process, a cooperative planning group was founded.

The methodology employed for a cooperative planning group follows, in general, the approach of participatory action research. Individuals from different sectors and organisational levels met on a regular basis in order to develop and implement an action plan on a predefined topic. In the first meeting, the cooperative planning group agreed on the following regulations:

1. Each meeting is facilitated by a moderator. The moderator structures the contents of each meeting, and regulates verbal contributions of all participants. The moderator safeguards equal contributions of each participant.
2. Participants attend every meeting of the group. Substituting participants would hamper progress during meetings and should therefore be avoided.
3. Every participant has equal say in all steps of the work of the group.

Six meetings of the group were scheduled. In the first two meetings, ideas for actions were brainstormed. In the next two meetings ideas for actions were structured and discussed. In the last two meetings, a time schedule for the implementation of actions was developed, and responsibilities for different implementation tasks are agreed upon. At the last meeting, the action plan was approved by all participants.

11.5.2 Implementation of Asset Application

The planning group consisted of women and experts of the two focus groups. Project staff were employed as moderators. At the first meeting, participants were informed about the purpose of the cooperative planning group and its regulations. Furthermore, results of the workshop and some results of the qualitative interviews with women of the target group were presented. The meeting concluded with a discussion about the results of the workshop brainstorming session. At the second meeting, the group separated into small work groups in order to elaborate on ideas generated during brainstorming. Project staff joined these groups and consulted group members on the identified assets for movement. While project staff had the primary function of moderating meetings, they were also asked to consult participants about ideas for developing health promotion interventions. In the next meetings, the cooperative planning group developed and approved an action plan for interventions to promote movement among women of the target group.

Table 11.1 Outcomes of the cooperative planning process: actions agreed upon in the cooperative planning group to promote movement among women from low-income background and ethnic minorities

Establishing exercise programmes	Organise taster days featuring different exercise classes
	Organise one low-intensity exercise class
	Organise one moderate-intensity exercise class
Creating new opportunities for movement	Organise "women only" opening hours in public indoor pool
	Establishing a meeting room for women in a public building of municipality
Educating women of the target group	Train women of the target group to become PE/exercise instructors
Running an information/marketing campaign	Form a marketing group to develop and distribute advertisements for actions
Developing infrastructures	Establishing a project office in the neighbourhood

11.5.3 Results of Asset Application

The cooperative planning group agreed upon several actions to promote movement among women of the target group. These actions included establishing new exercise classes, creating new opportunities for movement, educating women of the target group to become exercise instructors, running a marketing campaign to promote actions among the target group, and creating organisational infrastructures for sustainable project development (Table 11.1).

All interventions took into consideration the needs of women of the target group. For example: exercise classes and taster days included child care, and were either low or free of charge (taster days).

11.6 Evaluating the Use of Assets for Movement for the Development of the Interventions

11.6.1 Methodology of Evaluation

The evaluation of the use of assets in the process of developing and implementing interventions for movement posed to be a challenge. The following methodology was employed to evaluate the use of assets.

Firstly, project staff presented the identified organisational and infrastructural assets to the cooperative planning group at the group's first meeting. This was done by a slide presentation, additionally all participants received handouts charting the identified assets. During the successive meetings of the cooperative planning group, project staff encouraged the group to use these identified assets in the planning process.

This was again done by referring to the assets verbally and with handouts. Regarding the individual level assets, some of the named people were invited to join the planning process and did so from the first meeting on (e.g. staff of office of sociocultural work in neighbourhood, migrant women), Other individual level assets (e.g. female exercise instructor) were not invited, but were presented to the cooperative planning group on the handouts.

Secondly, the potential impact of assets for movement on the development of interventions was documented by project staff during the implementation and follow-up phase of the project. Project staff: documented the action plan that was approved by group participants; joined and documented meetings of the city council (at which aspects of the project implementation were discussed); engaged in informal conversations with some of the participants of the planning group; and organised and held a follow-up workshop where issues of project sustainability were discussed.

The goal of the evaluation was to generate hypothesises about the impact of assets for movement on the development of meaningful interventions for movement among women in difficult life situations. The recording of assets was motivated by the following research questions:

(a) Which (overlapping) assets for movement are identified by the different groups (experts, target group)?
(b) Which assets for movement are employed/are not employed in the process of developing interventions to promote movement?
(c) Which assets for movement generate an impact/generate no impact on interventions to promote movement?

11.6.2 Results of the Evaluation

Table 11.2 depicts an overview of some of the identified assets and their impact on the development of interventions. On the individual level, staff of the office for sociocultural work and the migrant women actively engaged in and had a high impact on project implementation. The exercise instructor conducted one of the exercise classes that was founded, and thus supported the project. The head of the elementary school initially did not support project work, but in the later stages of the project allowed the project to conduct exercise classes in the school. On the organisational level, the community centre in the neighbourhood supported the project by providing on various occasions meeting rooms. The protestant church and the "Anger Initiative" social organisation also assisted in promoting the project and offered their facilities for project meetings. The Turkish cultural club supported the project at the beginning of the implementation phase, but later ceased to cooperate actively. Interestingly, the sport club in the neighbourhood rejected any approach from project staff and did not engage in the project. On the infrastructural level, the gym of the elementary school, and the indoor pool hosted important project activities.

Table 11.2 Evaluation of assets for movement in the process of developing actions for promotion of movement among the target group

Level of asset for movement	Identified asset for movement	Referred to by	Impact on development of interventions
Individual			
	Staff of office for sociocultural work in neighbourhood	Both focus groups	• Participant in cooperative planning group • Participant in marketing group • Organised room for project office in neighbourhood • Recommended commercial artist for marketing group • Distributed posters and flyers in neighbourhood • Organised collection of registration forms for exercise classes in his organisation • Provided room for project office • Highly supportive of planning and implementation process
	Exercise instructor in local sport club	Both focus groups	• Instructor for taster day • Instructor for low-intensity exercise class • Supportive of implementation process
	Migrant women in neighbourhood	Both focus groups	• Participant in cooperative planning group • Multiplier for project activities in neighbourhood • Organised meeting room for women in public building • Joined meeting with local press • Participated in meeting with operator of public indoor pool to implement"women only" hours • Participant in marketing group, distributed posters and flyers in neighbourhood • Organised child care • Highly supportive of planning and implementation process
	Member of local sports association, responsible for women in sports	Experts focus group	• Participant in cooperative planning group • Moderately supportive of planning and implementation process
	Head of elementary school in neighbourhood	Target focus group	• Not supportive of planning and implementation process, later supported the process

(continued)

Table 11.2 (continued)

Level of asset for movement	Identified asset for movement	Referred to by	Impact on development of interventions
Organisational Level			
	Community Centre in neighbourhood	Both focus groups	• Provided meeting room for women • Provided room for meetings of marketing group • Supported marketing activities (distribution of flyers and posters) • Supported renting of gym in Pestalozzi elementary school for exercise classes • Highly supportive of planning and implementation process
	Protestant church in neighbourhood	Both focus groups	• Recruited participants for cooperative planning group • Offered room for exercise classes • Supported marketing activities (distribution of posters and flyers) • Supportive of planning and implementation process
	Sport club in neighbourhood	Both focus groups	• Not supportive of planning and implementation process
	"Anger initiative" social organisation in neighbourhood	Experts focus group	• Provided room for focus group meeting and child care • Recruited participants for focus group of target group • Participated in cooperative planning group • Highly supportive of planning and implementation process
	Turkish cultural club in neighbourhood	Target focus group	• Participated in cooperative planning group • Recruited women for exercise classes • Offered room for various activities of women in new building of cultural club • Cooperation cessed in later stages of project • Supportive of planning and implementation process
Infrastructural level			
	Gym of elementary school in neighbourhood	Both focus groups	• Used for exercise classes
	Room in meeting point for citizens living in neighbourhood	Both focus groups	• Used as meeting room for women
	Public indoor pool	Target focus group	• Operated opening hours for "women only"

11.7 Conclusions

The present study used a "health asset" model to promote healthy behaviour among women in difficult life situations. In order to promote movement among the target group, assets for movement were collected through qualitative interviews, focus group discussions, and a workshop with women of the target group and local experts. In a second step, a cooperative planning group was set up with women of the target group and local experts in order to plan and implement interventions for the promotion of movement using identified assets. Thirdly, project staff tracked identified assets for movement and its impact on the process of developing and implementing interventions.

Project results might indicate that the assets model can be employed to promote healthy behaviour. Assets were identified in focus group discussions, and were used by the cooperative planning groups in the process of developing and implementing interventions for the promotion of movement. While, at first glance, a number of these assets seemed to be important to the implementation of project activities, a sound evaluation of the impact of these assets posed to be difficult. Those difficulties might have been partially related to the lack of adequate methods and tools to evaluate the potential impact of assets. Additionally, it might be reasoned that some of those assets that were identified might have also made important contributions to the project even if the assets model had not been employed. The analysis of the process of asset assessment, assets application, and assets evaluation raises a number of questions that might be of importance for future projects that utilise the assets for health model to promote healthy behaviour:

- What is an asset for healthy behaviour? This question relates to the process of assets assessment. In the present study, both focus groups identified relatively large numbers of individual, organisational, and infrastructural (overlapping) assets. Research staff adopted the role of defining and documenting assets in the process of assets assessment. Nevertheless, it can be assumed that women and experts in the focus groups defined assets for healthy behaviour in different ways and this might have influenced outcomes of the process of collecting assets.
- On which dimensions should assets for healthy behaviour be identified? Within the methodology employed, identification of assets for movement was limited to the individual, organisational, and infrastructural level. The decision to focus on these levels was based on existing evidence on determinants for movement. However, it proved to be difficult to distinguish these levels, since participants often referred to individuals as members of organisations which feature certain infrastructures. Additionally, other potential dimensions of assets (e.g. past experience with health promotion activities) that might have had an impact on the development of health promotion strategies were, in the present study, not considered.
- How do we assess assets for healthy behaviour? While women of low-income groups and ethnic minorities were receptive to the process of assets assessment employed, experts voiced some criticism. For experts, mapping assets for movement was partially seen as a time consuming and superfluous task, resulting in

discussions of the purpose of asset assessment in the focus groups. This raises the question as to whether different methodologies for assessing assets in the group of experts and the target group should have been used.

- How do we apply assets for healthy behaviour to the development of health promotion strategies? In the present study, project staff encouraged participants of the cooperative planning group to adopt identified assets for movement for the development of intervention strategies. Project staff functioned as moderators and consultants of the cooperative planning group, this might have affected the development of interventions. Presumably, a more structured approach to the implementation of identified assets in the process of developing interventions for promoting movement might have produced different outcomes.
- How do we evaluate the use of assets for healthy behaviour? Within the present study, documentation of employed assets was used to evaluate assets for healthy behaviour. This methodology is clearly explorative in its character, and might be reconsidered by future projects.

Besides such questions that should be addressed by future studies, the application of an asset approach to the promotion of healthy behaviour seemed to be beneficial for the overall success of the project. The assessment of assets for movement in the first phase of a project with the purpose of the development of interventions for health promotion resulted in an efficient identification of individuals, organisations and infrastructures that were supportive of the project. Secondly, focus groups conducted for asset assessment provided research staff with in-depth information about individual and organisational relationships in the neighbourhood that turned out to be useful in the later stages of the project. Thirdly, focus groups were useful to disseminate the project and its goals within the neighbourhood, and thus served as a catalyst for future project activities. Fourthly, and most importantly, discussion about assets for movement with women of the target group paved the way for a trusting relationship between researchers and women that was fundamental to the overall success of the project.

References

American College of Sports Medicine. (1978). The recommended quantity and quality of exercise for developing and maintaining fitness in healthy adults. *Medicine and Science in Sports*, 10:VII–X.

American College of Sports Medicine. (1990). Position stand: the recommended quantity and quality of exercise for developing and maintaining cardio respiratory and muscular fitness in healthy adults. *Medicine and Science in Sports and Exercise*, 22:265–274.

Balfour, J. L., & Kaplan, G. A. (2002). Neighbourhood environment and loss of physical function in older adults: Evidence from the Alameda County Study. *American Journal of Epidemiology*, 155(6):507–515.

Ball, K., Bauman, A., Leslie, E., & Owen, N. (2001). Perceived environmental aesthetics and convenience and company are associated with walking for exercise among Australian adults. *Preventive Medicine*, 33:434–440.

Bauman, A., Smith, B., Stoker, L., Bellew, B., & Booth, M. L. (1999). Geographical influences upon physical activity participation: evidence of a 'coastal effect'. *Australian and New Zealand Journal of Public Health*, 23:322–324.

Bauman, A. E. (2004). Updating the evidence that physical activity is good for health: an epidemiological review 2000–2003. *Journal of Science and Medicine in Sport*, 7(1) Suppl:6–19.

Bensinhom, D. R., Kraus, W. E., Donahue, M. P., & Durham, M. D. (2006). Obesity and physical activity: a review. *American Heart Journal*, 151:598–603.

Berkman, L. F., & Syme, S. L. (1979). Social networks, host resistance and mortality: a nine-year follow-up study of Alameda County residents. *American Journal of Epidemiology*, 109:186–204.

Blair, S. N., Kohl, H. W., Gordon, N. F., & Paffenbarger, R. S. (1992). How much physical activity is good for health? *Annual Review of Public Health*, 13:99–126.

Booth, M. L., Owen, N., Bauman, A., Clavisi, O., & Leslie, E. (2000). Social-cognitive and perceived environment influences associated with physical activity in older Australians. *Preventive Medicine*, 31:15–22.

CDC. (1999). Neighbourhood safety and the prevalence of physical inactivity – selected states 1996. *Morbidity and Mortality Weekly Reports*, 48(7):143–146.

Cohen, S., & Syme, S. L. (1985). *Social Support and Health*. New York: Academic.

Dishman, R. K., Berthoud, H. R., Booth, F. W., Cotman, C. W., Edgerton, E., Fleshner, M., et al. (2006). Neurobiology of exercise. *Obesity*, 14:345–356.

Estabrooks, P. A., Lee, R. E., & Gyurcsik, N. C. (2003). Resources for physical activity participation: does availability and accessibility differ by neighbourhood socioeconomic status? *Annals of Behavioural Medicine*, 25(2):100–104.

EU. (2006). *EU Platform on Diet, Physical Activity and Health*. Synopsis: Commitments 2006. Brussels: European Union.

EU. (2008). *EU Physical Activity Guidelines. Recommended Policy Actions in Support of Health-Enhancing Physical Activity*. Brussels: European Union.

Eyler, A. A., Brownson, R. C., Donatelle, R. J., King, A. C., Brown, D., & Sallis J. F. (1999). Physical activity social support and middle- and older aged minority women: results from a US survey. *Social Science & Medicine*, 49:781–789.

Frank, L. D., & Engelke, P. O. (2001). The built environment and human activity patterns: exploring the impacts of urban form on public health. *Journal of Planning Literature*, 16:202–218.

Frumkin, H., Frank, L., Jackson, R. (2004). *Urban Sprawl and Public Health*. Washington, DC: Island.

Fuchs, R. (1997). Psychologie und körperliche Bewegung [Psychologie and Physical Activity]. Göttingen (Germany): Hogrefe.

Giles-Corti, B., Donovan, R. J. (2002). The relative influence of individual, social and physical environment determinants of physical activity. *Social Science & Medicine*, 54:1793–1812.

Haskell, W. L., Lee, I., Pate, R. R., Powell, K. E., Blair, S. N., Franklin, B. A., et al. (2007). Physical activity and public health: Updated recommendation for adults from the American College of Sports Medicine and the American Heart Association. *Medicine and Science in Sports and Exercise*, 39:1423–1434.

Hillsdon, M., Foster, C., Cavill, N.,Crombie, H., & Naidoo, B. (2005). *The Effectiveness of Public Health Interventions for Increasing Physical Activity among Adults: A Review of Reviews*. London: Health Development Agency.

Humpel, N., Owen, N., & Leslie, E. (2002). Environmental factors associated with adults' participation in physical activity. *American Journal of Preventive Medicine*, 22:188–199.

Kawachi, I., Kennedy, B. P., & Glass, R. (1999a). Social capital and self-rated health: a contextual analysis. *American Journal of Public Health*, 89(8):1187–1193.

Kawachi, I., Kennedy, B. P., Lochner, K., & Prothrow-Smith, D. (1999b). Social capital, income inequality, and mortality. *American Journal of Public Health*, 87(9):1491–1498.

Kawachi, I., & Berkman, L. (2000). Social cohesion, social capital, and health. In: Ed. Kawachi, I., & Berkman, L. *Social Epidemiology*. New York: Oxford University Press.

King, A. C., Bauman, A., & Abrams, D. B. (2002). Forging transdisciplinary bridges to meet the physical inactivity challenge in the 21st century. *American Journal of Preventive Medicine*, 23(2S):104–106.

Lindström, M., Hanson, B. S., & Östergren, P. (2001). Socioeconomic differences in leisure-time physical activity: the role of social participation and social capital in shaping health related behaviour. *Social Science and Medicine*, 52:441–451.

Margetts, B. M., Rogers, E., Widhal, K., Remaut de Winter, A. M., & Zunft, H. J. F. (1999). Relationship between attitudes to health, body weight and physical activity and level of physical activity in a nationally representative sample in the European Union. *Public Health Nutrition*, 2(1a):97–103.

Matthews, S., Stansfeld, S., & Power, C. (1999). Social support at age 33: the influence of gender, employment status and social class. *Social Science & Medicine*, 49:133–142.

Munro, J., Brazier, J., Davey, R., & Nicholl, J. (1997). Physical activity for the over-65s: could it be a cost-effective exercise for the NHS? *Journal of Public Health Medicine*, 19(4):397–402.

Pate, R. R., Pratt, M., Blair, S. N., Haskell, W. L., Macera, C. A., Bouchard, C., et al. (1995). Physical activity and public health: a recommendation from the Centers for Disease Control and prevention and the American College of Sports Medicine. *JAMA*, 273:402–407.

Ross, C. E. (2000). Walking, exercising, and smoking. Does neighbourhood matter? *Social Science and Medicine*, 51(2):265–274.

Rütten, A., von Lengerke, T., Abel, T., Kannas, L., Lüschen, G., Rodriguez Diaz, J. A., et al. (2000). Policy, competence and participation: empirical evidence for a multilevel health promotion model. *Health Promotion International*, 15(1):35–47.

Rütten, A., Abel, T., Kannas, L., von Lengerke, T., Lüschen, G., Rodriguez Diaz, J. A., Vinck, J., et al. (2001). Self-reported physical activity, public health, and perceived environment: results from a comparative European study. *Journal of Epidemiology and Community Health*, 55(2):139–146.

Rütten, A., & Abu-Omar, K. (2004). Prevalence of Physical Activity in the European Union. *Sozial- und Präventivmedizin*, 49(4): 281–289.

Rütten, A., Abu-Omar, K., Lampert, T., & Ziese, T. (2005). *Gesundheitsberichterstattung des Bundes. Körperliche Aktivität.* Heft 26. Berlin: Robert Koch-Institut.

Rütten, A. (2006). Beyond sport and physical activity: the concept of movement in health promotion. Sozial- und Präventivmedizin 51:252–253.

Sallis, J. F., & Owen, N. (1998). *Physical Activity and Behavioural Medicine*. Thousand Oaks: Sage.

Sallis, J. F., Hovel, M. F., & Hofstetter, C. R. (1990). Distance between homes and exercise facilities related to frequency of exercise among San Diego residents. *Public Health Rep*, 105:179–185.

Sallis, J. F., Linton, L., & Kraft, M. K. (2005). The first active living research conference. Growth of a transdisciplinary field. *American Journal of Preventive Medicine*, 28(2S2):93–95.

Singh-Manoux, A., Hillsdon, M., Brunner, E., & Marmot, M. (2005). Effects of physical activity on cognitive functioning in middle age: evidence from the Whitehall II prospective cohort study. *American Journal of Public Health*, 95(12):2252–2258.

Sooman, A., & Macintyre, S. (1995). Health and perceptions of the local environment in socially contrasting neighbourhoods in Glasgow. *Health & Place*, 1(1):15–26.

Stahl, T., Rütten, A., Nutbeam, D., et al. (2001). The importance of the social environment for physically active lifestyle – results from an international study. Social Science & Medicine, 52:1–10.

Taylor, W. C., Baranowski, T., & Rohm Young, D. (1998). Physical activity interventions in low-income, ethnic minority, and populations with disability. *American Journal of Preventive Medicine*, 15:334–343.

US Department of Health and Human Services (1996). *Physical Activity and Health: A report of the Surgeon General*. Atlanta: Centres for Disease Control and Prevention.

U.S. Department of Health and Human Services. (2008). *Physical Activity Guidelines Advisory Committee. Physical Activity Guidelines Advisory Committee Report, 2008.* Washington, DC: US Government Printing Office.

US Department of Health and Human Services. (2000) *Healthy People 2010*. 2nd Edition. Washington, DC: US Government Printing Office.

Weuve, J., Kang, J. H., Manson, J. E., Breteler, M. M. B., Ware, J. H., & Grodstein, F. (2004). Physical activity, including walking, and cognitive function in older people. *JAMA*, 292(12):1454–1461.

WHO. (1948). Preamble to the Constitution of the World Health Organization as adopted by the International Health Conference, New York, 19–22 June, 1946; signed on 22 July 1946 by the representatives of 61 States and entered into force on 7 April 1948.

WHO (1986). *Ottawa Charter for Health Promotion*. First International Conference on Health Promotion. Ottawa, 21. November 1986. WHO/HPR/HEP/95.1.

WHO. (2002a). *The World Health Report 2002. Reducing Risk, Promoting Healthy Life*. Geneva: World Health Organisation.

WHO. (2002b). *A physically active life through everyday transport with a special focus on children and older people and examples and approaches from Europe*. WHO Regional Office for Europe.

WHO. (2006). *Promoting physical activity and active living in urban environments. The role of local governments*. WHO Regional Office Europe.

WHA. (2004). *Global Strategy on Diet, Physical Activity and Health. Resolution WHA55-23*. World Health Assembly.

Wieland, H., & Rütten, A. (1991). *Sport und Freizeit in Stuttgart. Sozialempirische Erhebung zur Sportnachfrage in einer Großstadt*. Stuttgart: Naglschmid Verlag.

Yen, I. H., & Kaplan, G. A. (1998). Poverty area residence and changes in physical activity level: evidence from the Alameda County Study. *American Journal of Public Health*, 88(11):1709–1712.

Zaza, S., Briss, P. A., & Harris, K. W., Eds. (2005). *The Guide to Community Preventive Services. What Works to Promote Health?* Task Force on Community Preventive Services. New York: Oxford University Press.

Chapter 12
Sustainable Community-Based Health and Development Programs in Rural India

Alok Mukhopadhyay and Anjali Gupta

Keywords India • Khoj • Inequalities • Community • Women • Infant mortality • Rural

12.1 Background

The 'Khoj' project is an initiative of Voluntary Health Association of India (VHAI), to bring about a holistic change in the lives of its beneficiaries by uplifting the socio-economic and health status of vulnerable communities. The Khoj project operates in the remote parts of the country and equitably involves the community members, organizational representatives, and other local bodies in all aspects of the project activities (see Table 12.1). The partners contribute unique strengths and shared responsibilities to enhance the health and development of the population. One of its objectives is to build on the inherent capacities of the community and create an enabling environment by incorporating the interrelated components of participation, networking and action. Khoj is based on the premise of developing healthy alliances with the community and creating conditions that allow people to improve their health and quality of life with a broad view of health encompassing social and environmental factors. Fundamental to the Khoj program's approach has been identifying important stakeholders for all health promotion initiatives and community involvement in each place and building on their strengths.

12.2 Introduction

Reaching out to the unreached is a global challenge and of a larger concern in India with one third of its population, constituting 250–300 million, living in remote, difficult and vulnerable areas and whose basic needs are not fulfilled. Despite

A. Mukhopadhyay (✉)
Voluntary Health Association of India, B-40, Qutab Institutional Area, New Delhi-110016, India
e-mail: ceo@vhai.org

A. Morgan et al. (eds.), *Health Assets in a Global Context: Theory, Methods, Action*,
DOI 10.1007/978-1-4419-5921-8_12,

Table 12.1 Statistical profile of some of the Khoj Projects – Health Indicators

	IMR (per 1000 live births)		No. of maternal deaths		% of women receiving complete ANC		% of deliveries conducted by TBA		Immunization coverage	
PROJECT	2000	2006	2000	2006	2000	2006	2000	2006	2000	2006
SHHC, Bihar	62	25	10	4	64	86	63	95	74	92
PANI, Uttar Pradesh	44	34	5	1	78.8	83.1	72.8	96	78.7	94.1
MSK Chandauli, Varanasi, Uttar Pradesh	50	53	1	1	68	100	76	98	50	75
ECAT Karauli, Rajasthan	36.8	50.6	1	NIL	85	95	83	81	74	80
Shramjivi Unnayan Chattisgarh	52	30	5.2%	2.3%	53	94	61	98	53	98
CREFTDA Orissa	72	68.9	NIL	NIL	56	71	96.6	97	67.7	83
SURE, Barmer, Rajasthan	85.5	25.7	-	1	83.4	92	92.7	98	53.8	82.2
Nagaland VHA	46	32	2	1	56	85	20	50	52	80
Arunachal VHA	52	20	7	2	38	53	45	41	27	56

ANC antenatal care, *IMR* infant mortality rate, *TBA* traditional birth attendant

Source: The table is cited from VHAI Report (2007), "Khoj-A Search for Innovations and Sustainability in Community Health and Development, VHAI, New Delhi, pp. 25.

Box 12.1 Jodhpur

In 1993, life for 50,000 inhabitants of twenty project villages spread over 12,000 km^2 in Osian block of Jodhpur district in the heart of the inhospitable Thar Desert, was undeniably very hard. In addition to harsh climatic conditions, the area lacks adequate infrastructure. Water shortage is a serious problem all the year round. Summers are very hot with temperatures going as high as 50 °C. Furthermore, the population is widely scattered and there are very few roads and little public transport, which makes people highly vulnerable to worsening health and socioeconomic situation. When the Khoj project began, health situation, especially women's health and social status was appalling in the twenty project villages. Poverty and unemployment were extensive and literacy level was dismal. Many villagers suffered from cholera, malaria, leucorrhoea, anemia, and other infectious diseases. Virtually no women used family planning or had any antenatal care. Serious pregnancy-related complications were common, and maternal death rates were high. This called for focused health intervention.

A decade later, the picture has changed dramatically. Antenatal care was introduced for the first time in the area. Morbidity has reduced considerably. In 2002–2003 itself, more than 4,500 patients were treated in OPDs[1] for a variety of ailments and special camps like malaria camps were also organized. Laboratory facility is available for pathological tests.

Much of the improvement is credited to the community centric approach of the Khoj Project "Gramin Vikas Vigyan Samity (GRAVIS)," the vision of Voluntary Health Association of India (VHAI) trying to improve the lives of the rural poor.

Khoj is a concept of community based health care being implemented by VHAI through partner organisations. The project related conceptual thinking as well as the mid course correction is done by VHAI through the empowerment of the local groups. GRAVIS who knows the pulse of the local community develops and upscales the programme keeping in context the local realities. The community-based health program that began in 20 villages in 1993 now concentrates on other villages, which were falling within a radius of 250–300 km in Jodhpur.

several achievements and efforts, the 50 years of development plan has not changed the lives of almost half of India's population. As per the United Nations Development Programme's (UNDP) Human Development Report 2001, India still ranks at 115th place (UNDP 2001). As far as women are concerned, the Gender-related Development Index (GDI) for India is 105, a rating classed by the United Nations as "medium human development."

[1]Out Patient Department (OPD) in hospitals provides health promotion diagnostic and therapeutic services to patients who need hospital services without; the need to be admitted. It includes references made from outside doctors, patients coming on their own, references from private clinics investigations recommendations and civil hospital references, etc.

The continuing poverty of the rural poor is mainly due to structural constraints in improving their livelihood and securing their well-being in terms of parameters of health, education and gender equity. Analysis of available qualitative and quantitative data clearly shows extremely uneven health and development progress in various parts of the country. Even within the states that are doing reasonably well, there remain regions where little has changed since independence. Much of this deprived population lives in remote, difficult and vulnerable areas. Findings of a district level survey by VHAI (Health For the Millions 2004 and ICDHI Monograph, VHAI 2004; 2007), to assess the extent of state variations in regard to health indicators based on the data generated by National Family Health Survey 2005–2006 (IIPS 2007), Census of India 2001 (Office of the Registrar General & Census Commissioner 2001), and Rapid Household Survey 1998–1999 (IIPS 2001), Government of India (GOI), further confirm the widespread impoverishment of the masses in terms of health care education, basic needs and income insecurity. *The survey suggested a three-sector model 'GOPIN' where 'GO' stands for Government departments, 'PI' for Panchayati Raj Institutions*[2] *and 'N' stands for non government groups (NGOs). Confluence of all these three bodies at the district /constituency level can bring about a tremendous improvement in the daily lives of masses* (VHAI 2004).

These vivid differences along with the wide variations in the health situation in various states, suggest that there is no simple, central solution for India's health challenge. Numerous programs, which oriented Government and other development agencies to take initiatives in these areas, have not been able to make any significant change. It has remained a challenge for serious minded organizations to evolve a strategy and process, addressing the various social determinants affecting the health of the population, to make a paradigm shift. NGOs are expected to perform a significant role including: mobilizing local initiative and resources; building self reliant sustainable social capital; moderating between government and people; transforming the attitude of people; facilitating development education; building on the assets of the individuals communities, etc. Hence it is important to study the functioning of NGOs and governmental organizations in using the asset model to address the health inequities. Asset model as particularly defined in the Ottawa Charter (WHO 1986) emphasizes the need to strengthen local communities – the model through asset mapping promotes the process of community empowerment to encourage their ownership and control of their own endeavors. It also supports the development of personal skills through its salutogenic approach to health development. This asset model promotes a multi method approach to evaluation using a set of salutogenic indicators to measure the effectiveness of programs and initiatives aiming to contribute to the reduction of health inequities.

[2]Panchayati Raj is a system of governance in which gram panchayats are the basic units of administration. It has 3 levels: village, block and district. At the village level, it is called a Panchayat. It is a local body working for the good of the village. The number of members usually ranges from 7 to 31; occasionally, groups are larger, but they never have fewer than seven members. The block-level institution is called the Panchayat Samiti. The district-level institution is called the Zilla Parishad. (http://en.wikipedia.org/wiki/Panchayati_Raj).

In this broader context of Indian state's commitment to achieve "health for all," this chapter attempts to study the cross cutting intervention of an NGO to bring about a holistic change in the lives of the communities by uplifting their socioeconomic and health status. The success story of Khoj, a VHAI project operational in the remote rural parts of the country is discussed. This chapter tries to establish the fact that *"we cannot achieve health for all without building on the strengths of the people."*[3] In the Khoj project there is no concept of recipients as the community is involved in managing the development efforts, as well as figuring out how to obtain the resources needed, (locally if possible). With a vision to create an enabling climate for an overall sociopolitical development of the community in the difficult terrains of the country, Khoj begins with developing an understanding of the social, economic, cultural and political dynamics of the community, and integrates the knowledge gained with action to improve the health and well-being of community members.

The chapter is divided into three parts. The first part of this chapter briefly outlines the Health Sector in India – status and trends with a focus on the health inequities in the country. The second part discusses in detail the community-centric sustainable strategy of Khoj in three difficult settings, and its impact on the overall well being of the population. The final part contains major findings and concluding remarks.

12.3 Health Inequities in India

Health is an important factor in development and is closely related to socioeconomic and other factors. India is undergoing a dramatic demographic, societal, and economic transformation. However, the health status of the residents of India still lags behind relative to other populations, and the health gains in each country have been uneven across subpopulations. Although they have achieved substantial advances in life expectancy and disease prevention since the middle of the 20th century, the Indian health systems provide little protection against financial risk, and most importantly there is widespread inequity in the health status of the population. It is now clearly indicated that the poor have much higher levels of mortality, malnutrition and fertility than the rich; the poor–rich risk ratio is 2.5 for infant mortality, 2.8 for under-five mortality, 1.7 for underweight children and 2 for total fertility rate (Peters et al. 2001). Childhood diseases like diarrhea, anemia, etc., are also more prevalent among low-income households compared to high income households (IIPS 2000). The health sector in India is still characterized by sharp socioeconomic, rural-urban and gender inequalities.

It is essential to thus understand that the all India health scenario disguises the most important feature of the population's health status – that there are significant

[3]Quote from: Baba Amte, Ramon Magsaysay Award Winner for Public Service during his meeting with Alok Mukhopadhyay in Hemalkasa project in Maharashtra.

differences in the patterns of morality, fertility and morbidity within regions and states. Progress has been uneven, and has been confined to advanced, approachable and progressive areas. Vulnerable areas which are hilly, tribal, arid, drought prone, flood prone, marshy and coastal continue to make a slower rate of progress. The more remote, sparsely populated and resource poor an area is, the greater the chances of its neglect in terms of availability and effectiveness of health services. The consequence of this has been neglected areas, forgotten populations and overlooked issues. For instance, the stretch of tribal areas extending from West Bengal to Maharashtra and Gujarat record high levels of morbidity, arising out of poor nutrition, forced displacement and changes in trade lifestyles. The population in the desert and arid zones of the Western frontier, sub-Himalayan hilly and Teri tracts in Bihar, Jammu & Kashmir and Uttar Pradesh – be they tribals, scheduled castes, displaced or migrant population in search of work, remained under-served, ignored and are forced to meekly accept a lower quality of life. These wide variations across the country further add to the task at policy level. It's clear that it is important to develop an appropriate strategy, which addresses these variations while achieving its objectives for the country per se. Prognosis for the health sector in India is thus a challenging task.

12.4 Policy Environment

During the last few decades, the country has failed in its effort to reach out to the people living in the vulnerable areas. This inequality greatly impairs successful outreach of social, economic and political benefits to a large sector of our citizens. It was realized that many facets of inequity need to be addressed, to successfully bring social, economic and political benefits to a large sector of India's vunrable population.

Inequity that affects the health sector in India could be broadly categorized as follows:

1. Economic – In spite of focused and priority steps to address the problems of the poor, the nation still has 32% of the population living below the poverty line.
2. Political – In spite of adult franchise, representation of the poor families in governance in India has been limited.
3. Social – Distorted cast system has put a very large section of our population in considerable disadvantage vis-à-vis their social and economic mobility.
4. Gender Issues – Like most developing countries, the gender inequity has been a considerable impediment towards the progress in health and development in India.
5. Locational Problems – Far flung, cut off areas and ecologically vulnerable areas where large section of the population live.

India realizes that a paradigm shift in the prevailing situation of inequity is only possible if there is a change in the fundamentals of legal, social and political rights of the poor and under-privileged. The situation in India is also complicated by the fact that we are an extra-ordinarily heterogeneous nation with people from a variety of cultural and ethnic backgrounds. Being a democratic pluralistic nation, it is impossible to thrust a particular view of social transformation quickly and assertively. It is essential for the country to carry its people along in major decisions of social, economic, and political development, which means a long and sometimes frustrating consensus building process.

To address these issues of inequity in the recent times, some very radical measures have been taken by the GOI. These measures include: the 73rd Constitutional Amendment giving the responsibility of local level governance and development to the elected representatives of the people both in the rural as well as urban areas; special quota for employment for scheduled castes and scheduled tribes; active involvement of civil society in fulfilling the promises of health and development to the citizens. Despite such policy measures, the abysmal health and development indicators confirm the need for some innovative community based approach.

After many years of government under funding, India has committed to sizable increases in government investment in health. Although the public expenditure on health is still low – 0.85 of the Gross Domestic Product (GDP), there are now launches of ambitious programs like the National Rural Health Mission. It has been also recognized that the poor and rural populations are particularly disadvantaged in obtaining access to health care and face major financial risk in the event of illness. Thus, explicit policies are being developed to target the government's funding towards the poor and rural populations.

To date, however, the country doesn't have a systematic policy for reducing the inefficiencies in service provision and managing health spending inflation – a fundamental cause of unaffordable health care and heavy financial risk. It is still too early to know whether the additional government investment (channeled through insurance coverage and health facility infrastructure strengthening) will produce benefits for the people, in terms of increasing access to healthcare, reducing financial risk, improving health status, and reducing inequalities in health and healthcare. However, our view is that money alone will not be sufficient to deliver effective, high-quality care. Unless we make the health system community oriented by making the target group i.e., the community itself the subject of process. The existing policies still focus on the needs of the community whereas the conceptual framework gaining ground in rural development is "asset based" development (Allen 2007). In the asset based community development, as followed by Khoj projects in various rural settings, community members were purposively grouped together based on their needs and existing capabilities. The communities were found to be flexible and welcoming towards any support aimed at improving their basic situation. This has been identified as an important asset helping the projects like Khoj to work constructively on the existing skills in the community members and providing them new avenues to grow. With some initial support community members have the ability to organize amongst themselves to work towards common goals more proactively. Communities build personal and community capital through an efficient management of their traditional skills, improved farming methods, and a natural resource base such as enhanced water use capacity, irrigation systems and forestry.

In India nearly 70% of the population lives in remote areas/villages, these people are often the most under privileged section of the society. The aim is to reach this segment of the population with a multi faceted approach aimed at an overall development of the individual and the community at grassroot level. Community involvement, self reliance and sustainability through efficient NGOs are the key factors.

The chapter focuses on the efficiency of Khoj, alternative strategies for health promotion and overall development, successfully practiced in villages/remote/difficult terrains of the country. Khoj strategies have been in implementation in more than 20 different locations of the country since 1993 and have helped create replicable examples that can be quickly adapted to a variety of contexts. The following section discusses in detail this community based health and development project in the unreached areas of India.

12.5 Community-Based Health and Development Programme – Khoj: An Innovation for Further Adoption

Against this backdrop, an innovative approach called Khoj, was developed to tackle health and development issues. The approach evolved from VHAI's deep concern to find the breakthrough to improve the health status of people living in remote and difficult areas and generally having extremely low economic status. Khoj is a Hindi word, which literally means 'search'. The philosophy of Khoj is to search for innovative methods and strategies to combat community health related problems. Khoj also aims to search for viable alternatives to the existing health care development model being followed by the government and also some voluntary organizations. Khoj puts this philosophy into practice by building upon the strengths of community and lending support to innovative projects by small voluntary organizations in neglected areas which can be replicated elsewhere without the recurring requirements of heavy infrastructure or investment which besiege some of the larger projects. This approach perhaps is an extension of the salutogenic model of health promotion based on the key premise of *involving community in improving health situation and an overall development.* The project helps the community to move towards better health as a facilitator.

Khoj is one of the long-term initiatives of VHAI, being implemented since 1993. The Khoj project is located in some of the most remote and difficult areas of our country. These areas have high mortality and morbidity rates and practically no semblance of health services. The overall concept and framework of Khoj – a community based health and development programme was carefully planned on the premise of having greater relative advantage, *compatibility*, potential for *replicability*, minimum or *no complexity* and *observability* (Tandon et al. 2007).

Box 12.2 Definitions of Key Characteristics Ensuring Community Health and Development

- *Relative Advantage*: The degree to which an innovation is perceived as better than the idea it supersedes
- *Compatibility*: The degree to which an innovation is perceived as being consistent with existing values, past experiences, and needs of potential adopters
- *Complexity*: The degree to which an innovation is perceived as difficult to understand and use
- *Replicability*: The degree to which an innovation may be experimented elsewhere
- *Observability*: The degree to which the results of an innovation are visible to others

With these key characteristics Khoj has proven to be a successful example in the field of community health and development for improving the health status of the entire community through an integrated approach.

12.6 Khoj Initiative – Programme Approach and Outreach

Following various parameters outlined in Box 12.3, VHAI identified 21 pockets in the country to initiate the Khoj project. While identifying these locations, it was ensured that they sufficiently represent social, economic, political, geographical and ethnic varieties of the country. These locations are broadly in the physically hard areas like the remote mountains and desert areas, areas mainly inhabited by the indigenous people, and heartland India. In these areas, social, economic and gender status are highly polarized and the overall feudal infrastructure is still not dismantled. Our premise was that the experience of working in these diverse areas will give us enough experiential learning to upscale similar initiatives in most of the vulnerable pockets of the country.

12.6.1 Khoj Strategies

At the conceptual level, the project emphasized development that was truly participatory and sustainable in nature. Direct health related activities were given primary importance during the initial years and gradually, with improvement in the health patterns, other developmental activities were focused upon. While finalizing the approach to our work for these pockets, we felt that (1) we should go with an open mind and develop the project depending on the local basic needs as expressed by the people; (2) utilize the existing government infrastructures as optimally as possible;

Box 12.3 Khoj – A Vision for Progress in Community Health and Development Partnerships

1. *Khoj Initiative – Programme Approach and Outreach*
   - Partnership challenges and relationship to health and development
   - Khoj strategies
   - Experimental designs to assess Khoj impact
   - Outcomes
   - Sustainability
2. *Work-in-Progress and Lessons Learned*
   - Building community partnerships
   - Engaging community members in implementation
   - Training community partners
   - Challenges in working in difficult terrains
   - Sustainability, community ownership
   - Formative work
   - Sustainability
3. *Practical Tools*
   - Resources/tools to develop community partners' skills
   - Monitoring and Evaluation strategies
   - Systematic guidelines for project implementation and validating
   - Behavioral intervention to culturally diverse groups
   - The success/failure of community based approach
   - How to use local, state, and national data sources to help community partners with their service delivery and grant opportunities – sustainability
   - How to provide effective feedback and communication
4. *Systematic Review*
   - Reviews of Khoj methods
   - Review of Khoj effectiveness
   - Role of Khoj in empowering community and making the project sustainable
   - Community perspectives on role of Khoj projects

(3) identify and build local health and development skills and expertise; (4) use sustainable initiatives, from financial as well as human resources; and (5) ensure that on the whole it not only affects health and development status of the people, but ensures a permanent capacity building of the community. The initial phase involved mapping the existing services and potential of the community members. Another critical aspect was to identify local project partners in the voluntary sector, who may not have tremendous experience, but are motivated and are also rooted in the local community.

12.7 Work-in-Progress and Lessons Learned

VHAI in close collaboration with its state voluntary health associations (SVHAs) after the identification of the project area and the implementing agency performed the following key tasks:

Practical Tools to develop community Khoj partners' skills:

- Help in selecting of staff and their orientation
- Microplanning
- Assisting NGOs in the preparation of action plans based on the needs identified and also the narrative reports
- Providing support in setting up project management and financial management information systems
- Reporting format on the progress of the project
- Actively support the Khoj project in times of crisis or emergency
- Participating actively in monitoring and evaluation of the project in collaboration with VHAI
- Conducting relevant training programs for the project partners who in turn provide training to grassroots level workers
- Advising the project partners to comply with the project agreement particularly project related accounting and reporting based on the agreement between VHAI and the project partners
- Reminding the project partners of reporting in case of delays and ensuring that the request documents are submitted
- Visiting projects periodically for monitoring and evaluation and providing appropriate technical support to project partners
- Considering flexibility in the case of unforeseen deviation from the original action plan and implementing certain activities, which may not have been envisaged earlier, but have later became necessary

12.8 Khoj Thrust Areas of Work

The thrust areas of work of development initiative taken up under this programme can be classified as follows:

- Health
- Community development
- Gender rights – women empowerment
- Right based approach
- Environment

Over a period of time, a marked change has been seen in the previously mentioned areas in the Khoj project. However, all the project areas are at different stages of achievement due to differences in the time of their initiation and considerable variations in local geography, culture, political scenario, and law and order situation.

12.9 Health Interventions

Since the beginning, health interventions were used to develop rapport with the community so as to ensure their fullest participation in the overall development process for the area. Health interventions were mainly used as an entry point. From the baseline in most of the project areas, it was apparent that there was not any access to quality healthcare. In such projects, the emphasis in the initial phase was much more on provision of curative services. The curative services were provided by a team comprising of village health workers, a trained supervisor, and a medical doctor. To take care of emergencies and provide supervised care, a small Khoj health centre has been established in most of the projects for indoor admission and a small field laboratory managed by a qualified doctor and nurse. In most of the places, villagers or panchayats provide land either free or at a nominal cost. In addition, health camps and relief camps in epidemic like situations such as malaria, diarrhea, etc. are organized from time to time. Each project has developed linkages for proper referral of complicated cases. The projects have also developed rapport with some of the local doctors to provide specialized care on a regular basis.

12.9.1 Women and Health

In the development of community health, priority has been placed on addressing the entire range of women's health needs; both for their own sake and for the effects that women's health has on community health. Women's health status has been given due consideration throughout their entire life span from young girls to reproductive age women, to menopausal and postmenopausal women. Khoj projects have adopted a holistic approach to reproductive health. This has enabled the projects to initiate an attitudinal change towards women's health not just in terms of their reproductive capacity but also in terms of their basic rights.

12.9.2 Specific Health Issues

In almost all the areas, malaria, diarrhea and measles were extremely common. All three were the major cause of not only high morbidity, but also high mortality. Almost 40% of child deaths were due to these problems. Now each project has been able to control mortality and morbidity because of these diseases. In most of the areas, there were no epidemics in 1999. Similarly, most of the projects did not have deaths due to diarrhea or malaria.

12.9.3 Health Promotion

In the Khoj projects, curative component is an important but small component. The major focus is on health promotion and prevention of diseases by improved communication through village health workers as well as Mahila Mandals and Youth Clubs members. Right from the beginning, the efforts were made to develop need based area specific communication strategy. Different tools more suitable for the particular area were used for government health services and health education.

12.10 Community Organization

With a focus on the existing assets of the community, all the projects have taken effective steps to organize people's groups at different levels in the project villages. The formation of these groups has ensured a comprehensive relationship between the project and the community. These groups are mainly in the form of:

Village health committees (VHC) – composed of representatives from different groups who come together and decide the future plans and strategies for health and development-related work to be undertaken in the villages. This process has also ensured that community has a say in the decision making process. This has also given a strong feeling of ownership to the community and has enhanced their involvement in all stages of the project.

These community groups have been women's groups (Mahila Mandals), youth groups and farmers groups, self help groups (SHGs), village development committees (VDCs); village education committees; village old people's associations (VOPAs). The people's organizations are democratic and engage people from all sections of the community to manage the development efforts, as well as figure out how to obtain the resources needed, locally if possible. The communities are thus endowed to carry on the development initiatives without further assistance from VHAI – and are able to attain self-reliance.

Each community has its own assets like traditional healing, local artisans and above all a desire to work together. Khoj projects looked at these assets and helped the communities in overcoming the initial hindrances and made the various groups which have been instrumental in sustaining the project and bringing about a holistic change in the socioeconomic situation of the masses.

The deficit model as mentioned in Chap. 1 focuses more on the needs of the community. Khoj, working with the asset mapping approach instead, calls them the key focus areas which need to be improved through the efforts of the community (see Box 12.4). This has been done in various settings like Kashmir/Orissa, where the untapped local skills of the artisans were promoted through the right channels and helped the community in generating self revenue and thus bringing an overall improvement in their health and living conditions.

Box 12.4 Needs and asset based approaches to community development

Traditional Model: Need based Community Development:
Based on – Needs
Goal – Institutional Change
Conversation – Problems and Concerns
Change Agent – Power
View of Individual – Consumer/Client
Needs are based on Community Problems:
Broken families, child abuse, crime, gangs, housing, illiteracy, school drop outs, unemployment, etc.
Alternative Model: Asset Based Community Development:
Based on – Assets
Goal – Building Communities
Conversation – Gifts and Dreams
Change Agent – Relationship
View of Individual – Producer/Owner
Assets are based on Community Treasures:
Artistes, clubs, community groups, cultural groups, farms, hospitals, parks, youth, senior citizens, etc.

Source: Allen (2007)

12.10.1 Education

Some of the Khoj projects have initiated non-formal education centres for school dropouts. It has helped not only in improving the literacy level but also developing rapport between the community and the project.

12.10.2 Community Development

Khoj is a health initiative which tries from the beginning to address the conditions responsible for ill health. Major strategies adopted for community development are capacity building, income generation programmes and education.

12.10.3 Capacity Building

The process of capacity building involved vocational training, training for other income generation activities, more effective utilization of locally available resources and entrepreneurship development.

12.10.4 Income Generation Programme

These include vocational trainings, promotion of local crafts (training/marketing support) and entrepreneurship development.

12.10.5 Formation of Self Help Groups

SHGs are usually groups of seven to ten women who are encouraged to make periodic savings, and are linked with banks. Women use this money either to initiate some income generation activity or to take a loan for the treatment of sickness or buying seeds, etc.

12.10.6 Livestock Improvement

Since most of the Khoj projects are in rural areas, artificial insemination was used to help communities improve livestock breeds. Projects also provide technical support on how to maintain the animals.

12.10.7 Environment

Improving the village environment, sanitation, and drinking water. Related project activities including proper care of drinking water sources and village drains by villagers themselves, aforestation, prevention of deforestation, preservation of natural resources, kitchen gardening and horticulture.

12.10.8 Collaboration with the Government

The trend towards collaboration with the government is increasing. The following activities are the mainstay:

- Health: Immunization programme, family planning programme, health camps, workshops (as resource persons from the government), referrals
- Sanitation and drinking water: linkages with government funding agencies, block offices and panchayats
- Direct benefits under various government schemes
- Training of panchayat members

- Recognition of the projects by state governments as seen by handing over of primary health centers (PHCs)[4] in Arunachal Pradesh, Orissa, etc., training of animators and direct financial support to projects for specific activities.

12.10.9 Sustainability

Sustainability is an essential feature of the Khoj project. Right from the very beginning, conscious efforts were made to select sustainable interventions. Some of these efforts are in the direction of:

- Sustainable income generation programs
- Emphasis on human resources development
- Strengthening local panchayats
- Developing local leadership and linkages with government and other agencies

Ensuring sustainable impact requires consistent efforts over considerable time periods. In the case of Khoj initiatives in rural settings, this has meant concerted efforts at a grassroots level before the results and subsequent impact on the quality of life is visible.

12.10.10 Monitoring, Reporting and Evaluation

Systematic guidelines for project implementation and validating have been developed. The evaluation strategy for the Khoj project is precisely based on asset mapping of the community. It is target free and carefully designed, comprising of both qualitative and quantitative aspects.

Systematic reviews of the Khoj methods; effectiveness of Khoj intervention and the role of Khoj in empowering community and making the project sustainable are undertaken on a regular basis. Monitoring of the Khoj projects is a participatory and ongoing process in which VHAI, state VHAs, project staff, and village committees are involved. Professionals from VHAI visit these projects on a regular basis. To assess the community perspectives on the role of Khoj projects, the process of project evaluation and impact assessment involves intensive interactions with the community, the village committees, people's groups, and the project staff. The project records and reports are also scrutinized.

Findings of the baseline survey act as the reference point to be checked after a considerable duration for the changes brought in various health and social indicators

[4]Primary Health Centers are the first contact pint between the village community and the medical officer. It is manned by a Medical Officer and 14 other staff. It acts as a referral point for six subcentres and has 4–6 beds for patients. It performs curative, preventive, promotive and family welfare services. Each PHC is targeted to cover a population of 30,000 in plain area and 20,000 in hilly/tribal area.

like infant mortality rate (IMR), maternal mortality rate, SHGs formed and savings of SHGs.

The village health workers maintain monthly records and vital statistics that are checked by the supervisor who reports to the programme coordinator. Doctors maintain clinical records and morbidity profile. Quarterly, half yearly and annual narrative and financial reports are sent to VHAI. A meeting of all the Khoj partners and VHAI is also held annually. This is followed by a mid-term evaluation in all the projects. This includes a scrutiny of the statistical figures and also focus group discussions, adding a qualitative dimension to our evaluation of the project.

12.10.11 Impact and Achievements

The impact of the strategy tried out by the Khoj project should be assessed seriously. As discussed previously the Khoj project has successfully enhanced the knowledge, attitude and practice of community members on health, nutrition, water and sanitation. To bring in women empowerment, SHGs have been formed and linked with banks. Non-formal schools operated by projects have created an opportunity for the deprived children to achieve their right to primary education. Some of the current activities include capacity building of the state VHAs, local NGOs partners and the second line management staff through exposure visits to other development projects and training workshops on various health and development issues by VHAI. Some of the positive outcomes of initiatives towards community organisation are:

- Mobilization of village committees
- Formation of social action groups to optimize government resources
- Effective linkages with panchayats

The health impact of the Khoj project can be summarized as:

- Increased health awareness reflected by reduced time lag between onset of symptoms and reporting to health functionaries
- Increased utilization of available government health services
- Significant improvement in antenatal care, natal care and post natal care
- Reduction in mortality, especially due to communicable diseases like diarrhea, malaria, acute respiratory infections (ARI), as well as due to pregnancy and associated complications
- Effective diseases surveillance leading to prevention of epidemics from taking place
- Significant reduction in health expenditure as the quality health services including laboratory services are available within a reasonable distance and reasonable cost

In the annexure section we have discussed briefly the strategy, impact and learning gained in two areas of the Khoj project in different and difficult settings; in Shivpuri, a tribal belt of Madhya Pradesh and in the post disaster Orissa.

12.11 Key Learnings

The Khoj project focuses on asset building, and has been successful in achieving a holistic change in the lives of communities in some of the most remote and underserved rural areas of the country. This was possible only because of the following key factors:

- Strategic planning – Planning needs to be done from the onset with the local community
- Identification and building on the community's strengths
- Multidimensional approach – responding to various socio-economic determinants to bring about a change in the health and general condition of the population
- Creative partnering within the community and external environments need to be forged. Most importantly, communities need to control the process. The ultimate goal is for communities to have the confidence and competence to make informed choices from a range of appropriate options for sustainable and equitable development

Two key themes that emerged in this project were the importance of engaging community in positive activities, and providing opportunities for development. Positive activities ranged from: learning about their culture; forming village development committees and SHGs, especially of women; and networking with the local leaders, government, and organizations. The opportunities include: participation training and skill-development; promoting indigenous medicine; promoting community networking with the government and other agencies; and educational workshops on various schemes and programs.

In the early stages of the project's development it became apparent (mainly because of the team members comprised of local residents) that certain environmental realities had to be addressed. For example, the Khoj project in the Faizabad district of Uttar Pradesh state, known for the endemic caste conflict, intense gender stratification and political unrest, worked intensely to empower the community for its own development. A maternal and child health program was the core point of focus during project implementation with the vulnerable community. The source of the project's success was the formation of SHGs of women in this environment. Under the project, various activities were taken up and the nature, dimension and magnitude kept on changing as project progressed with time. For sake of simplicity, these activities were categorized in two major programme sectors: (1) community health promotion and (2) community development programme. In the first category, Khoj has initiated various activities like: activating and supplementing health facilities; maternal and child health programme; organization of a health camp; health education programme; training of traditional birth attendants (TBA); training of health monitors; preparation and distribution of information education and communication (IEC) material; school health programme; creating a cleaner health environment; promotion of personal hygiene; open well care; and hand pump maintenance. The community development programme also included school health programme as well as: community based organizations[5]; income generation activities; promotion of self help groups; activating existing institutions like panchayati raj institutions (PRIs); capacity building activities; and linkages with other programmes.

The project has been able to achieve these objectives by strengthening and activating community health systems. The project innovated and adopted strategic approaches like taking low cost traditional agricultural practices among small and marginal farmers on one hand and emphasized new agricultural practices on the other. The project provides routine motivation for entrepreneurship development of a target community through a motivator. During 2005–2006, a total of 60 entrepreneurs were facilitated through Rs. 10,77,000 micro-finance mobilized through banks, which has led to an improved quality of life.

As a principle it has been important to shift ownership of projects to the community to ensure sustainability. The process was important and flexibility was essential to the overall outcome. It was also important to understand that circumstances within each community were dictated by its particular socio-economic and cultural issues.

For example, the problems of the communities in the Thar Deserts of Rajasthan were different from those of a cyclone affected community, or the tribals. A Khoj project in the valley of Kashmir with long standing armed conflicts, had a culturally sensitive approach while discussing issues of health, family planning and safe deliveries. The project area remains cut off due to snow for almost six months in a year, thus careful planning for health and medical services was required. Since the community has faced hardships for many years due to the armed conflicts in the state, an integrated health and development program was initiated by the Khoj project, gradually involving the local community and NGOs. It addressed the issue of chronic poverty and started appropriate income generation, literacy, women's empowerment and vocational training programs, thus building upon the capacities of the community for their overall development.

The feasibility of long-term partnerships with targeted local small scale organisations across the country needs to be scoped. This should take into account the fact that a significant number of these organizations have limited capacity to develop, implement and sustain reconciliation initiatives at the local level. To ensure sustainability, it is imperative that strategic alliances are identified at a national, state, regional and local level, and that community participation examples are explored. The Khoj projects creatively pooled the community's physical and financial resources, along with human and social capital. We focused earlier on building the capacity of the organiza-

[5]"Community Based Organizations (CBOs) are grassroots organisation, locally based membership organisations that work to develop their own communities. The most common types of CBOs are local development associations, such as village councils which represent an entire community and interest associations such as women clubs which represent a particular section of the community. Third group includes borrowers' groups, cooperatives which may make profit but are different from the private business due to their community development goals." (The challenge of slums: global report on human settlements, 2003, United Nations Human Settlements Programme (UN-Habitat), Nairobi, 2003, pp.151).

tions, and the local communities. That meant entering into relationships and partnerships being clear that Khoj was not going to run the projects forever, but build upon the capacities of the local organizations and the communities to do so.

Most importantly the value of women in the overall community development has been realized. Empowered women are able to contribute fully to the development process and should not be seen as a side issue, but central to and in the process. In all the different Khoj settings women's groups have been formed, trained, and involved in the income generation activities and health improvement efforts.

Another most important lesson learnt was need of perseverance in face of challenges. Challenges were not unexpected in the steps towards improving community health and an overall development: however, these challenges served to highlight the need for this project. In the beginning there were some difficulties experienced as a consequence of the community members reluctant to get involved or take any initiative. However, as time passed, the community and the Khoj project workers got to know each other and began working together. The need for consistency in all the programs is of utmost importance to bring about the desired impact. People are a part of the solution, not just the target. Their vulnerability needs to be reduced by building on their capacities and developing thier skills. Social mobilization can be a very effective tool of reaching and involving individuals, families, communities and government at various levels. This is only a part of the project, however; it does not show the background to the process of creating an empowered community in some of the most deprived, difficult terrains of the country. The project has been an innovative community based health and development tool in itself as it has facilitated and pioneered the development of good governance models based on community ownership in the country.

12.12 Conclusion

> "Development really is the process of expansion of individual freedom, which, in turn, is a function of people's capabilities and opportunities."

Amartya Sen, winner of the 1998 Nobel Prize for Economics. (Agarwal and Sarasua 2002)

In a large, complex yet vibrant country like India, promoting health is a challenging task, but given the size of the population of the country it also holds the key to dramatic change in global health situation. Happily, the solutions to these complex problems clearly exist in many innovative successful experiments within the country itself. It is a matter of concern that a large part of the existing health structure of the government within the country is operating in an unimaginative manner, which does not inspire confidence about their ability to cope effectively with the current problems and future challenges. Restructuring and revitalizing the sector is an urgent need.

In most parts of the country, the key to improving people's health lies in larger areas of social and economic development. Therefore, policy makers, health professionals and activists need to take a more committed interest on these issues in every possible complex setting. Involvement of the larger civil society including the community, traditional healers, NGOs and private sector can make significant difference in all aspects of health and development. Until now, serious pro-active efforts have not been made towards their larger involvement.

In most of the rural communities of India, health and social infrastructure is inadequate and the governance has been poor, affecting the overall well being of communities. Thus proactive efforts are required to ensure that the benefits of various government policies and programmes reach the expected beneficiaries. It has been noted that the government approach has been insensitive and missing a creative dimension to address the developmental problems. Therefore our effort has been to provide an ingenious dimension by involving the community and helping them to build on their assets/capabilities in order to bring an overall improvement in their health, social and economic status. This approach makes the effort sustainable in the long term and provides an example for the government system to follow elsewhere.

Success has been shown over the years through an overall improvement in the various health and development indices of India's underserved communities living in difficult and remote parts of the country. Khoj exemplifies the need of identifying and building on the capabilities of the communities, unlike most other development projects based on the problems and needs of the community. The Khoj project is based on the following key premises:

1. Focusing and reinforcing the local capabilities, especially of the underprivileged sections, has been an integral component of the project.
2. Exploring the untapped potential of the smaller grassroots level projects that have been working towards the promotion of community health and development, but have been hindered from attaining excellence either due to paucity of resources or capabilities.
3. VHAI has taken up the "scaling up" of the beneficiary coverage, activity portfolio and the institutional sustainability as one of the core concerns in all its Khoj projects. In many ways scaling up has been a natural, almost organic, process for most of the Khoj projects. The motive remained to scale up the impact rather than making the organization larger.

We obviously need a new paradigm of healthcare, far removed from the current bio-medical model and closer to a sociopolitical and spiritual model. The "germ theory" needs to be replaced by a model where the human being is regarded as central and helped to regenerate a sense of well-being and fitness in his or her life situation. Interestingly, most of the traditional systems approach health from this holistic perspective. Human society must know how to deal with such biological occurrences as birth, death, pain, etc. Perhaps the solution to an enormously critical health and development problem lies in serious reflection on some of these issues.

The health of any nation is the sum total of the health of its citizens, communities and settlements in which they live. A healthy nation is, therefore feasible only if there is total participation of its citizens towards this goal.

12.13 Annex: Success Stories

12.13.1 Towards a Culture of Preparedness and Sustainability

12.13.1.1 Aparajita Orissa

The super cyclone struck coastal Orissa in the year 1999 and left the households, communities and the state exposed to the disastrous impact of the calamity. The loss of lives and property could have been reduced substantially if the system of disaster management and preparedness to face natural disaster were in place at both the household and community level. This realization brought out the idea of continuing an innovative long-term development initiative for an integrated development model.

To give this idea substance and meaning, the Khoj project is being implemented in the Kujanga Block of Jagatsinghpur district. The block consists of 27 gram panchayats (local government) and 169 revenue villages. Due to its coastal location, the area is highly disaster prone.

Currently no plans have been made to establish development linkages with the disenfranchised people. Unfortunately, the government and the policy makers have yet to establish a link between disaster preparedness and poverty alleviation. Furthermore, no initiative has so far been taken to integrate relief, disaster mitigation and preparedness into normal development plans. Normal development plans are poorly formulated, too loosely integrated with other programs and haphazardly implemented.

Aparajita's strategy, right from the onset is to strengthen the capacity of the affected community and minimize their vulnerability. Aparajita's program focuses on livelihood restoration, healthcare, capacity building of the community, self help, coordination and networking. The provision of livelihood focused inputs had a direct bearing on the earning opportunities of the beneficiaries and accelerated their journey to economic recovery. The healthcare package developed by Aparajita empowered the community in meeting their basic healthcare needs and promoting health status of the community. The coordination and networking have helped Aparajita to avoid duplication, unhealthy competition and conflict, and helped to use its resources, time and energy to reach out to a large number of people with significant inputs.

Aparajita is continuing its efforts to develop, manage and sustain disaster mitigation, preparedness and response planning. However there is a need for implementing more systematic survival strategy and effective coping mechanism to face the future emergencies. It is felt that the Khoj based community initiative will facilitate a long term planning for hazard mitigation, preparedness and capacity building of the community.

Agriculture and animal husbandry are the main occupations of the people. Since the arable land is single cropped, it does not provide sustenance to a family for more than three to four months in a year. Therefore the male population has to migrate to other areas to work as contract labor, road construction workers or to urban areas to undertake sundry activities. Due to the absence of male members in the family, the women have to look after the agricultural activities and animal husbandry. The women also look after the aged and young members of the family, collect wood and drinking water and performing other household chores. This leaves them with little scope for taking care of their own health even during the advance stage of their pregnancy, leading to pregnancy related complications. The reach of health services is inadequate; which compel people to rely on traditional healers, quacks and diviners.

Women and child health is a major focus area of the project. The services are provided through project medical officers, auxiliary nurses, village health workers (VHWs) and trained traditional birth attendants (TBAs). During April 2005–August 2006, 176 antenatal cases were registered and 164 cases were provided complete antenatal care including tetanus immunization. Twenty-one high risk cases were identified and referred to district hospital. Total of 169 births were recorded out of which 162 were conducted by trained personnel, including trained TBAs.

To spread and disseminate the health and development messages to the community, the appropriate mode and suitable media is required. Through the information education and communication (IEC) activities, the project disseminates the development messages to the community. Street theatres and cultural groups are the major media that have been formed and trained to perform on different subjects. In all the five panchayats, these groups have performed on different issues such as mother and child health care, nutrition, sanitation, school health, environment, etc. The health awareness and education program has been attended by more than 15,000 people.

Several initiatives have been started with the SHGs to carry out and expand their livelihood program. One hundred sixty-five SHGs have been formed with a total membership of 2029. A holistic approach has been adopted to set up units of such activities where there is scope for the involvement of more number of women SHGs. Units of stitching and sewing, spices making and bamboo seasoning, and making of products have been supported through this initiative. The women SHGs are also involved in dry fish business, tent house management, agriculture, floriculture, etc.

The Khoj project essentially covers various population groups. There are specially designed program for schools as well as adolescents. The school health programme has different components to serve the health need of the school students of adolescent age group. Health promotion activities, safe drinking water, healthy sanitation conditions are maintained with the available facilities and infrastructure.

To address the specific issues of adolescents, regular monthly meetings amongst them are organized. Their need for education and awareness are very important as they are in the formative stage of their lives. Aparajita addresses these groups by dividing them into two parts, one is the school attending section through its school health program and the second one for the school drop outs. The school dropout adolescents are not only provided education and awareness on health issues; but are also provided with adequate and timely health services, vocational guidance and support to start their own group enterprises for earning livelihood. They have been formed into SHGs. There are 34 such SHGs consisting of 423 members. These groups maintain their group records and have opened banks accounts, so they have savings both in hand and in the bank.

All the initiatives under the Khoj program are regularly reviewed and assessed. Based on the feedback and suggestions of the field and core staff, the plan of action and priority area of intervention is decided.

The village level health workers have emerged as the most active health cadre in the villages of the Khoj operational area. Along with the health team of Aparajita, they are actively taking part in organizing the health activities in their respective areas. With adequate training, now they are well versed with different health issues which are commonly seen in their villages in different seasons. They are also trained to treat common diseases and provide first-aid.

Marginalised and vulnerable groups and individuals have been supported to initiate and sustain their livelihood activities. These marginalized families are identified after intensive interaction with the community, consultation with the panchayats, village leaders and community heads. After a through interaction with the family, their vulnerability is assessed. The support is extended, keeping in view the capacity of the person to take up and manage the activity. Appropriate follow up is done by the volunteers and supervisors.

A rescue equipment demonstration programme has been initiated in five panchayats of the operational areas of the Khoj programme, where five disaster shelters have been identified. These are the focal points of the gram panchayats for the purpose of disaster management and preparedness activities. Regular activities such as mock drills, meetings of disaster management team are organized in these shelters. In the previous year rescue equipments were procured and kept in these shelters.

Hema Manjari Behera, aged 45 years, belonged to a very poor family in the village Ameipala of Kendrapara district. Being part of the fisher folk community, she learnt about group cooperation from the beginning: the men would go fishing while the women would process and dry the fish for selling. When the boats and nets were damaged by the super-cyclone, the male population could not go fishing anymore and thereby women's work was also interrupted. It became difficult to meet the needs of the families. Hema Manjari and three of her friends went to Paradeep port where bigger boats and trawlers did the fishing, but they were disappointed as the fishermen would only sell in bulk. She realized that they would have to increase their investment capacity. Hema Manjari discussed the matter in a community meeting organised by Aparajita and learnt that women of the village could be formed into self help groups (SHGs) and thus make bigger. She managed to convince all the women and thus four SHGs were formed in the village. They collected money among themselves and went to Paradeep to purchase two truckloads of fish. There was a massive activity of dry fish processing and the women learnt the process of group enterprise. They underwent training for adding value to their products by processing them in a hygienic manner. They also went for an exposure visit to the Integrated Coastal Management Institute at Kakinada. With value-added production, they were able to increase their income and profit. Hema Manjari says "*our income was never enough to meet the basic needs of the family. We were not able to think about the education and health of our children. For a set of bangles and few yards of sari, we were dependent on our husbands. But today, we are earning, having our own savings. We care for our children and their future.*" Khoj builds on the potential of the community and makes them self sufficient.

Aparajita, Orissa: Impact Assessment

Particulars	Base line year 2004	Year 2000	Year 2006
No. of villages	24	24	24
Health Indicators			
(a) Morbidity			
Diarrhoea (%)	12.5	14	5.6
ARI (%)	7.8	8.5	5.7
Malaria (%)	6	7	3.9
TB (%)	1.3	1.5	0.1
Aneamia (%)	61	68	38
(b) Mortality			
IMR per 1000 live births	62	68	43
Maternal deaths (Total no. of cases)	12	14	4
(c) Maternal and Child Health			
Complete ANC Coverage (%)	36	21	89
TT immunization	22	18	92
Primary immunization	46	41	86
Births by TBAs	32	25	76
(d) Community Organization (No. of groups)			
SHGs	11	None	96
VHCs/VDCs	None	None	24 (VDC) 24 (VHC)
Youth Groups	8	4	21
Any other type of organizations. (Male SHGs)	None	None	19
(e) Income Generation Programme (IGP)			
Total No. of programmes	5	5	36
Type of activities	Agriculture Fishery Goatery Poultry Petty trade	Agriculture Fishery Goatery Poultry Petty trade	Agriculture Fishery, Goatery Poultry, Handicraft Activities – Agarbati making, Spices making, Food processing, Floriculture, Vegetable Cultivation, Dairy farm, Petty trade,
(f) Capacity Building			
No. of VHWs trained	None	None	52
No. of TBAs trained	21	21	58
No. of persons trained for IGPs	None	None	52
No. of participants in health education	No record	No record	12,345

ANC antenatal care, *ARI* acute respiratory infection, *IGP* income generation programme, *IMR* infant mortality rate, *SHG* self help group, *TB* tuberculosis, *TBA* traditional birth attendant, *TT* Tetanus, *VDC* Village Development Committee, *VEC* Village Education Committee , *VHW* village health worker.

12.13.2 Long Term Development Through Community Participation

12.13.2.1 Sambhav Social Service Organisation, Shivpuri, Madhya Pradesh

The Khoj project was initiated in 1993 in 20 villages in the Shivpuri block of Shivpuri district in Madhya Pradesh for the benefit of Saharia tribes, which belong to one of the most deprived communities in the state. The block is barely 125 km from the Gwalior city and 300 km from Delhi and yet it had remained resource poor and marginalized for years. Lack of appropriate health services and communication facilities were the major problems. Besides, there were a host of other problems including land alienation, exploitation, illiteracy, and lack of safe drinking water and sanitation. Saharias live under extreme poverty. There is rampant malnutrition especially among women and children, and alcohol was a serious social problem. The resultant effect was a self-perpetuating indebtedness. Khoj project in Shivpuri has been actively involved in the organizing Sahariya tribal communities to assert their rights of equality, health, food and secured livelihood and a respectful place in the society. Since health was a major concern, health services and health education was given top priority. Right from its inception, the project laid emphasis on a participatory approach. Various village based groups, VDCs, youth groups, SHGs, etc., were formed, duly trained and involved in the project. This gave the community a sense of ownership and confidence. While community capacity was thus being built, rapport was established with the district administration. This had a very desirable effect and the community began to demand proper health services from the government. Gradually, the ambit of health services was enlarged to include referrals, pathology tests, immunization, ante and postnatal clinics. A well developed planning and management system, with clearly defined parameters for monitoring, evaluation and a functional management information system[6] has seen to a very efficient implementation of project.

There has been a tremendous impact of the project on the health and overall development of the people. *Improvement in health care* has been significant and can be judged by a constantly declining trend in the Infant Mortality Rate (IMR), which from 124 in 1993 has declined to 50 in 2003. Better antenatal and postnatal care coverage (79% as against 16% in 1993), skill enhancement trainings of Dais and better immunization coverage have reduced maternal and infant mortality rates. Now, 100% deliveries are conducted by trained personnel.

There has been an *overall reduction in morbidity and mortality* due to increased awareness and knowledge about various diseases, their causes, prevention and management, for example, diarrhea related morbidity is well under control and there has

[6]Management Information System is a planned system of the collecting, processing, storing and disseminating data in the form of information needed to carry out the functions of management.

been a declining trend in mortality related to the same. No diarrhea deaths were reported during the previous year, against 30 in 1993. Furthermore, increased health awareness has encouraged people to come forward to seek treatment for tuberculosis (TB), which was very difficult for them earlier due to stigma attached.

Local capacity building with a view of long-term sustainability was a very important component. Thus, due emphasis was laid on local capacity building of village health workers (VHWs) and trained birth attendants (TBAs), etc. on regular basis. Village panchayats have been fully involved. Building linkages with the government departments has improved health services, encouraged peoples groups like SHGs, etc. to avail of various income generating schemes of the government. Beginning with nil in 1993 in 2003 there were 64 SHGs, 20 Mahila Mandals and 20 VDCs which helped in raising awareness about existing government schemes and facilities and raised voice for bridging the gaps. This is reflected in various memorandums submitted by people to the government. Promotional programs like education and school health, etc. have resulted in better attendance, increased health and environmental awareness.

Various *village development and income generating activities* like kitchen gardening; livestock farming, poultry, etc. are being implemented through the above people's organization. New technologies have been introduced in agriculture. Mahila Mandals have created a conducive atmosphere towards gender equity and overall empowerment of women. They also take care of programmes for adolescent girls. Women actively participate in advocacy campaigns through SHGs and Shabri Mukti Morcha, etc.

After the successful completion of 10 years, to make the programme financially sustainable in future, several funds like a health fund, TB fund, and education fund were set up. There has been an increased collaboration with the government and panchayats for future support to the development programs. There is full community support for TBAs, village meetings and cultural programs, and SHGs have already made rapid advancements towards self support.

One can say with confidence that the project has entered the phase of self-sustenance with due preparation. There is now a strong network of VHWs, Dais, animators and panchayat workers. Health workers are well versed to identify common ailments, their treatment and referrals as well as disease surveillance. It has also a functional training center at Shivpuri. With years of hard work, the project enjoys very good relationship with various government departments.

Sambhav

Particulars	Baseline Year 1993	Year 2000	Year 2003
No. of villages	20	20	20
Health			
(a) Morbidity % of total cases			
Diarrhea %	10.8	6.5	4.6
ARI %	14.7	4.1	2.3
Malaria %	19.4	9.2	10.4
TB %	2.8	1.2	1.2

(continued)

(continued)

Particulars	Baseline Year 1993	Year 2000	Year 2003
(b) Mortality % of total deaths			
Deaths due to diarrhea	30	7	Nil
Deaths due to ARI	25	6	8
IMR per 1000 live births	124	64	50
Maternal deaths (Total no. of cases)	15	Nil	Nil
(c) Maternal & Child Health			
Complete ANC Coverage %	16	81	79
TT immunization %	20	85	87
Primary immunization coverage %	4.9	68	78
Registration in first trimester	10	60	60
Deliveries/births	35–45% by untrained personnel	100% by trained personnel	100% by trained personnel
Community Organization			
SHGs	Nil	14	64
MMs	Nil	20	20
VDCs	Nil	20	20
Capacity building			
No. of VHWs trained	Nil	15	15
No. of TBAs trained	Nil	21	21
No. of people trained in health education	Nil	3219	2907
Income Generation Programs			
SHG Members	Nil	267	674
Agricultural program	Nil	327	400
Goat Breeding	Nil	10	40
Poultry	Nil	95	100

ARI acute respiratory infection, *ANC* antenatal care, *MM* Mahila Mandal, *IMR* infant mortality rate, *SHG* self help group, *TB* tuberculosis, *TBA* traditional birth attendant, *TT* Tetanus, *VDC* Village Development Committee, *VHW* village health worker.

References

Allen, J. C. (2007) Morphing Rural Community Development Models: The Nexus between the Past and the Future. *Community Investments*, Spring 2007 pp. 16-30. Available http://www.frbsf.org/publications/community/investments/0705/morphing_rural_community_development.pdf cited May 2009.

Agarwal, S., Sarasua, I. (2002). Community-based health financing: CARE India's experience in the maternal and infant survival project. *Research in Healthcare Financial Management, Annual 2002.* Available http://findarticles.com/p/articles/mi_hb1381/is_1_7/ai_n28930735/pg_7/ cited November 2009.

IIPS. (2007). *National Family Health Survey (NFHS-3), 2005-06,* Mumbai: International Institute for Population Sciences. Available http://www.nfhsindia.org/ NFHS-3%20Data/ VOL-1/ India_volume_I_corrected_17oct08.pd f]. cited December 2009.

IIPS. (2001). *Reproductive and Child Health –Rapid Household Survey (RCH-RHS-* Phase I & II*), 1998–99.* Mumbai: International Institute for Population Sciences. Available http://www.rchi-ips.org/pdf/rch1/National_Report_RCH-1.pdf] cited December 2009.

IIPS. (2000). *National Family Health Survey 1998–99 (NFHS-2).* Mumbai, India: International Institute for Population Sciences. Available http://www.nfhsindia.org/index.html cited December 2009.

Office of the Registrar General & Census Commissioner. (2001). Census of India 2001. Available http://censusindia.gov.in/ cited November 2009.

Peters, D., Yazbeck, A., Ramana, G., Sharma, R., Pritchett, L., Wagstaff, A. (2001). *India - Raising the Sights: Better Health Systems for India's Poor.* Washington DC: The World Bank.

Tandon, S. D., Phillips, K., Bordeaux, B. C., Bone, L., Brown, P. B., Cagney, K. A. et al. (2007). A Vision for Progress in Community Health Partnerships. *Progress in Community Health Partnerships: Research, Education and Action,* vol 1.1. 11–30. The Johns Hopkins University Press.

UNDP. (2001). *Human Development Report 2001. Making New Technologies Work for Human Development.* Published for the United Nations Development Programme. New York: Oxford University Press. Available http://hdr.undp.org/en/reports/global/hdr2001/ cited November 2009.

VHAI. (2007). *ICDHI Monograph. Update on Health and Development Status of India.* Independent Commission on Development and Health in India (ICDHI). New Delhi: VHAI.

VHAI. (2004). *Health for the Millions* April-May & June-July 2004, Vol. 30, No. 1&2. New Delhi: Voluntary Health Association of India.

WHO. (1986). Ottawa Charter for Health Promotion. Copenhagen: World Health Organization.

Chapter 13
The Application and Evaluation of an Assets-Based Model in Latin America and the Caribbean: The Experience with the Healthy Settings Approach

Maria C. Franceschini, Marilyn Rice, and Cristina Raquel C. Garcia

Keywords Latin America and the Caribbean • Social determinants of health • Healthy Municipalities, Cities and Communities • Regional Program for Action and Demonstration of Alternatives for Malaria Vector Control without the use of DDT • Tai Chi in the Parks

13.1 Introduction

One of the most outstanding characteristics that distinguish Latin America and the Caribbean (LAC) from the rest of the world is the social, cultural and economic diversity among and within its countries. Nevertheless, while not being the poorest set of countries in the world, LAC is one of the most unequal in terms of wealth and health (World Bank 2007).

How to decrease inequities in health through the reduction of poverty and inequality is one of LAC's biggest challenges, in the face of the enormous social, economic, political, climatic and ethnic variations present in these countries. The evidence indicates that the countries have significantly advanced in many aspects, such as the reduction of people living in poverty and increases in literacy rates and life expectancy at birth. However, this progress refers to average values for all the countries together and often hides great inequalities among and within countries (PAHO/WHO 2007).

Although it is recognized that inequity in health is a direct consequence of the inequitable allocation of resources, opportunities and power, the greatest share of the resources for health in LAC continues to be invested in health care alone. Policies and interventions in LAC have traditionally focused on disease prevention and treatment, following what Morgan and Ziglio in Chap. 1 call the deficit model of health promotion, as opposed to the promotion of factors that create and sustain health and development.

M.C. Franceschini (✉)
Pan American Health Organization
Area of Sustainable Development and Environmental Health
e-mail: francesm@paho.org

A. Morgan et al. (eds.), *Health Assets in a Global Context: Theory, Methods, Action*, DOI 10.1007/978-1-4419-5921-8_13, © Springer Science+Business Media, LLC 2010

Nevertheless, as the interest in the social determinants of health (SDH) has grown worldwide, addressing their impact on population health has become a priority in many LAC countries. Over the past few years, an increased emphasis has been placed on understanding how the SDH impact health conditions in general, as well as unfair and avoidable inequalities in health. As a result, LAC countries have experienced an increase in policies and activities that incorporate a SDH approach to tackle health inequalities (Comissão Nacional sobre Determinantes Sociais de Saúde CNDSS 2008), recognizing, strengthening, and utilizing a population's capacities and resources to improve health (what Morgan and Ziglio refer to as "assets" in Chap. 1).

The creation of healthy and supportive settings (municipalities, schools, workplaces, etc.), also known as the settings approach, has been one of the most used and successful health promotion strategies implemented in LAC in the past few decades. The settings approach is based on the belief that determinants of poverty and equity, and their influence on health, can be addressed through: the creation of sustainable public policies and laws; development of supportive environments; establishment of public–private partnerships; strengthening of networks; and the promotion of active participation of municipal and local governments in health promotion and development. Healthy settings interventions and policies build strongly on community, population, economic, social/cultural, environmental and institutional assets.

While healthy settings is widely considered to be a successful approach to mobilize intersectoral efforts around health goals and to promote health at the local level, the evidence base and generalization of accomplishments to various local settings remains unclear. Currently there is no consensus on the methods or recommendations for assessing the effectiveness of healthy settings and similar health promotion programs and policies. Furthermore, demands for greater "accountability" means that health promotion programs and evaluations are often driven more by public concerns related to the allocation of health resources and generating greater responsiveness of policymakers and health professionals, than by the creation of scientific evidence (Judd et al. 2001). While there is strong pressure to generate evidence of the effectiveness of health promotion interventions, the current medical framework commonly used to define "evidence" is based on methods that are not necessarily suitable for health promotion practices. This can lead to stakeholders drawing inappropriate negative conclusions related to health promotion as a viable approach to improve community and population health.

While most practitioners and decision-makers emphasize the need for a conceptually sound evidence base for health promotion initiatives, the current methods and strategies used to build that evidence often do not correspond with the community contexts in which they are applied. As a result of the use of inappropriate methods, the evidence base for health promotion often overemphasizes data related to health status outcomes and individual behavior change. This is to the detriment of producing evidence related to capacity building (community, institutional, individuals) and the benefits of addressing the broader social determinants of health. Therefore, the advancement of health promotion and assets-based models as effective approaches to improve health and to reduce health inequalities requires an adapted and balanced evidence-base. In addition, an approach to evaluation should incorporate a salutogenic perspective while accommodating stakeholders' concern for both evidence and accountability.

The use of assets-mapping, as proposed by Morgan and Ziglio (2007), can help to support the advancement and implementation of programs that incorporate an assets-based model by allowing communities and practitioners to identify and build an inventory of the strengths, resources and "wealth" (in terms of people, services, material, etc.) that communities possess and that could be drawn upon. Assets-mapping offers an opportunity to bring out in the open the knowledge, skills and capacities that can be used and developed for everyone's benefit. It also highlights the web of interconnections among these assets and the potential for accessing and improving them.

This chapter will discuss the development of the healthy settings approach in LAC and the application of a participatory evaluation methodology developed by the Pan American Health Organization (PAHO)/World Health Organization (WHO) to support the evaluation of health promotion programs in the Region. The experience with the participatory evaluation shows that such methodology can be a powerful tool to support the application of assets-mapping and to demonstrate the effectiveness and usefulness to health promotion and assets-based programs.

13.2 Background

Since the First International Conference on Health Promotion in Ottawa, Canada, in 1986 and the publication of the Ottawa Charter for Health Promotion (WHO 1986), health promotion has been increasingly utilized as a central strategy in community development initiatives. Over the last three decades, governments and international organizations worldwide have significantly increased their investments in health promotion programs.

From an approach focused on disease prevention in the 1970s, the concept of health promotion has evolved and broadened. During the 1980s and 1990s practitioners recognized the need for complementary interventions (such as healthy public policies), to incorporate other sectors and to create healthy environments, in order to make health promotion initiatives effective and successful. In the past few years, the concept of the social determinants of health has been incorporated into the health promotion approach, as global movements of social change and the need to invest and strengthen leadership in health promotion have became more prominent.

Salutogenesis, or the creation of health, is also a core value for the development, articulation and implementation of health promotion programs and policies. The adoption of a salutogenic perspective in health promotion highlights the importance of understanding how health is created and maintained; it establishes a link to the notions of social capital, capacity building and citizen engagement; and it focuses on the need to implement activities that seek to maximize the health and quality of life of individuals, families and communities (Judd et al. 2001).

The Latin America and Caribbean countries have a long tradition of social mobilization and community-driven movements to improve living conditions for their populations. Movements towards the adoption of salutogenic approaches to health have been taking place in the Region for decades. Starting in the 1950s, the concept of local development took hold in many countries as a way to improve the quality of life primarily in rural areas. These movements were characterized by efforts to organize and mobilize communities to implement health programs more effectively. However, most of these initiatives still implemented a top-down approach and assumed that communities would accept the ideas and health priorities as defined by outsiders. By the 1970s, as community resistance mounted, new integrated community development strategies that focused on promoting more active community participation and greater access to health services were introduced with varied results.

Since the 1980s, the LAC countries have experienced major democratization and decentralization processes that significantly re-shaped their social, political, cultural and economic profiles. Decentralization processes that took place in various degrees in the LAC countries have resulted in a territorial redistribution of power and resources through political-administrative reforms. This resulted in greater autonomy, decentralized decision-making power, and control of resources at the local level. Consequently, the concept of local and regional governments as facilitators of community participation and the mobilization of local resources and capacities have been greatly strengthened.

Concomitant to health sector reforms that took place during the 1980s and 1990s, a series of strategies have been put into place by countries in the Region aiming at improving health by incorporating more equitable, sustainable, participatory, and health promoting approaches. In the early 1980s, countries in the Region made a commitment to implement the Primary Health Care (PHC) Strategy, with a focus on community participation and improving access to health care by the most vulnerable population groups. By 1986, renewed emphasis was placed on strengthening Local Health Systems (known as "SILOS"), as a viable strategy to tackle health priorities among the most vulnerable populations. The SILOS strategy was characterized by a focus on decentralization and local development in order to contribute to sustainable democratization, social participation and social justice processes. It called for a shift from traditional approaches to health to one that incorporated health promotion and a focus on families and communities sharing the responsibility for their own health and their search for solutions for their own health problems.

By the 1990s, health promotion surfaced as a major strategy in the Region; one that fit the complex health profile of its countries, with feasible proposals for integral health and human development. Health promotion recuperated the importance of the social setting as a central element to achieve true equity in health by incorporating a positive concept of health and recognizing people as active participants in the process. In this context, interest in preventive and educational activities quickly spread throughout the Region, and particular emphasis was placed on promoting healthy lifestyles. Greater importance was placed on the importance of strengthening the social construction of health and the centrality of community participation in order to achieve better health (PAHO/WHO 1999).

13.3 The Healthy Municipalities, Cities and Communities Movement in LAC

Experiences from the last two decades in LAC countries demonstrate that the local level, represented by regional or local governments, constitutes an important asset when conditions are created that facilitate the implementation of health promotion actions and when other assets present at the local level (community, individual, environmental, etc.) are mobilized and strengthened. Local authorities are responsible for establishing policies for a specific territory and population (PAHO/WHO 1999), and therefore they have greater capacity to mobilize and integrate the action of the various sectors and actors present at the local level. Additionally, they can make health be a priority on their political agendas and they are strategically positioned to better adapt health programs and policies to the specific social, cultural and ethnic context of their communities.

Local governments and communities in LAC have demonstrated increasingly stronger motivation and social, political and technical commitment to initiatives aimed at promoting sustainable local development and improving living conditions of their populations. In particular, initiatives make use of community capacity, resources and potential; foster self-reliance; improve coping abilities; and raise individual and community self-esteem.

The Pan American Health Organization (PAHO) developed and introduced the Healthy Municipalities, Cities and Communities (HMC) strategy in the 1990s to improve and promote local health and development in the hemisphere of the Americas. This strategy is being actively implemented in 18 of the 35 countries and three territories of the Americas.

Based on the definition that health promotion is "the process of enabling and empowering people to take control over and improve the determinants of health" (WHO 1986), the orientation of the Healthy Municipalities, Cities and Communities Strategy is to ensure continuous improvements in the underlying conditions that affect the health and wellbeing of their members. It also focuses on improving health in the social context of people's daily lives by identifying, utilizing and strengthening communities' and population's assets. The improvements affect social conditions and life styles, which in turn have an impact on people's health and promote sustainable system changes.

Based on the notion that being healthy means having a good quality of life, the actions of the HMC strategy focus more on the underlying determinants of health than on their consequences in terms of diseases and illnesses (PAHO/WHO 2002). It also focus strongly on the notion that every community has assets and resources that, when strategically aligned around community-driven priorities, can lead to more effective change. This is achieved by facilitating joint action among local authorities, community members and key stakeholders, aimed at improving their living conditions and quality of life in the places where they live, work, study and play.

The HMC Strategy is based on the premises that (1) various systems and structures governing social, economic, civil and political conditions, as well as the physical environment, can affect individuals' and communities' health; and that (2) health is inherently linked to an individual's capacity to take action in the community and society to which he/she belongs. HMCs strive to create a synergy between these two premises: promoting individual actions and society's response.

The HMC Strategy incorporates an assets-based approach by:

- Emphasizing capacity building through (1) community empowerment, education, and participation; (2) strengthening individual skills and fostering critical thinking among those involved in the initiative; and (3) supporting the development of leadership, agents of change, and advocates.
- Promoting action by communities, institutions, and interserctoral organizational structures for action through (1) the identification of community resources and assets (assets-mapping, community assessments, etc.); (2) and the definition of priorities, strategic planning and the development of a responsive and appropriate action plan.
- Fostering sociopolitical action by (1) guaranteeing formal commitment by local governments, (2) forming community-based, intersectoral committees, and (3) utilizing participatory, community-based methodologies.

Municipal Governments as a Strategic Health Asset: The Experience of a Malaria Prevention and Control Initiative in Central America and Mexico[1]

Between September 2003 and June 2008, the *Regional Program for Action and Demonstration of Alternatives for Malaria Vector Control without the use of DDT* (DDT/PNUMA/GEF/OPS Project) was implemented in eight countries of Mesoamerica (Belize, Costa Rica, El Salvador, Guatemala, Honduras, Mexico, Nicaragua and Panama). The goal of the project was to prove the cost-effectiveness and viability of an integrated vector control model that utilizes alternative methods and techniques to control the malaria vector without the use of DDT or other persistent pesticides. Community participation and the incorporation of municipal governments was the key strategy of the model that was established in 202 pilot communities from 52 municipalities.

The project resulted in a 63% reduction of malaria cases in the pilot communities between 2004 and 2007, and an 86.2% reduction in the cases caused by *P. falciparum*, which is the type of malaria vector that causes the highest morbidity and mortality from the disease worldwide. It was the first time in the

[1]Pan American Health Organization (2009). El papel de los gobiernos municipales y la participación comunitaria en el manejo integral del vector de la malaria sin el uso del DDT en Mesoamérica. Washington, DC (To be published).

sub-region that municipal governments were successfully incorporated into local activities to combat malaria, a responsibility that was traditionally considered to be under the pervue of the Ministry of Health's mandate.

The participating municipal governments contributed to the success of this initiative by financing important infrastructure projects such as bridges, basic sanitation systems, recovering of river banks; provision of materials, supplies and personnel to assist in community cleaning brigades; creation of permanent committees or staff positions (with proper resources allocated to it) to address issues related to malaria; the creation and enforcement of policies aimed at improving environmental management (such as the regulation of waste disposal); and advocacy for and promotion of the participatory model at national and international levels. Another great achievement was the identification and training of community leaders to serve as a link between the community and the project's technical personnel. Community leaders assisted in the coordination of activities at the local level, which in turn resulted in an increase of up to 63% of community health agents in the pilot communities.

In this project, municipal governments demonstrated their capacity to act as agents of change. They achieved this through the development and implementation of public policies and innovative management mechanisms that produced sustainable changes in the social, cultural, and physical structure of their communities in order to prevent and control malaria. They successfully mobilized other actors, sectors and resources which resulted in better coordination of activities and more rational use of resources. The project also resulted in increased knowledge and improved skills in the population related to malaria-vector lifecycle and control. The population demonstrated improved community environmental management (e.g. proper waste disposal), changes in attitudes and behaviors (e.g. improved personal hygiene), greater sense of responsibility about their and their families' health (e.g. keeping their properties clean), and less dependency on the public sector for the implementation of malaria vector control strategies (e.g. organizing and participating in cleaning brigades independently of the presence of the health department technical team).

This experience demonstrates that municipal governments can play a key role in the implementation of health promotion strategies. They are in a privileged position to act upon a variety of factors and levels, and to create the appropriate setting for the successful implementation and sustainability of such initiatives. They are also able to place health and health promotion on the local political agenda, and to generate momentum for the discussion and resolution of community issues and problems without the creation of new or parallel structures. This indicates that municipal governments can be an important health asset, and that their incorporation into health promotion initiatives can be an effective and sustainable strategy.

13.4 Building the Evidence of the Effectiveness of Interventions that Incorporate an Assets-based Approach in LAC

Evidence-based policy-making to tackle health inequalities is greatly compromised by lack of good evidence on the effectiveness of policies and interventions. As noted in Chap. 1, policies and programs designed to promote health and tackle health inequalities are mostly based on evidence built on a "deficit model," The model defines communities and individuals in negative terms and greatly disregards existing positive and health-promoting factors. The alternative is the development of an evaluation approach that builds the evidence base from a "salutogenic" perspective of health and that aims to maximize key health promotion assets. This has been recognized by the international community as key to strengthening the capacity of institutions and communities to activate solutions that are effective, coherent, empowering, and that can contribute to the reduction of health inequities.

Health promotion interventions tend to be complex, context-dependent, occur at different levels (individual, lifestyle or behavioral, community, socioeconomic, environmental, etc.) and in diverse settings and groups. They also employ multiple strategies (healthy settings, healthy public policies, community empowerment, capacity building, behavioral changes, skills development, reorientation of health services, etc.), are large in scope, have extended timeframes and require many resources (Judd et al. 2001). They also need to be flexible and responsive to changing realities.

Practitioners working in countries in LAC have long highlighted the need to develop appropriate methods, indicators, and frameworks that can measure change in such multifaceted and evolving contexts. Appropriate evaluation will help governments, as well as decision makers and policy makers, understand the benefits of investing in approaches that focus on health-promoting factors and key health assets, and that can effectively tackle health inequalities. Existing evaluation tools and methodologies do not appropriately capture changes in essential health promoting factors and assets, nor do they provide insights into the multiplying effect of working with various assets and determinants of health in a coordinated manner. Furthermore, an intervention may not be equally effective for all population subgroups. The effectiveness for a disadvantaged population may be lower due to a number of factors such as place of residence, race/ethnicity, occupation, gender, religion, economic status, sexual orientation, etc. This requires the incorporation of a health equity approach into evaluation designs, methods, indicators and domains for data analysis.

13.5 PAHO's Evaluation Initiative

In an attempt to address these gaps, in 1999 PAHO established a Healthy Municipalities Evaluation Working Group formed by evaluation experts from leading institutions in the Americas working on issues related to health promotion, evaluation and local development. The Working Group was comprised of people from governmental, non-governmental and academic sectors from various countries in the hemisphere, including Argentina, Brazil, Canada, Chile, Colombia, Ecuador, and the United States. It developed a series of evaluation tools, among them, a *Participatory Evaluation Guide for Healthy Municipalities, Cities and Communities,* published in 2005.

Participatory evaluation was considered by the Working Group to be an appropriate methodology because of its potential to systematically generate new knowledge and social capital. Participatory evaluation recognizes the complexities of the HMC Strategy as a local development initiative, and facilitates the development of capacities for critical analysis and reflection, learning and empowerment. It is a methodology that involves key stakeholders in all phases of the process, including the design, implementation, management, interpretation, and decision-making about the evaluation and its results. As such, the process of conducting a participatory evaluation is a positive and inclusive endeavor, which stimulates autonomy and community self-determination. It can improve a community's ability to identify and activate solutions to its own problems, and it builds upon assets, strengths, and resources already in existence in the community (PAHO/WHO 2005).

The *Participatory Evaluation Guide for Healthy Municipalities, Cities and Communities* provides guidance and tools to evaluate healthy settings and health promotion efforts. The guide uses an evaluation framework that incorporates essential health promotion elements and assets such as intersectoral collaboration, social participation, capacity building, individual physical and material conditions, health determinants, and community capacity, among others. It aims to provide an alternative evaluation framework that reflects the underlying health promotion principles embedded in many long-term initiatives taking place in LAC countries while continually building on a community's assets and capacities through continued participation.

The participatory evaluation methodology proposed in the guide supports the documentation and analysis of changes and accomplishments in terms of processes, outcomes and results related to a series of domains, and it guides users on how to communicate and act upon the results to improve their initiatives. Although specific indicators are not proposed in the Guide, a compilation of possible indicators in each of the evaluation domains is included to orient the decisions about which ones are the most appropriate for the initiative being evaluated.

13.6 The Application of the Participatory Evaluation Guide in LAC

In recent four years, the Participatory Evaluation Guide has been introduced into and applied to several LAC countries. These experiences highlight some of the potential benefits that assets-based models and evaluation frameworks can generate and the challenges posed by the complex and multidimensional local and national contexts into which they are introduced. This section will present the lessons learned by applying the participatory evaluation methodology in Brazil, Dominican Republic, Honduras, Mexico, Peru, and Trinidad and Tobago.

Given the strong emphasis of initiatives such as HMC in the involvement of local governments and authorities, political context and timing were two of the main factors affecting the implementation of the participatory evaluation methodology in these countries. Election periods and political transitions often caused major delays (if not termination) of initiatives, shortage and/or change of personnel and funds, and great uncertainty about the future of the initiatives. Constant advocacy about their purpose and benefits, and the establishment of strong coalitions and support bases among all stakeholders was often an efficient strategy to provide continuity and sustainability to the evaluation initiatives during these transitional periods.

The establishment of intersectorial collaboration posed another challenge for most evaluation initiatives in LAC countries despite its centrality to the sustainability of health promotion efforts. It was reported that lack of support from critical stakeholders, such as municipal program managers or key personnel in public institutions, resulted in serious delays or isolation of the participatory evaluation initiative. In some cases, it also jeopardized the possibility that the evaluation results would be seriously considered by all relevant stakeholders, hence threatening the likelihood that the information generated would be utilized to improve health promotion programs and policies.

Various factors accounted for this resistance by key institutions and stakeholders to applying a participatory evaluation methodology. High among the concerns reported were those related to the benefits of conducting a participatory evaluation, particularly due to the time it takes to conduct the process and reservations about the usefulness of the data it produces. Difficulties also arose related to developing indicators, and to articulating which factors and variables were relevant and would be tracked and assessed, given the diversity and breadth of health promotion policies and programs. Such programs and policies are often based on notions of empowerment, community participation, intersectoral collaboration, capacity building, and equity. This emphasis was often perceived by some key stakeholders as being in conflict with established criteria and notions of evidence-based decision making and accountability, and with funders' and decision-makers' concerns with measuring outcomes and impact.

These are valid concerns given the challenges faced by stakeholders coming from institutions with rigid and bureaucratic structures. Such stakeholders often do not have a policy that enables or facilitates coordination with other institutions or intersectorial collaboration, yet are under great pressure to produce specific results in a short period of time. The implementation of the participatory evaluation methodology often required in-depth changes in how groups, organizations and institutions functioned, and, most importantly, in their expectations about the type of data such processes would generate. The countries that utilized the participatory evaluation reported that it was critical to recognize the need for institutions, organizations and individuals to understand, adapt, and accept a new methodology and paradigm to evaluate health promotion interventions. Achieving this acceptance, particularly from public institutions and their staff, is essential in order to be able to incorporate the evidence generated from this kind of evaluation into programs and policies. The acceptance therefore, leads to more effective implementation of health promotion practices and principles, more consistency with the communities' expectations and priorities, optimization of resources, and improvement in personal motivation among public staff and other stakeholders. Given the appropriate support, consideration and time, people from the countries involved became motivated and applied dedicated efforts to implementing the new methodology.

Coordinating the evaluation effort with public institutions also proved challenging due to lack of institutional support or excessive bureaucracy, lack of coordination among public sector institutions, strict guidelines regarding the use of funds, and conflicts among the different actors involved (federal, state, municipal level institutions). High turnover of personnel at all levels and institutions was particularly disruptive. On the other hand, most of the countries involved in this experience reported that the process of engaging public institutions in the participatory evaluation initiative improved channels of communication, resulting in other levels, institutions and sectors providing valuable inputs for the evaluation process. It also cleared the way for exploring new modes of intersectoral collaboration and provided an opportunity for involvement of institutions that could potentially have a far-reaching impact on promoting and supporting the implementation of new paradigms and methodologies, as well as the allocation of resources for them.

All experiences reported that the participatory evaluation process was lengthy and time consuming. This was due to various factors, such as bringing together a variety of stakeholders from various backgrounds, sectors and interests; reaching consensus on core concepts, indicators and paradigms; and working through institutions and organizations with rigid and bureaucratic structures and work cultures. The various levels of knowledge and literacy among those involved also affected the time it took to complete the process. The countries reported a general lack of understanding about health promotion and assets-based approaches (often considered as approaches to disease prevention), their principles (such as community participation) and the participatory evaluation methodology. This can have a direct impact on the planning of the evaluation since how people understand key concepts shape the design, data collection, analysis and presentation of evaluation results. The adoption of a participatory evaluation methodology can play an important role in addressing these issues by serving as a catalyst to engage people in a joint reflection and learning process.

It was also common for initiatives trying to apply the participatory evaluation to be confronted with the fact that their health promotion programs (objectives and definitions of success, expected results, strategies and activities employed, indicators developed and data collected) often were not operationally articulated in a transparent, measurable, or even logical manner. While most programs and policies had the stated purpose of impacting core health promotion principles and assets, accompanied by a more positive and salutogenic approach to health, the activities, strategies and indicators used often reflected disease prevention, individualistic and services-oriented approaches to community health.

As described previously, the Participatory Evaluation Guide was developed to respond to a direct need expressed by health promotion practitioners in LAC. However, once the methodology was made available and applied, most practitioners reported not being ready to implement such an innovative approach to evaluation, partly due to the disconnect between program planning and implementation described above. Primarily, stakeholders came to a realization that their health promotion initiatives had not appropriately taken into account key health promotion principles (such as intersectorial collaboration or community participation). As a result, many initiatives decided to re-examine their planning processes in order to make them more coherent with the conceptual models they intended to implement and the goals they planned to achieve. These experiences highlighted the need to address the different levels involved in these initiatives from a conceptual and planning perspective. In order to appropriately generate more useful evidence, evaluation domains that reflected health promotion and assets-based models should be used, with principles and values clearly delineated and incorporated from the outset of the process.

These experiences also indicated that conducting a participatory evaluation was an empowering and assets-building process by itself. These processes provided an invaluable opportunity to discuss and reflect on communities' experiences, challenges, assets and potentials. The experience brought to light the various interpretations that stakeholders gave to health promotion concepts and principles. It engaged them in a productive and positive dialogue to reach consensus on the various concepts and principles utilized in their health promotion initiatives and evaluation processes. They also shed light on the gaps in their efforts and mobilized those involved to confront the problems and reflect on how to address them. Merely by engaging in the planning and implementation of the participatory methodology, communities and stakeholders were more willing to and interested in participating. This in turn served as a catalyst for generating intersectoral and participatory processes.

Many countries reported that deep-rooted apprehensions arose about efforts conducted with community input, particularly in those countries in which, traditionally, decisions were implemented from the top-down with few mechanisms for meaningful community representation and participation. Concerns included an expressed fear of receiving negative comments, prejudice against actions taken with "too much" input from community members, and the possibility that the process would generate "unrealistic demands" for services and resources. In many cases, however, the process itself of conducting a participatory evaluation and having the opportunity to engage with other community stakeholders served as an eye-opener for stakeholders in these countries. The process resulted in positive changes in attitudes and perspectives related to the potential of community participation.

Having strong, sustained and dynamic leadership was central to the sustainability of a community-responsive evaluation initiative. Active commitment and engagement from institutions both at the local and national levels were key to the success of these initiatives, as well as the quality of the collaborative work among them. National and regional HMC networks effectively created and maintained such leadership, given their potential far-reaching connections to municipalities, institutions and key stakeholders throughout a country or region.

The Application of the Participatory Evaluation Methodology to the *Tai Chi in the Parks Program*, in Miraflores, Peru[2]

Since 1990, the "Tai Chi in the Parks" Initiative has been implemented in the municipality of Miraflores, in Lima, Peru. Its main objectives are to incorporate the practice of Tai Chi and its philosophy as a daily, voluntary and accessible habit in the life of Miraflores' elderly population; and to achieve physical, psychological, social and spiritual development of Miraflores' elderly population through the practice of Tai Chi.

The initiative offers free Tai Chi classes during weekdays in the municipality's parks, supports the creation Tai Chi clubs, maintains a "Tai Chi in the Parks" network, promotes community activities (such as Tai Chi championships), and trains community elderly to become Tai Chi instructors. Today, more than 20,000 elderly people practice Tai Chi in the municipality through this program.

During 2005, an Evaluation Subcommittee was formed comprised of technical staff from the municipality, the program coordinator, program participants and elderly members of the community in order to apply the participatory evaluation methodology to this Initiative. All participants received training in the participatory evaluation methodology through a series of meetings, guided by a trained facilitator, which included discussion among the group members in order to reach consensus on all of the methodology's core concepts.

Working with the elderly and mostly retired population proved to be advantageous as participants had more flexibility and availability to participate in the process. Most participants of the Evaluation Subcommittee were not involved with the health sector or were not health professionals. This was found to be beneficial because it allowed the group to more openly explore issues related to the social and psychological benefits of the program, and not focus exclusively on evaluating its health benefits in terms of disease prevention.

Based on the process and the steps proposed in the Participatory Evaluation Guide, the group developed an evaluation plan and defined key indicators, data collection methods and a work plan. During this process, the group came across some major issues which posed a challenge in applying the participatory evaluation framework: the Tai Chi in the Parks Program had not been planned and implemented in a participatory manner, and it had not fully taken into account core health promotion principles (such as intersectorial participation). However, simply engaging in the participatory

[2]Information about this experience was compiled from a report submitted by the Peruvian Network of Healthy Municipalities, Cities and Communities to PAHO/WHO (2005) that describes the application of the participatory evaluation guide to various HMC initiatives in Peru.

evaluation process highlighted these deficiencies and mobilized the group to search for solutions. The group approached its problems from different perspectives and took into account the factors that might have facilitated or hindered the participation of other stakeholders in their evaluation plan and analysis.

Among the challenges reported was the resistance by some participants to implementing a participatory methodology due to ingrained and negative preconceptions related to actions taken with community input. There were also fears of receiving excessive criticism and increased "demands" by the community if it was offered the opportunity to participate. Difficulties in coordinating the work with the technical staff from the Ministry of Health and a local university providing technical guidance, resulted in delays in the data collection and analysis phase of the process. Difficulties also resulted from discrepancies related to the various interpretations given by the group to the concept of health promotion and other core concepts related to the evaluation. This was compounded by inflexibility on the part of some group members to listening and engaging in a true dialogue. Having a good facilitator was reported as key to guiding the discussion and helping the group reach conclusions. In addition, turnover of key personnel in the municipality caused major delays in the evaluation process.

While collecting data the group observed issues that required immediate attention such as difficulties with sound systems and the need to limit the access of dogs to the parks during the Tai Chi classes. This information was quickly transmitted to the program coordinator and the issues were promptly resolved. Seeing the results of their efforts highly motivated the Evaluation Subcommittee participants to become more involved in the process, with many manifesting an interest in evaluating other aspects of the Tai Chi in the Parks Program and learning more about the participatory evaluation methodology. This resulted in a series of workshops aimed at identifying other key aspects of the program and priorities for the next round of evaluation.

These workshops were organized by the Evaluation Subcommittee itself and provided an important opportunity to bring together program managers and program beneficiaries to participate in the process. The strategies devised to broaden the evaluation initiative included: (1) incorporating the San Marcos National University to provide technical support in evaluation processes, and (2) engaging the current Evaluation Subcommittee in the evaluation of other municipal programs targeting the elderly population. As a result, the participatory evaluation brought about significant changes in how programs were planned and implemented in the municipality, particularly with respect to involving various stakeholders and sectors, and incorporating participatory planning into the process.

13.7 Discussion

Health promotion and assets-based approaches can greatly contribute to the development of programs and policies that support the preservation of health and the decrease of health inequities, rather than only the prevention of diseases. During the past few decades the implementation of the healthy settings approach in LAC countries have greatly advanced the cause for health promotion in the Region. Valuable experiences and information related to the process, outcomes, benefits and challenges of these approaches to community and population health have also been accumulated. Nevertheless, practitioners in the field are often concerned that health promotion programs and policies will not be continued due to a perception on the part of decision makers and funders that there is a lack of success and effectiveness. In order to highlight the positive results from health promotion initiatives, a new type of evidence base needs to be created that incorporates an inclusive, positive, and salutogenic orientation, while at the same time being consistent with the context and population in which such initiatives are implemented. Such an approach will help to produce arguments that might guarantee support from policy makers and funders for health promotion programs and policies.

This approach to building evidence can demonstrate how these participatory and assets-based processes help to enhance health, quality of life and wellbeing, while recognizing that health is a key asset to community development rather than just an end in itself. In order to achieve this goal, there is a need to shift from a view of evidence and evaluation based on a pathogenic, risk factor and outcomes-oriented perspective to a balanced, inclusive and positive approach to assessing change and success; one that can contribute to the production of knowledge and capacities to improve the health of individuals, families and communities.

Interest in building the evidence base of health promotion effectiveness has increased greatly in the past few years. However, these efforts have been hampered due to insufficient attention being paid to ensuring the presence of sufficient capacity, political will, resources and leadership in order to develop and apply appropriate frameworks and methodologies that will generate this evidence. The participatory evaluation methodology described in this chapter can help to generate such evidence and promote understanding of the barriers to taking effective actions that address health inequities and the promotion of more inclusive and positive approaches in LAC. It can also be a powerful tool when applied in conjunction with assets-mapping as it can help to demonstrate the value of approaching communities from a positive, salutogenic perspective, and building on their strengths and resources.

Factors affecting the successful implementation of the HMC Strategy and the participatory evaluation methodology in LAC were identified at various levels (individual, institutional, political, community, etc.). These factors overlapped and impacted each other in very complex ways. These experiences indicate that "re-dressing the balance between an assets and a deficit model evidence base", as discussed in Chap. 1, requires taking into account these challenges, which are inherent in most collaborative and participatory efforts.

When they were conducted in a truly participatory manner, HMC and other settings-based health promotion initiatives, accompanied by the use of the participatory evaluation methodology, promoted accountability, motivated continuous and active participation from all stakeholders, and created a sense of common interest among those involved. The approach encouraged community participation, the development of personal skills and the understanding of the key assets that created supportive environments for health development. It also helped to uncover hidden assets and resources in the community, as well as potential connections and possibilities for improvement and growth. As such, the participatory evaluation can be an important tool for assets-mapping as it can be implemented in various stages of an initiative and involve a variety of stakeholders.

Engaging in the participatory evaluation was highly motivating and revitalizing, concretely stimulating those involved to look at their actions more consistently and promoting interest in issues related to health promotion, community assets and equity. The participatory evaluation experience strengthened capacities among those involved, generated commitment to adhering to health promotion principles, and strengthened alliances among key stakeholders. The experience also emphasized the potential of "salutogenic approaches," such as using participatory evaluation as a decision-making tool.

There are complexities inherent in building the evidence-base of the effectiveness of these initiatives, and practical barriers for conducting evaluation studies as described by the experiences of LAC countries with the participatory evaluation methodology. Therefore it is essential to create opportunities for mutual learning, exchange of experiences and the pro-active identification and dissemination of evidence and "good practices," taking into account the complexity of communities and decision-making processes. In doing so, it is important to articulate the definition of success in health promotion initiatives, and redefine the criteria to judge the evidence generated in these efforts in order to improve programs and policies aimed at improving community health and reducing health inequalities.

Well designed evaluations can assist funders, policymakers, practitioners and communities in linking the success of specific programs and policies to broader contextual, economic, environmental and social issues. It can also help with the development of rational strategies for tackling health inequalities that can be understood by policy and decision makers and applied to policies and interventions at the national and local levels.

References

Comissão Nacional sobre Determinantes Sociais de Saúde (CNDSS). (2008). *Relatório final. As causas sociais das iniqüidades em saúde no Brasil.* http://www.determinantes.fiocruz.br/comissao.asp cited Jun 24, 2008.

Judd, J., Frankish, C.J., Moulton, G. (2001). Setting standards in the evaluation of community-based health promotion programmes – a unifying approach. *Health Promotion International* Vol. 16 No. 4 367–380.

PAHO/WHO. (1999). *Planificación Local Participativa: Metodologías para la Promoción de la Salud en América Latina y el Caribe.* Washington DC: Pan American Health Organization/World Health Organization.

PAHO/WHO. (2002). *Mayor's Guide for Promoting Quality of Life.* Washington DC: Pan American Health Organization/World Health Organization.

PAHO/WHO. (2005). *Participatory Evaluation for Healthy Municipalities, Cities and Communities.* Washington DC: Pan American Health Organization/World Health Organization.

PAHO/WHO. (2007). *La salud en el contexto del desarrollo. In: Salud en las Américas.* Washington DC: Pan American Health Organization/World Health Organization.

World Bank. (2007). Economic growth, inequity and opportunity creation in Latin America and the Caribbean. Available at: http://web.worldbank.org cited Jul 14 2008.

WHO (1986). Ottawa Charter for Health Promotion. *The Move Toward A New Public Health, Ottawa 17-21 November 1986.* World Health Organization.

Chapter 14
Parents and Communities' Assets to Control Under-Five Child Malaria in Rural Benin, West Africa

David Houéto and Alain Deccache

Keywords Sub-Saharan Africa • Child malaria • Benin • Community • Fever • Millennium Development Goals

14.1 Introduction

Malaria continues to be the principal cause of morbidity and mortality in sub-Saharan Africa (SSA) countries (Breman et al. 2004; Hay et al. 2009) (Fig. 14.1). Each year, 350–500 million people suffer from it in the world, generally in its severe form (WHO 2005). Nearly three million children and adults continue to die of this disease in the world each year in spite of the existence of effective preventive and curative measures (Greenwood et al. 2005). Approximately 94% of these deaths due to malaria in the world occur in SSA (Bryce et al. 2003, 2005). The victims are mainly children under 5 years of which at least one dies every 30 s (WHO 2003a). This large prevalence of malaria translates to a situation of poverty and the health services inadequacy (Barat et al. 2004; Keiser et al. 2004; Malaney et al. 2004; Panosian-Dunavan 2006). Furthermore, the consequences of malaria contributes to maintaining the populations in a state of poverty, generating for the SSA countries a total loss of more than 12 billion dollars US each year through the loss of incomes, foreign investments and resources related to tourism (Greenwood et al. 2005; Panosian-Dunavan 2006). At households' level for instance, Malaria decreases the resources intended for the expenditure of first needs (food, expenses of schooling, etc) and supports the multiplication of the births because of the logic which is often evoked: "*it is necessary to make some sufficiently in forecast on behalf of death*" (Panosian-Dunavan 2006).

D. Houéto (✉)
Health Promotion, Agence de Médecine Préventive (AMP), Cotonou, Benin
e-mail: dhoueto@yahoo.fr

A. Morgan et al. (eds.), *Health Assets in a Global Context: Theory, Methods, Action*,
DOI 10.1007/978-1-4419-5921-8_14,

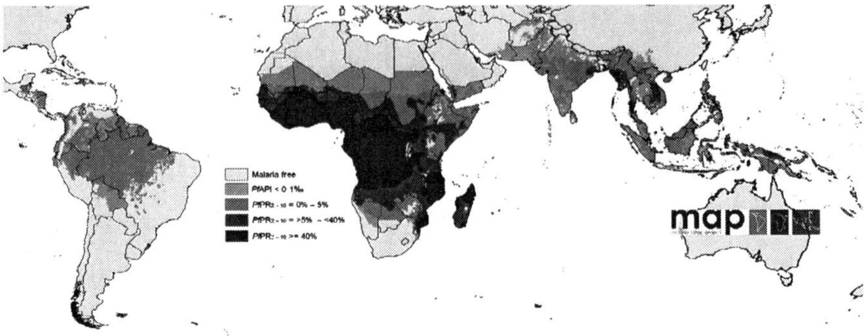

Fig. 14.1 (Hay et al. 2009). The spatial distribution of P. Falciparum Malaria PfPR2_10 predictions stratified by endemicity class. They are categorized as low risk PfPR2_10 – 5%, light red; intermediate risk PfPR2_10 – 5–40%, medium red; and high risk PfPR2_10 – 40%, dark red. The map shows the class to which PfPR2_10 has the highest predicted probability of membership. The rest of the land area was defined as unstable risk (medium grey areas, where PfAPI, 0.1 per 1,000 pa) or no risk (light grey).

Vis-a-vis malaria, several uncoordinated actions have been undertaken for already several decades with the support of several development partners. However, this known situation of malaria has little change in terms of prevalence (Houéto 2007) and continues to challenge the whole of the actors engaged in the process of its control (Greenwood et al. 2005; Panosian-Dunavan 2006). It is in this context that we initiated an experiment to show the node of the failure of the various actions undertaken to date. We evoke some actions undertaken and/or in progress at the time of our study.

14.2 International and National Context at the Time of the Study

At the time of carrying out the present study, Heads of State and Government of the SSA, on many occasions, have paid attention on the malaria issue and have worked with the adoption of many declarations for its better control. Among these declarations we mention that of Abuja and the Millennium Development Goals (MDGs).

14.2.1 The Heads of State and Government Summit in Abuja on Malaria

Being aware of the malaria issue, SSA Governments gave a priority to the fight against this disease in interventions aiming at the people's wellbeing in the region (WHO 2000). A particular emphasis is put on child malaria; children constitute one of the vulnerable populations to Plasmodium falciparum, the principal pathogenic agent in the region (Greenwood et al. 2005). This concern of the African leaders had led them to meet in Abuja (Nigeria) in 2000 when it was expected that at the end of the year 2005:

- At least 60% of those suffering from malaria have prompt access to, and are able to correctly use affordable and appropriate treatment within 24 h of the onset of symptoms;
- At least 60% of those at risk of malaria, particularly children under 5 years of age and pregnant women, benefit from the most suitable combination of personal and community protective measures such as insecticide treated mosquito nets and other interventions which are accessible to prevent infection and suffering (WHO 2000).

To achieve these goals, Governments of the SSA region initiated, within many other actions, the strengthening of the community base interventions with mainly the Home Malaria Management initiative (HMM) (WHO 2003b), the Integrated Management of Childhood Illness (IMCI) (Breman et al. 2004), and the generalized use of the impregnated mosquito nets (Abdulla et al. 2005; Lengeler 2005; WHO 2004). Several studies were conducted with encouraging results in communities in many countries of the region, such as Kenya (Marsh et al. 2004), Ethiopia (Kidane and Morrow 2000), and Burkina Faso (Sirima et al. 2003). Some of these experiments are only locally realized, while others cover whole regions of the countries concerned, but none are replicated to across an entire country (Yamey 2004; Ahorlu et al. 2006). It is thus not surprizing that at the end of the year 2005, the commitments of Abuja Declaration are not reached (Ahorlu et al. 2006; Butler 2007; Molyneux and Nantulya 2004; Yamey 2004).

However, one can wonder, if the generalization of these studies had taken place, would it have made them possible to achieve the goals of Abuja? If one considers the analysis of Adongo et al. (2005), Baume (2002a, b), Jones (2006), Jones and Williams (2004) and Williams and Jones (2004), one should anticipate the failure of the Abuja Declaration even with the implementation of the HMM initiative and alike. According to these authors, malaria care requires the intrinsic consideration of factors such as those socioeconomic, cultural, environmental and others factors which underlie this disease. Beyond these factors, there is the whole health system in SSA countries which constitutes a potential barrier to the attainment of these goals (Panosian-Dunavan 2006; WHO 2004). In other words, several factors are to be considered simultaneously for an effective malaria control in general, and child malaria in particular, which imply a comprehensive approach and perfect community participation (Jones 2006; Jones and Williams 2004). Interventions implemented in order to attain Abuja goals did not take into account these intrinsic aspects of broad determinants of malaria prevalence (Panosian-Dunavan 2006; Molyneux and Nantulya 2004; Yamey 2004). At the international level, the persistence of the malaria prevalence is acknowledged through its inclusion in the MDGs. Although the MDGs include at the same time some social aspects e.g. poverty reduction, primary education for all etc, with the principal diseases that are causing more deaths worldwide, they are not conceived in the way it should be with the health promotion concept.

14.3 The Millennium Development Goals

Beyond the African continent, the malaria issue is a concern at the international level expressed through the MDGs. MDGs are expressions of the international community recognizing the importance of malaria on the poor economic level of SSA countries (Lapeyre 2006; Panosian-Dunavan 2006). In other words, MDGs are making the link between certain diseases including malaria and the development of victim communities. However, MDGs as goals, targeting some particular diseases without considering them in the specific contexts which generate them, seems to put the resolution of the malaria issue under the biomedical vision of health (Lapeyre 2006). The link that is supposed to exist through the MDGs between specific diseases and the development status is not obvious within these goals. According to Lapeyre (2006), this form of resolution regarding these issues is far from supportive to the attainment of the MDGs. Murray et al. (2007) affirm, by examining the MDG 4: "*Globally, we are not doing a better job of reducing child mortality now than we were three decades ago…*" If therefore nothing is done in order to take correct actions adapted to the malaria reality such as the one experimented by communities in SSA region, "*MDGs should fail certainly*", said many authors (Bryce et al. 2006; Campbell 2007). African children under five will continue dying from malaria (Werner and Sanders 2006). In other words, malaria control programs should consider the perceptions and representations of communities that are suffering from Malaria. To do so it is to put into their hands the development of these programs, what we shall call "people-centered malaria control programs". This is completely different from the way the MDGs are approaching the disease issue.

14.4 Approaches Used in Benin to Control Malaria

In Benin (West Africa), malaria is the main cause of under-five children morbidity and mortality. In 2005, 49% of under-five children consultations and 50% of hospitalizations were due to malaria. Malaria is a major priority of action for the country leaders through the Ministry of health (MS/Benin 2006). Several actions have been initiated in link with the policies that are progressing at the regional and international levels to control malaria, including: use of impregnated mosquito nets (IMN) and malaria cases management using Artemisinin Combined Therapy (ACT) (MS/Benin 2006). The Malaria Program has a lot of resources (human, material and financial) and is dealing with the equity issue by providing free IMN to all vulnerable populations. In spite of all these efforts, when one considers for instance the decade from 1996 to 2005, one can notice that malaria remained the first cause of morbidity and mortality in Benin, with a trend of increased prevalence (MS/Benin 1997–2006). The persistence of the malaria situation despite the many efforts and resources, has led some health actors in Benin to say that "*Malaria is feeding more than it kills*".

14.5 How to Deal with the Persistence of Malaria?

Is malaria an invincible disease in spite of the existence of effective curative and preventive measures? One can say that these measures have to be delivered with the right access, equity, coverage and quality. But we know that in possession of these, people continue to not use them properly or refuse to use them because of their social and/or cultural conditions (Houéto et al. 2007b). It is also possible to imagine that the vaccine is the ideal solution. Yet the recent events as regards immunization on the continent recall that the vaccine is not always the best solution for populations that are not convinced of the biomedical logic on the same basis as the health professionals (Helman 2007). The malaria issue invites, according to us, a revisit to the traditional strategies to control diseases. For Alilio et al. (2004), Jones (2006), Jones and Williams (2004), strategies currently used against malaria are not adapted. According to them, malaria in SSA is characterized by its anchoring in a cultural, socioeconomic, environmental particular context. Also, with malaria and more precisely with fever which is the main sign, there are particular perceptions and representations from individuals in communities depending on each sub-region of SSA (Adongo et al. 2005; Baume 2002a; Helman 2007, p. 412; Jones and Williams 2004; Kamat 2006). All this has led communities in the region to get an "indigenous knowledge" in the field of malaria in particular and that for fever in general. Thus, because there is no link established between fever and child malaria, parents have recourse to some therapeutic practices to control fever using e.g. anti-pyretic and/or anti-malarial drugs, but with inadequate dosage and duration of the treatment (Baume 2002a; Helman 2007, p. 412; Kamat 2006; Marsh et al. 2004). The majority of the campaigns against malaria have often little or no aspects which deal truly with these various factors (Houéto et al. 2007a; Baume 2002b; Helman 2007). One of the possible reasons is that medicine manages disease with a biomedical vision which leads health professionals to bring solutions to the populations without seeking a true collaboration of these populations in order to systematically identify the various above-mentioned factors and to work with them (Alilio et al. 2004; Baume 2002b; Helman 2007; Jones and Williams 2004; Kamat 2006). Dealing with the malaria issue by taking into account populations' perceptions and representations would be a way of empowering them. This is because taking into account their "indigenous knowledge", their assets, would shift an amount of power that was previously with the health professionals. This approach also conforms to the Primary Health Care declaration (WHO 1978) which stated: "*A strong participation of the people is essential and social autonomy and conscience are key factors of the human development*". This has nothing to do with the Information, Education and Communication (IEC) method some health professionals try to use, thinking that by adding to this a kind of participation (that is not empowering), people can take responsibility for prevention and treatment of disease in general and malaria in particular.

In other words, when it comes to strategies that lead to more positive results within the framework of the fight against malaria, to work with the populations' characteristics, knowledge and practices (good and bad according to the biomedical vision of disease) could play an important part in their empowerment to control malaria. To improve this, communities must be put at the centre of the intervention for they are the ones who know their conditions more than the external people such as health professionals. That is what we call a "people-centered malaria control program". When health professionals can acknowledge that public health programs such as the malaria program do not work this way, it is time to reorient the basic strategies in this field so that health action becomes more effective. In other words, there is a need to come back to the new public health that is health promotion (Kickbusch 2007).

We have, on the basis of this principle of populations' assets and especially because the characteristics of malaria seem to us to depend on it, initiated the intervention about which we are going to report in this chapter for an effective fight against under-five child malaria in Benin. We will discuss:

- How assets based policy has worked to improve malaria control and reduce inequalities;
- The critical conditions required to ensure the effective implementation of assets based policy at a community level;
- New methodologies for constructing the evidence base on assets approaches to health and development; and
- How assets based policy has worked to improve malaria control and reduce inequalities.

14.6 Intervention (Houéto and Deccache 2008)

The intervention took place in Benin (West Africa) in a rural area. It lasted 27 months, and involved a village of around 1,000 inhabitants in developing a program to control under-five children malaria based on their assets through participation and empowerment. The process is reported here after.

1. *Identification and description of the health priority problem*: With the community, we did a baseline study after several contacts and discussions with the village leaders, notables and the whole community in a general assembly.
2. *Expressed problem*: A feedback session of the baseline study results was organized. Its aim was to establish a general community understanding of the cause of fever in children. The various health or non-health factors of fever, in connection with the realities of the village, were identified. The problems to be resolved for the organization of the fight against fever were identified.
3. *Reformulation of problems*: The main problems identified were reformulated after their validation, according to the community's understanding and based on locally available means.
4. *Prioritisation*: The problems identified were ranked according to the importance placed on them by the community members.

5. *Resources inventory*: The community discussed the issues around the resources needed for the resolution of the identified problems as well as the potential collaborations with health professionals and other professionals according to the needs identified.
6. *Desirable and feasible changes*: The community identified various actions to be taken. They identified the need for, and set up a steering committee, which decided on several main lines of action.

Here are the actions implemented by the steering committee:

- *Early home treatment of the child fever by mothers.* On the community initiative, training was organized for mothers in different hamlets of the village. This was ensured by the principal investigator, in collaboration with the departmental management of health, which gave a material support to this activity and the entire process. At the end of each training session, mothers established their criteria and unanimously chose a community health worker (CHW). Mothers proposed to add vermifuge, because according to them, intestinal worms worsen child fever. The doses of treatment were pre-packaged in reconditioning sachets. Supply of medicines and prices are managed by the steering committee.
- *Use of impregnated mosquito nets (IMN).* The steering committee, after discussion with the community, decided to use IMN. They estimated that 300 IMNs were required, which the Ministry of Health provided within one week.
- *Parents' income improvement.* Two very important income-generating activities came into force. There was the installation of two grain mills for processing corn, beans and other cereals, and also cassava. For the farming activities, contacts were made with the International Institute of Tropical Agriculture (IITA) in order to improve agricultural practices. This was made possible via the former Director of IITA who is naturalized Benin citizen and an inhabitant of the village.
- *Setting up of a micro-insurance for health.* The community agreed upon some methods of the micro-insurance: 100F CFA ($US0.2)[*] as membership fees and a monthly contribution of 200F CFA ($US0.4) by household ($US4.8 per year). The contribution covers 100% of care at the CHW level and at the district health centre. The steering committee committed itself to supervise a regular (quarterly) deworming programme through the micro-finance scheme, in order to reduce children "susceptibility" to fever according to the belief in the village. [*$US1 = 500F CFA]
- *Environment cleanliness and creation of mosquito-free habitat.* According to the understanding of the community after discussions, there is a model of habitat in the village which provides protection from mosquitoes' bites. Community members adopted a new model of habitat with regards to this understanding with appropriate measures to maintain and clean their environment.
- *Systematic schooling of children and adult literacy.* The process of discussion in order to understand under-five children fever led the community to the conclusion that literacy was related with a better health attitude and behaviour. They decided to ensure the schooling of all the children of the village. Mobilization of children

for school started from the following academic year, while the elimination of adults' illiteracy was also planned in order to help the rest of the village.

- *Implementation*: The steering committee played the leading role during the implementation of the identified activities. It created and maintained informal relations with the community mainly through the community leaders, the notables, and periodic village meetings.
- *Assessment*: An evaluation of the intervention was done after 27 months. It involved the steering committee and community members as well as the principal investigator. At this evaluation, the results below were noted as the fruits of this intervention based on the community's assets.

14.7 Results

Many changes were noted from before and after the intervention regarding cognitive information:

14.7.1 At the Individual Level

- *Causal attributions of under-five child fever*: Correct attributions before and after intervention were respectively 6 and 15 among 18 households interviewed. Incorrect attributions were respectively 12 and 3 among 18 households. One of the interviewees stated before intervention: "natural fever never worsens, but when caused by the witchcraft, always becomes complicated". After intervention, he said: "mosquitoes and houses insalubrities" cause child fever.
- *Knowledge of prevention methods*: Before intervention, 8 amongst 18 households knew malaria prevention practices. After intervention, 16 amongst 18 households knew adequate methods for malaria prevention and practised them.
- *Parents' practices of recourse to health centre in the case of child fever*: Table 14.1 presents practices of recourse to adequate health care in the intervention village before and after the intervention ($\chi^2=48.07$, $P=0.000000$). One of

Table 14.1 Recourse to adequate health care in the intervention village before and after intervention

Recourse to adequate health care	Intervention village			
	Before intervention		After intervention	
	n (%)	*N*	*n* (%)	*N*
Active screening of malaria	6 (12)	52	19 (66)	29
In-depth interviews	2 (11)	18	16 (89)	18
Total	8 (11) [5–21]	70	35 (75) [60–86]	47

N number of households interviewed, *n* frequencies of adequate recourse to health care, *[ ]* 95% confidence interval.

the households interviewed was asked "does child fever require recourse to modern care?" They answered: before intervention: "yes, but after at least three days, because if it is natural, it will give up with the house remedies." After intervention: "Yes, because not treated by them (health professionals), fever can lead to anaemia and even the loss of the child. It will be without conditions. The ideal to be reached will be that parents contribute in advance in order to have recourse to health centre without worrying about the price to pay".

Community participation and actions implemented: According to in-depth and group interviews, about 80% of the community members participated in the intervention through the different actions implemented. The interviewees confirmed that the high level of participation was due to the fact that community members were the authors of the proposed interventions.

14.7.2 At the Community Level

- Community behaviours, through participation in meetings, gradually developed informed decision making and readiness to be engaged in the project activities;
- Competence to treat child fever adequately is developed very quickly (see details in Houéto 2007; Houéto and Deccache, 2008), contributing to the development of people's self-esteem;
- Skills to establish partnerships were also developed;
- Communication through a positive interaction, and the confidence to express divergent points of view was developed during the intervention;
- Development of a critical conscience through the manifestation of collective, social, political conscience, engagement towards the other members of the community, and the acceptance of a personal liability for change were noted.

14.7.3 Health Data

We have, for active screening of malaria as well as the registers analysis, obtained modifications of the health data.

- The prevalence of fever and other signs of malaria were significantly reduced (before: 34% [27–42], after: 20% [14–28], $P=0.008$);
- The recourse to the health facilities in the case of fever increased, in particular an early and adequate home treatment of fever as showed on Table 14.1;
- Consequently, there is reduction in severe cases of fever compared to the year before the intervention (13% [7–22] in 2003–2004, and 7% [3–15] in 2005–2006, $P=0.18$, this reduction is not statistically significant); and
- A statistically significant reduction in the deaths caused by malaria (4 in 27 months of intervention versus 15 in 2004, the year just before our intervention, $P=0.001$).

These successes require certain conditions that are indispensable for a successful community-led development based on their assets.

14.8 The Critical Conditions Required to Ensure the Effective Implementation of Assets Based Policy at a Community Level

The very strong support obtained from the community seemed to be related to the process which we followed in this intervention, summarized below:

- No action was taken without considering the local context of the intervention community;
- The issue approached has priority for the intervention community;
- Participation, giving real capacity to the community to take all the possible and suitable actions, according to the members community's assets, for the fever control;
- We (professionals) acted as a referent, guiding the process and contributing to actions under consideration by the community;
- Expanded beyond the health sector to use several types and strategies of action against malaria concerning various aspects of the community's life; and
- Confidence in the community (their assets) contributed to the development/increase of their self-esteem, in turn acting as motivation to make their own suggested actions successful.

We summarise all these aspects in Fig. 14.2 and name it "The principle of the crank" in order to figure out the roles of the community and of the professionals, the former being at the centre of the process using its assets and the latter just

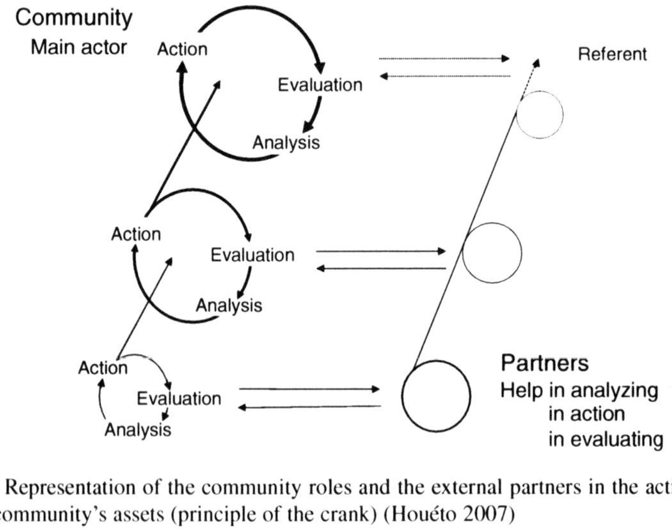

Fig. 14.2 Representation of the community roles and the external partners in the action process based on community's assets (principle of the crank) (Houéto 2007)

accompanying the process (mainly at its beginning), being confident in the community's assets and progressively taking distance and becoming a "referent". This role of referent will disappear with time according to the characteristics of each community as stated by Boyte (1989). According to McFarlane and Fehir (1994), it will take two to 5 years for the community to get control of the whole process. We think, as far as we are concerned, that this time will also depend on the initial level of powerlessness of each community or the quality of its assets and its will to change its health status and quality of life. The time required will also depend on the strength of the role the professionals have played at the beginning of the intervention process (the force of the crank) by really giving power to the community (Raeburn and Corbett 2001). According to Arole et al. (2004) from whom we have drawn this "principle of the crank", and Raeburn and Rootman (1998), the role of the professionals in achieving this goal, will have to be located in the logic of a guide and an adviser which supports community control through three lines of action, namely:

1) To take care that health interventions/programs lie within the framework of health and wellbeing of the populations concerned, while aiming at a community control from the very beginning;
2) To support community's development initiatives which contribute to the improvement of the quality of life of the partner populations;
3) To nuture the community competences and skills development, i.e. the development of their assets.

Through the "principle of the crank" we are acknowledging some new methodologies to construct sustainable results in community interventions that lead to community development. Here after we are attempting to present the new methodologies as we perceived them in our malaria control experience in a rural area.

14.9 New Methodologies for Constructing the Evidence Base on Assets Approaches to Health and Development

To construct evidence base on assets approaches, we found through this intervention that community participation is central. There is evidence as stated by Raeburn (2005) that community participation, as experienced within this intervention, is the core process of using and developing people's assets. This kind of participation is compared to the crank as it's important at the beginning of a health/development action where professionals help start the reflexion and the enlightenment of the issue in a specific community. By doing so, professionals are not the principal actors for they are not going to replace the community, but just help them solve the problem. It is for the community to continue doing things with new resolutions. Through community participation based on community assets, it was possible to the community in our intervention to discover the biomedical reality of child fever and to adopt behaviours favourable to its control. This form of participation is possible, only when programmes focus on the local contextual factors and not on some generic actions, as it is the case in many national malaria control programs in SSA (Houéto et al. 2007b). Community involvement is necessary for ensuring equity in health care, as well as the sustainability of the health action (Raeburn 2005; Ridde et al. 2007). Without doing so, how can one assume to control successful child malaria in SSA where communities have many assets by living for many decades in their environment knowing some other cultural aspects of their life related to malaria, for instance, that health professionals do not know? It is to say in other words that health systems in SSA cannot "roll back malaria" without a health promotion approach which values people's assets through participation, empowerment, and contextualism (WHO 1998). The role of researchers/actors appears to us as the major factor in such an approach, for its capacity to be both "present and not", for the benefit of "indigenous knowledge", by keeping only a status of a guide/mentor and resource persons. Why professionals would like to be "gods" for communities when they have also knowledge, and are the ones living in their own context? One can imagine what we should gain in this particular intervention if we go beyond 27 months, as it was the case in the community empowerment projects reported by Raeburn (2005).

Speaking generally way, for the national health system, regarding interventions which ensure people's health and wellbeing, it seems necessary to us to mention essential attributions that professionals must have. We have drawn these attributes from the role that we played as health professional and researcher in this particular study based on population's assets. Care must be taken that health interventions/programs lie within the framework of health and the global wellbeing of the populations concerned while aiming at the community control from the early beginning of their development. Professionals take a role of:

- Guides for the establishment of the process of the intervention while aiming at the empowerment of the partner communities; and
- Advisers who are solicited according to the needs identified by the community itself within the framework for the program, neither imposing their points of view nor giving particular instructions.

Support the initiatives of community development which contribute to the improvement of the quality of life of the partner populations. The professionals are then:

- Guides of the communities in the development of social cohesion, mutual support, networking, cooperation, friendship, and the improvement of their quality of life; and
- Facilitators for the establishment of partnerships and other links between communities and the other potential actors.

Take care of the development of the community competences and skills. The professionals contribute to:

- The reinforcement of community competences through trainings and explanations on topics identified by the community itself in the course of the action,
- The development of the self-esteem and critical conscience at individual level, bringing them to more participation in the community action,

- The valorization of the positive community practices for health and wellbeing and encouragement of the community initiatives,
- Advocacy and negotiation with regard to the community's harmful practices.

The whole of these attributions shows the importance of the multisectoral work that is centered on specific contexts with its related realities. These realities are not sufficiently perceived without the full participation of the members of community, using in consequence various strategies. All this leads to the sustainability of the action through the process of implementation and evaluation and contributes to the resolution of specific health problems and to the reduction of the social inequalities of health (Fig. 14.3).

The example of malaria in SSA is a real case which shows the inefficiency in the traditional way of solving health and development problems of the populations. To base intervention on the populations' assets is certainly the best way to "roll back malaria" because of the multiple cultural and socioeconomic implications which rather make it an issue of community development. Indeed, it is known that malaria is not prevalent in the environments whose standing is average or top-of-the-range in terms of urbanization, healthiness and thus of a minimum of wealth within the populations. That implies that this work is made beyond the health system since the causes of malaria are associated with sectors outside of the health system and the community in particular. To work with the populations' assets, is to give them the possibility of putting forward all their competences and improving them in order to be able to continue implementing effectively the necessary steps for a sustainable fight against malaria. In other words, in the current situation of malaria in the SSA countries, the national malaria control program, in a global vision based on the

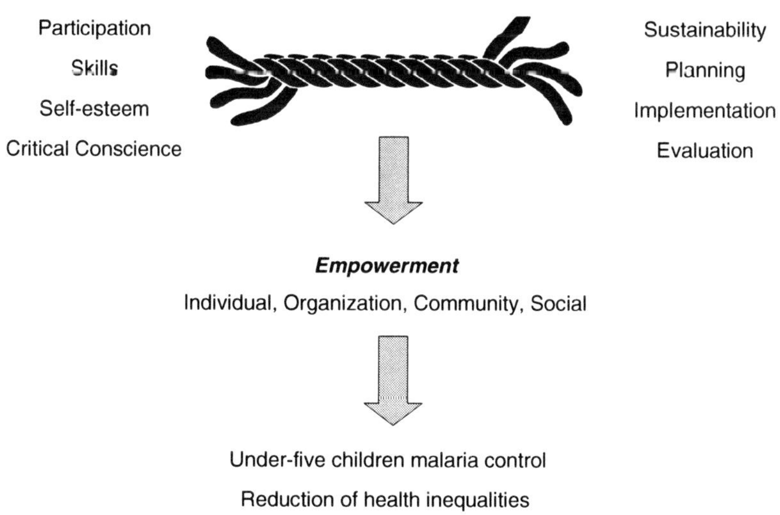

Fig. 14.3 Illustration of the process, effects and impacts of malaria control intervention based on population's assets (Adapted from Ridde et al. 2007)

populations' assets, should be sheltered by any other department rather than the Ministry of Health. Indeed, the curative aspect of malaria program will remain on the hands of the Ministry of Health because health professionals are experts in this field. This needs to be organized in the health promotion perspective in order to avoid the problems raised by a similar approach in HIV/AIDS prevention. The department to steward the malaria program could be the Presidency of the Republic or the Prime Minister in order to be able to influence the various factors that underlie malaria by giving power to those who really need it for their control. Alternatively make the Ministry of Health a Ministry delegated to the President of the Republic, as the majority of the health problems need a strategy which goes beyond the biomedical approach of disease. There is a need for the reorientation of the health system even of the system of government in the region's countries in order to be able to contribute to the improvement of health and wellbeing of the populations which suffer too much from misery and disease. Endorsing this is to work from the health promotion perspective which recognizes the important role of the individual and the community in the resolution of their health and development issues.

14.10 Conclusion

Our experience underscores the importance of using an assets based approach in the fight against child malaria. Many health problems, like malaria, are rooted in several other sectors, whose involvement is necessarily in order to reach a solution. The community in many cases also has to play an important role. So it is worth basing interventions on what the community has as resources. This has the advantage of entailing the community to be managed by the awakening of its critical conscience, but to also contribute to the resolution of other problems and to its own development. Such action deserves to be taken on a larger scale to examine more of the various methodological and operational outlines. At the current stage of health promotion status in the SSA region, the issues could be situated at the level of the availability of competent human resources, as well as the capacity of the current health systems to bring about a successful conclusion. Such an action would nevertheless turn out to be indispensable if we want to achieve the Millennium Development Goals and targets for the Health for All policy.

References

Abdulla, S., Gemperli, A., Mukasa, O., Armstrong Schellenberg, J. R. M., Lengeler, C., Vounatsou, P., et al. (2005). Spatial effects of the social marketing of insecticide-treated nets on malaria morbidity. Tropical Medicine and International Health, 10(1), 11–18.

Adongo, P. B., Kikwood, B., & Kendall, C. (2005). How local community knowledge about malaria affects insecticide-treated net use in northern Ghana. Tropical Medicine and International Health, 10(4), 366–378.

Ahorlu, C. K., Koram, K. D., Ahorlu, C., de Savigny, D., & Weiss, M. G. (2006). Socio-cultural determinants of treatment delay for childhood malaria in southern Ghana. Tropical Medicine and International Health, 11(7), 1022–1031.

Alilio, M. S., Kitua, A., Njunwa, K., Medina, M., Rønn, A. M., Mhina, J., et al. (2004). Malaria control at the district level in Africa: the case of the Muheza district in north-eastern Tanzania. American Journal of Tropical Medicine and Hygiene, 71(Suppl. 2), 205–213.

Arole, R., Fuller, B., & Deutschmann, P. (2004). Improving community capacity. In: R. Moodie, & A. Hulme (Eds.), Hands-on Health Promotion (pp. 130–145). Melbourne: IP Communications.

Barat, L. M., Palmer, N., Basu, S., Worrall, E., Hanson, K., & Mills A. (2004). Do malaria control interventions reach the poor? A view through the equity lens. American Journal of Tropical Medicine and Hygiene, 71(Suppl. 2), 174–178.

Baume, C. (2002a). Comparing care-seeking for childhood malaria: lessons from Zambia and Kenya. Arlington, Basic Support for Institutionalizing Child Survival (BASICS II) for the United States Agency for International Development. Arlington, Virginia.

Baume, C. (2002b). A Guide to Research on Care-Seeking for Childhood Malaria. Published by the Support for Analysis and Research in Africa (SARA) Project and the Basic Support for Institutionalizing Child Survival Project (BASICS II) for the United States Agency for International Development. Arlington, Virginia.

Boyte, H. (1989). Common Wealth: A return to Citizen Politics. New York: Free Press.

Breman, J. G., Alilio, M. S., & Mills, A. (2004). Conquering the intolerable burden of malaria: what's new, what's needed: a summary. American Journal of Tropical Medicine and Hygiene, 71(Suppl. 2), 1–15.

Bryce, J., el Arifeen, S., Pariyo, G., Lanata, C., Gwatkin, D., & Habicht, J. P. (2003). Reducing child mortality: can public health deliver? Lancet, 362, 159–164.

Bryce, J., Boschi-Pinto, C., Shibuya, K., Black, R. E., & the WHO Child Health Epidemiology Reference Group. (2005). WHO estimates of the causes of death in children. Lancet, 365, 1147–52.

Bryce, J., Terreri, N., Victora, C. G., Mason, E., Daelmans, B., Bhutta, Z. A., et al. (2006). Countdown to 2015: tracking intervention coverage for child survival. Lancet, 368, 1067–1076.

Butler, D. (2007). Poor follow-up hampers malaria projects. *Nature*, 450, 144–145.

Campbell, P. (2007). Millennium development holes. Nature, 446(7134), 347.

Greenwood, B. M., Bojang, K., Whitty, C. J. M., & Targett, G. A. (2005). Malaria. Lancet, 365, 1487–1498.

Hay, S. I., Guerra, C. A., Gething, P. W., Patil, A. P., Tatem, A. J., Noor, A. M., et al. (2009). A World Malaria Map: Plasmodium falciparum Endemicity in 2007. PLoS Medicine, 6(3), e1000048.

Helman, C. G. (2007). Culture, Health and Illness. 5th Edn., London: Hodder Arnold.

Houéto, D. (2007). Prévention et traitement du paludisme de l'enfant au Bénin: Empowerment communautaire et participation des parents. Thèse de Doctorat en Santé Publique, option promotion de la santé. Ecole de Santé Publique, Université Catholique de Louvain, Brussels, Belgium.

Houéto, D., & Deccache, A. (2008). Child malaria in Sub-Saharan Africa: Effective control and prevention require a health promotion approach. The International Quarterly of Community Health Education, 28(1): 51–62.

Houéto D, D'Hoore W, Ouendo EM, Deccache A. (2007a). Fièvre chez l'enfant en zone d'endémie palustre au Bénin: analyse qualitative des facteurs associés au recours aux soins. Sante publique, 19: 1–10.

Houéto, D., d'Hoore, W., Ouendo, E.-M., Charlier, D. & Deccache, A. (2007b). Malaria control among children under five in sub-Saharan Africa: The role of empowerment and parents' participation besides the clinical strategies. Rural and Remote Health, 7(4), 840. Available from: http://www.rrh.org.au.

Jones, C. O. H. (2006). Hitting malaria where it hurts: household and community responses in Africa. Id21 Insights Health, 9, 1–2.

Jones, C.O.H., & Williams, H.A. (2004). The social burden of malaria: what are we measuring? American Journal of Tropical Medicine and Hygiene, 71(Suppl. 2): 156–161.

Kamat, V. R. (2006). Seeking treatment for childhood fevers in Tanzania. *id21 Insights Health*, 9, 4.

Keiser, J., Utzinger, J., Caldas de Castro, M., Smith, T. A., Tanner, M., &. Singer, B. H (2004). Urbanization in sub-Saharan Africa and implication for malaria control. American Journal of Tropical Medicine and Hygiene, 71(Suppl. 2), 118–127.

Kickbusch, I. (2007). The move towards a new public health. Promotion & Education supplement 2, 9.

Kidane, G., & Morrow, R. H. (2000). Teaching mothers to provide home treatment of malaria in Tigray, Ethiopia: a randomized trial. Lancet, 356(9229), 550–555.

Lapeyre, L. (2006). Objectifs du Millénaire pour le développement: outils de développement ou cheval de Troie des politiques néolibérales? Alternatives Sud, 13-2006 (1), 9–26.

Lengeler, C. (2005). Insecticide-Treated Bed-Nets and Curtains for Preventing Malaria. Oxford, UK: Cochrane Database System Review CD000363.

Malaney, P., Spielman, A., & Sachs J. (2004). The malaria gap. American Journal of Tropical Medicine and Hygiene, 71(Suppl. 2), 141–146.

Marsh, V. M., Mutemi, W. M., Willetts, A., Bayah, K., Were, S., Ross, A., et al. (2004). Improving malaria home treatment by training drug retailers in rural Kenya. Tropical Medicine and International Health, 9(4), 451–460.

McFarlane, J., & Fehir, J. (1994). De madres a madres: a community, primary health care program based on empowerment. Health Education Quarterly, 21(3), 381–394.

Ministère Béninois de la Santé (MS/Bénin). (1997–2006). Annuaire des statistiques sanitaires 1996-2005. SNIGS/DPP/MS.

Ministère Béninois de la Santé (MS/Bénin). (2006). Annuaire des statistiques sanitaires 2005. SNIGS/DPP/MS.

Molyneux, H. D., & Nantulya, M. V. (2004). Linking disease control programmes in rural Africa: a pro-poor strategy to reach Abuja targets and millennium development goals. BMJ, 328, 1129–1132.

Murray, J. L. C., Laakso, T., Shibuya, K., Hill, K. & Lopez, D. A. (2007). Can we achieve Millennium Development Goal 4? New analysis of country trends and forecasts of under-5 mortality to 2015. Lancet, 370, 1040–1054.

Panosian-Dunavan, C. P. (2006). La lutte contre le paludisme. Pour la Science, 343, 42–48.

Raeburn, J. (2005). Community capacity building and mobilization: Current dimensions of community action in health promotion. A discussion paper within Track 2 Sustainable Action: Leadership, Partnership and Mobilization. Sixth Global Conference on Health Promotion, Bangkok.

Raeburn, J., & Corbett, T. (2001). Community development: How effective is it as an approach in health promotion? Paper prepared for the Second International Symposium on the Effectiveness of Health Promotion, University of Toronto, May 28–30, 2001.

Raeburn, J., & Rootman, I. (1998). People-Centred Health Promotion. Chichester, UK: John Wiley & Sons.

Ridde, V., Delormier, T., Goudreau, G. (2007). Evaluation of empowerment and effectiveness. Universal concepts? In: McQueen DV, Jones CM (Eds). Global Perspectives on Health Promotion Effectiveness. New York: Springer, 385–399.

Sirima, S. B., Konate, A., Tiono, A. B., Convelbo, N., Cousens, S., & Pagnoni, F. (2003). Early treatment of childhood fevers with pre-packaged antimalarial drugs in the home reduces severe malaria morbidity in Burkina Faso. Tropical Medicine and International Health, 8(2), 133–139.

Werner, D., & Sanders, D. (2006). Vie et mort des soins de santé primaires. In: A. Katz, & J. Duchatel (Eds.), La santé pour tous! Se réapproprier Alma Ata (pp. 27–37). People's Health Movement, Geneva: CETIM.

Williams, H. A., & Jones, C. O. H. (2004). A critical review of behavioral issues related to malaria control in sub-Saharan Africa: what contributions have social scientists made? Social Science and Medicine, 59, 501–523.

WHO (1978). Alma Ata Declaration on Primary Health Care. Geneva: World Health Organization.

WHO (2000). The African summit on Roll Back Malaria, Abuja, Nigeria. Geneva: World Health Organization (WHO/CDS/RBM/2000.17).

WHO (2003a). Malaria Is Alive and Well and Killing More Than 3000 African Children Everyday. Geneva: World Health Organization: 3. Consulté le 2 juin 2004 au http://whqlibdoc.who.int/press_release/2003/PR_33.pdf cited May 2009.

WHO (2003b). The Africa Malaria Report. Geneva (WHO/CDS/MAL/2003.1093).

WHO (2004). Scaling up Home Management of Malaria: from Research to Implementation. Geneva, World Health Organization (WHO/HTM/MAL/2004.1096).

WHO (2005). World Malaria Report 2005. Geneva: World Health Organization. http://www.rollbackmalaria.org/wmr2005 cited May 2009.

WHO (1998). Health Promotion Evaluation: Recommendations to Policy Makers: report of the WHO European working group on health promotion evaluation. Copenhagen: World Health Organization/Europe.

Yamey, G. (2004). Roll Back Malaria: a failing global health campaign. BMJ, 328, 1086–1087.

Part IV
Health Assets and Public Policy

Chapter 15
Strengthening Asset Focused Policy Making in Hungary

Péter Makara, Zsófia Németh, and Ágnes Taller

Keywords New Hungary Development Plan • Linking health and development • Health promotion in Hungary • Serfdom • EU Structural Funds

15.1 Introduction

Hungary is entering a new phase of public health development. The challenges of facing the social and health impact of the economic and financial crisis require a redressing of the balance between the assets and deficit models for evidence based public health. A greater focus on assets based approaches could help unlock some of the existing barriers to effective action on health inequities. Hungary has a history of asset approach in local communities but not always and appropriately supported by policy making at the national level. If an asset approach is to be realised, a number of things need to be in place to ensure that the aims and objectives of the New Hungary Development Plan (NHDP) can be reached. This chapter sets out the lessons learnt from the past and highlights the critical conditions for policy to assure they take account of the country's assets at the national, regional and local level.

15.1.1 Health Policy Environment

At the present situation in Hungary, the key elements of the macro-policy environment influencing the chances to promote health can be summarised as follows:

P. Makara (✉)
Master School of Health Policy, University of Debrecen, Hungary
e-mail: makara.peter@oefi.antsz.hu

A. Morgan et al. (eds.), *Health Assets in a Global Context: Theory, Methods, Action*,
DOI 10.1007/978-1-4419-5921-8_15, © Springer Science+Business Media, LLC 2010

- The present government undertook important new steps to carry out health care reform. The leadership of the Ministry of Health (MoH), for politically understandable reasons, paid more attention to the key elements of the reform (co-payments, restructuring of the care system, new system of insurance etc.) and had less energy and motivation to focus on long-term issues of health promotion.
- The complicated economic situation of the country is characterised by a considerable twin deficit of the state budget and the foreign debt of the country. Moreover a low rate of growth and from the second half of 2008 an explicit recession restricts the possibilities of public funding. This rather difficult financial situation requires innovative ways of thinking to use the assets of the country and a closer linkage of health and development.
- In the medium-term perspective, the European Union (EU) Structural Funds offers a historically unique opportunity of investment in building new capacities for disease prevention and health promotion.
- Inequities in health in Hungary are much greater than the EU average and they continue to increase. The present situation challenges policy development to use new techniques to efficiently tackle social and economic determinants of health inequalities in Hungary.

15.1.2 Main Characteristics of Health Promotion in Hungary

Health promotion has a long history in Hungary, the first programmes were established in the 1980s. The system is well developed, but not consistent, with fragile processes and capacities. The present Hungarian Public Health Strategy, "Johan Béla National Programme for the Decade of Health" (MoH 2003) has an uncertain sustainability due to its marginalization in health policy, limited government level political commitment and declining public funding. At the same time, there is a relative stability in institutional human resources and a number of action areas, such as non-communicable disease prevention, fight against harmful lifestyle habits, and HIV/AIDS prevention. Equity is a horizontal dimension of every programme planning and evaluation in public health in a mandatory way, an explicit concern on reducing health inequities is the prerequisite of any government based target founding. There are specific programmes matched to the needs of different marginalized groups, like the Roma population and poor children. However, inequity in health is still increasing in Hungary and the equity focus of the Public Health Strategy, despite of the explicit concern, is not a success area.

Examples of good practice appear mainly in communities and settings at regional and local level. There are a large number of outstanding programmes, successful initiatives and prime-movers in the different settings, such as workplaces and schools and at the community level. There are also a limited number of recent successful experiences in cooperation with the private sector (Healthy Settlement Association 2006; Healthy Settlement Association 2008).

The question that arises is how to put health, equity in health, and health promotion, higher on the policy agenda of a country in which economic circumstances and weak advocating power lead to a rather unfavourable context. The challenge in Hungary is similar to that of a large number of low- and medium-income countries in Europe. It is clear that the argument for a needs-based approach with a risk focus, despite all the moral considerations, may be insufficient in the given context. The experience of Hungary may offer an example of linking health and development at central, regional and local levels based on the assets of the country.

15.1.3 The Main Assets of Promoting Health in Hungary

In a Hungarian-specific situation for developing a successful health promotion strategy there are a number of organisational and infrastructural assets to take in consideration:

- In Hungary there is a rather well-developed legislation and institutional basis for equity and equal opportunities
- Strong representation of social scientists among health promotion professionals, with sensitivity to equity issues
- There is an existing and well-developed general nursing network, which has access to practically to all families with children
- There is a developing tradition of local health planning: more than 500 settlements have health plans and the Healthy Cities Network is well functioning
- The new legislation prescribes to each school to prepare a health plan
- In the last few years the, "health promoting workplaces" has been quite a successful initiative and has become a real movement (Association for Healthier Workplaces website; ENWHP 2004; Füzesi et al. 2008).

15.2 Setting the Scene

15.2.1 Background, Main Trends of Economic Development

After four decades of state socialism Hungary became a parliamentary democracy and a market economy in 1990. It was admitted to NATO in 1999 and joined the EU in May 2004.

After an economic and social crisis following the transition there was a period of growth in the economy between 1996 and 2005. The public debt was decreasing and the country seemed to be becoming competitive, attracting direct foreign investments. This trend has turned around 2004–2005. The last few years have seen significant economic problems with economic growth restrained by unfavourable international inflation trends and high taxes, which have reduced the competitiveness of enterprises and curbed employment. Although the causes of the difficulties and failures and possible reform solutions are still subject of public debates, there seems to be a consensus, that the roots of the current problems are deep and lie within the structural problems of the economy and society.

Opportunities for development are determined and limited to a significant degree by the tensions in the government sector. The increase in welfare spending and an overstretched pace of investment led to a budget deficit which exceeds that of most of the accession countries. Therefore Hungary's current economic policy priority is to reduce both its budget deficit and foreign debt. As a consequence of failing to meet the Maastricht convergence criteria, the adoption of the Euro has been postponed.

15.2.2 Budgetary Restrictions

Health promotion activities depend primarily on financial resources from the state budget. Coupled with rather marginal advocating possibilities, this dependency led to a decrease in funding and political support which can be clearly documented in the history of the Hungarian Public Health Strategy adopted by the Parliament in 2003 (MoH 2003). State budget restrictions have been on the agenda since 2004. Measures to reduce the budget deficit in 2006 were mainly aimed at raising incomes and less at reducing expenditures. Restrictions affect the degree of financing of government-based institutions and the employment level of public employees. (For example, the number of staff at the National Institute for Health Development in Budapest was reduced from 87 persons in 2005 to 29 in 2008, and the target funding of the Public Health Programme followed a similar trend from a starting budget of 2 billion Forint in 2004 to 600 million in 2008.) In the conditions of a financial crisis, an effective use of the EU Structural Funds for health aims, linking health and development and adopting an assets approach might be an appropriate way of tackling the challenges of a economic and social crisis.

15.2.3 Facing the Uncertainties of an Economic and Financial Crisis: The Nature of Challenge

The impact of the economic and financial crisis on the health of the Hungarian population will certainly be negative, however, we have a very limited knowledge on the nature, size and the exact mechanism of the effects we have to face. The main challenges at the moment seem to be as follows:

- The impact of economic crisis on the social and economic determinants of health
- Crisis and inequities in health
- Labour market changes, unemployment, job insecurity and health
- Crisis and mental health
- The impact of deteriorating living standards on consumption (for example, changing patterns of nutrition and use of leisure time and health)
- Health of socially excluded groups facing crisis
- The impact of the economic and financial crisis on the health system

For the short and medium term future of health promotion in Hungary, the real basis is the NHDP and using the assets of local communities.

15.3 The New Hungary Development Plan as an Asset for Promoting Health at Central Government Level

The NHDP presents a historic and unique opportunity for Hungary to catch up with more developed member states of the EU. Extraordinary financial resources are provided by the Structural Funds and Cohesion Funds of the EU for the NHDP. According to the decision of the European Commission Hungary will be eligible between 2007 and 2013 for EUR 22.4 billion to accelerate the economic improvement. This remarkable amount itself represents a great asset to ensure the necessary resources to finance and implement various development programmes.

The most important objective of NHDP is to expand employment and to create the conditions for sustainable growth (Government of the Republic of Hungary 2007). New workplaces and greater employment rate will be crucial assets for the social and economic development of the country. Six priority areas are integrated in the NHDP: the economy, transport, for the renewal of the society, environment and energy, regional development and state reform. An important asset of the NHDP is that many elements of the priorities are strongly interlinked and they build a great platform for enhanced intersectoral cooperation. Moreover, the NHDP creates a dynamic process of development and keeps these objectives on the agenda. The attention of the government will be focused on the smooth implementation of the programmes.

In general, the NHDP is an extremely important asset specifically for tackling social and economic determinants of health. Public health and health promotion received a much higher priority and more significant budget than in other countries from the new member states of the EU. The NHDP explicitly underlines the importance of promoting healthy lifestyles, developing social services and reducing child poverty. The social integration of marginalised groups such as the Roma people is targeted through actions for fighting discrimination, creating more services in local communities and strengthening the activities of non government groups (NGOs).

In the present situation the implementation process of the NHDP has started. The concrete measures related to health are mainly, but not exclusively, integrated to the operative programmes for social renewal.

The key messages in the planning process of the operative programme for social renewal are that the planned development activities should contribute to:

- Realization of the aims and objectives of the National Public Health Strategy (MoH 2003)
- Increase of healthy life expectancy
- Decrease of differences between regions
- Structural changes of the health system

The action plan was adopted in July 2007, and the implementation is currently at the start of the bidding process. The plans foresee the participation of all the partners of health promotion including government-based agencies, local governments, universities and research institutions, NGOs, and private expert agencies, mainly in the form of consortiums.

In the period 2008–2010 the key activity areas of implementation should be:

- Evidence based health curriculum development for the different levels of the educational system
- Early childhood programmes
- Programmes for healthy lifestyles
- Country-wide health monitoring system on regional basis

Most of the tenders are focused on the different settings in health promotion: schools, workplaces, and local governments, with special focus on deprived areas and socially excluded populations. The communities of most disadvantaged areas without real assets and having no skills and capacities are at high risk to be excluded from the development funding. Another open question is the sustainability of increased capacities and actions after the implementation period of the NHDP. The potential for long-term sustainability is a critical element in the decision-making process of the funding allocation, but there are a number of controversial past experiences where the development processes in public health collapsed after the end of a target funding mechanism. The most characteristic lesson learnt is the lack of sustainability of the different health promotion components in the frame of the Hungarian World Bank Loan for health services in the second half of the 1990s when, with the end of the funding, most of the important achievements were lost. Building on real existing assets might be the best guarantee for the expected sustainability.

Health promotion in Hungary is now at a critical point. If the implementation process of the NHDP is successful we can hope medium-term important outputs, outcomes, processes and results in promoting health. Also the health impact of the overall development process and the different components should be assessed. This is a task for the negotiations in the near future.

15.4 Specific Features of Community Development in Eastern Europe

In evaluating the assets of Hungarian and also Central and East European communities, their specific features and different way of functioning, as compared to Western Europe, have to be taken in consideration.

The causes of difference are historical. Throughout much of the history of European civilisation, two basic concepts of individuals dominated the way of thinking about the organisation of public life. One of them is marked by a stress on the individual as a sovereign human being who is fully competent and responsible for managing his or her own affairs, having equal abilities and inalienable rights for taking part in public decision making process. Citizens in societies based on this concept may exercise their abilities and pursue their ambitions within political, social and economic spheres of life relatively freely. These societies tend to create a liberal environment which is generally embodied and fixed in laws and an institutional infrastructure characterized by pluralist democracy and a free market economy.

The other concept emphasises a naturally unequal distribution of abilities among individuals and the inability of most people to solve their own problems themselves; it is therefore seen as appropriate to assign most if not all social competencies and responsibilities to an elite, a privileged group of people endowed with certain extraordinary qualities. Societies founded on this concept tend to build a paternalist environment in which citizen's political, social and economic activities are more strictly controlled and, as a compensation for this, most responsibilities are undertaken by state administrated or collectivist institutions which guarantee to citizens a basic economic and social security. These two concepts of individuals and the societies are "ideal types" as defined by Max Weber (1968).

The Western and rather protestant part of Europe can be associated with the first pathway. On the contrary, the communist regimes in East-Central Europe before 1989 represented the more typically paternalist societies. It is important to emphasize, however, that the communist regimes were not the original creators of the paternalist orientations. These regimes built upon and strengthened such tendencies which were already to be found at the time they came to power.

Serfdom in Western Europe came largely to an end in the 15th and 16th centuries, because of changes in the economy, population, and laws governing lord-tenant relations in Western European nations. With increased usage of money, paid labour, industrialization and urbanisation Western Europe followed a different pathway than Eastern Europe. Serfdom reached Eastern European countries later than Western Europe – it became dominant around the 15th century. Through increased demand for agricultural production in Western Europe during the later era when Western Europe limited and eventually abolished serfdom, serfdom remained in force throughout in Eastern Europe during the 17th century so that nobility-owned estates could produce more agricultural products for the profitable export market. This also led to the slower industrial development and urbanisation of those regions. Generally, this process, referred to as "second serfdom" or "export-led serfdom", which persisted until the mid-19th century, became very repressive and substantially limited serfs' rights.

The "second serfdom" was, according to the Marxist view, a return to the most primitive form of peasant service and a retreat from a market-based and money-based economy. Marxist historians further argued that it led to the gradual destruction of both peasant and urban economies, because it deprived urban craftsmen of markets for their products by hampering the growth of an affluent rural population and by fostering the self-sufficiency of landed estates. The second serfdom is seen to reflect the underdevelopment of Eastern Europe (Baldersheim et al. 1996).

As for Hungary, major elements contributing to this pathway in history are the following:

- The feudal and semi-feudal institutions were weaker than its Western-European versions, but they survived longer and hindered the development of new structures including a Western type development of local communities

- Middle classes appeared later and were not so strong. There was no homogeneous middle class culture as in developed industrial countries
- Achievements of the industrial revolution and capitalism were imported in a very rapid way and the adoption of them happened in a few decades, lacking the relevant social and economic antecedents and traditions
- The adaptation of socialism even strengthened the survival of the former patterns of historical development and also limited the development of local community and society

The strictly centralised structure of political power and the economic system resulted in a top-down structure of society, meaning that local power was the least influential in the system (Hankiss 1982).

Within these circumstances, civil activity appeared already in the 1970s rather as kind of resistance mentality, for example, in the economy as "second alternatives" and later in environment protection, anti-nuclear protestation, etc.

On the contrary, the community assets approach is based on positive incentives. So, for reasons deeply enrooted in Central and East European history, concepts like community resilience and citizens' participation in local community life have a very different content from the Western standards, also reflected as norms in international documents. Taking all this in to consideration, community level health promotion has been a success story in Hungary in the last two decades (Gergely 1993).

15.5 Integrating Health in Local Development Plans

15.5.1 The City Health Promotion Plan of Békéscsaba

The following case study aims to demonstrate a good example of a local health plan developed by Békéscsaba, a Hungarian city, located in a less developed, economically deprived region of the country Békéscsaba is one of the few Hungarian cities that have developed a long-term health strategy. The health plan is based on a thorough situation analysis, has set clear targets and is successfully embedded into the general, comprehensive development framework of the city.

15.5.2 The Socioeconomic Profile of Békéscsaba

Békéscsaba is the seat of the Békés county which is situated in South-East Hungary, close to the Romanian border. This region has always had a strong agricultural profile and has never been economically well-developed. Since the economic and political transition in the 1990s, the marginalised position of the region in terms of industrial production and the export in services has not improved. The gross domestic product (GDP) in Békés county is 59.5% of the national average and 38.8% of the EU-27 average (KSH 2007). Regarding employment, the inactivity rate is 64% and the unemployment rate is four times greater than in 1990 (Békés megye területi jellemzői az európai uniós csatlakozáskor 2004). The county is characterised by a low density in population and negative demographic trends. In Békés county the birth rate is the third lowest among all Hungarian counties, yet has the highest mortality rate leading to the highest natural demographic decrease compared to other counties.

Békéscsaba has 67,000 inhabitants and, due to the number of administrative bodies, transport junctions and developing infrastructure, it is the most important and biggest city in Békés. The city is characterised by long historical traditions, a notable cultural heritage and a strong local identity.

15.5.3 Experience in Health Promotion Prior to the City Health Promotion Plan

Békéscsaba has been a member of the World Health Organization (WHO) Initiative "Network of Healthy Cities" since 1998. Thanks to a group of committed and skilled health professionals and especially a strongly engaged, charismatic expert, Békéscsaba has been an active member of the Hungarian Healthy Cities Association.

One of the key achievements of the last decade has been the establishment of the Intersectoral Committee on Health, composed of 21 members from different sectors and administrative bodies such as the public health office of the county, the local government of the city and the county, the district nurses, the family counselling centres, the police, various health care units, environmental authorities, and so on. The work of the Intersectorial Committee is coordinated by the health office of the local government. Among others this office is responsible for the implementation of the programmes linked to the Healthy Cities Network.

In 2000 a "Health Profile" was carried out by the local government to assess the health status of the population and to map the health assets of the city. This report later served as a starting point and provided baseline measures for the development of the City Health Promotion Plan.

15.5.4 The Development Plan of Békéscsaba: A General Framework

Before 2004, when Hungary joined the EU, some cities launched development plans for the application of EU grants, most importantly to the Structural Funds. The local government of Békéscsaba also prepared a so-called City Development

Plan (Városi Egészségfejlesztési and Békéscsaba 2004) for the city. The Plan consisted of several sub-programmes such as an Environment Protection Plan, a Housing Programme, a Social Policy Service Planning Concept and an Education, Culture, Sport Concept. With special respect to the objectives and activities of these sub-programmes the Settlement Development Plan was completed by a Health Promotion Plan.

15.5.5 Setting up the City Health Promotion Plan

The City Health Promotion Plan (Városi Egészségfejlesztési and Békéscsaba 2004) was prepared in 2003 and set objectives for a time frame of ten years, from 2004 to 2014. The Intersectorial Committee on Health was responsible for defining the fundamental priorities and key objectives of the Plan. Strong links were established with other sub-programmes within the comprehensive Settlement Development Plan, and the objectives were built upon the programmes of the Healthy Cities Network as well as upon the aims of the National Public Health Strategy (MoH 2003).

As a next step working groups elaborated each objective and provided a detailed description about the activities. The first draft was commented by the corresponding expert committees of the local government. This amended version was launched on the website of the self governance for a public debate. Based on the citizens' opinions and comments the second draft was launched by the Intersectoral Committee. After a final approval of the Health Committee of the local government the General Assembly accepted the plan.

15.5.6 Key Objectives of the City Health Promotion Plan

The objectives were defined along the principle that promoting and maintaining health has to be based on partnerships and multisectorality. It is clearly stated in the document that developing health is the most effective investment for the future. Therefore it is a fundamental task and interest of the local government to strengthen the assets of individuals and communities, and to foster existing programmes and structures in health development. It is strongly emphasised that promoting health goes beyond the health sector, thus all objectives have to be linked with work programmes of other sectors such as environment, education, and so on.

The plan declares medium-term and long-term objectives. On long-term, until 2014 the plan aims:

- To visibly improve the quality of life of the population
- To increase the number of healthy life years by 3–4 years
- To decrease premature mortality by 5%
- To reduce the number of people suffering from addictive behaviours by 7%
- To decrease the smoking prevalence by 5%
- To reduce fat consumption by 10%

- To decrease the prevalence of abortions by 10%
- To close the health gap for marginalised people
- To make healthy lifestyles a social norm
- To establish and to foster intersectorial cooperation in health
- To develop health prevention services and to increase the number of community-based leisure time health promotion programmes by 40%
- To improve the cost-effectiveness and the quality of health care

These objectives should be implemented through five programmes:

Programmes for creating a supportive environment for a better health.These programmes address in particular youth and the elderly in various settings. Several programmes aim to tackle health inequalities and target discriminated and marginalised groups, especially Roma people, unemployed, homeless people, disabled people and youth-at-risk.

1. Programmes for healthy lifestyles. These programmes cover smoking cessation, prevention of drug use and excessive alcohol consumption. Fostering healthy nutrition and strengthening physical activities are also integrated into the programmes.
2. Programmes for environmental health. These programmes are strongly linked to other developmental projects of the city such as creating a new system of waste management, building bypass roads to avoid the built-up area of Békéscsaba, and the eradication of ragweed or to improve drinking water quality. Moreover, the programmes also include education programmes for school children and establishing a population-based information system on environmental health.
3. Programmes for preventing premature mortality. The programmes are implemented against four major non-communicable health threats: cardiovascular diseases, cancer, mental health problems and musculoskeletal disorders. Certainly all programmes are interlinked to other programmes on smoking cessation, prevention of drug and excessive alcohol use, promoting healthy nutrition and physical activity as well as strengthening environmental health.
4. Programmes for screening tests. Information campaigns are organised to increase the participation in screening tests such as cancer screening, blood pressure screening, mammography and cervix screening.

15.5.7 Main Assets of the City Health Promotion Plan

Applying the concepts of Kretzmann and McKnight 1993, the assets tackled by the City Health Promotion Plan of Békéscsaba can be described as follows:

1. *Primary building blocks*: referring to the assets and the capacities located inside the neighbourhood and largely under neighbourhood control.
   In Békéscsaba there have been a number well-functioning services and organisations in place representing the positive capability of the city to identify key challenges and to activate solutions in health promotion.

First, the city has always shown a true commitment towards promoting health and tackling health inequalities. A series of examples illustrate these efforts, as described above, such as the active membership in the Healthy Cities Association, carrying out a situation analysis in health, etc. The leadership of the city showed a generally positive approach towards health promotion which was proved by establishing an Interesectorial Committee on Health, supporting the work of the expert team and maintaining a good relationship with civic organisations.

Second, probably due to the long historical traditions and the notable cultural heritageof Békéscsaba, its citizens have developed a strong local identity and social cohesion. It should be emphasised that this positive cooperative attitude was an important pre-requisite for launching the Settlement Development Plan. The sub-programmes of the plan from other sectors served as an essential reference point and created crucial links with the health targets: for instance reconstructing the waste management system has clearly a decisive impact on health.

Third, a number of civil organisations, local foundations and clubs play an essential role in health promotion in Békéscsaba and they are integrated in the implementation of the City Health Promotion Plan. A voluntary peer group, "Támasz–Téka", and a so-called self-knowledge programme, "Érted! Érted?" both target youth. A pregnant women club, a telephone hotline for the elderly and a cooking club are also important instruments in reaching the goals of the City Health Promotion Plan. Two foundations, the Dr Baly Mental Health Foundation and the SOS Teenager Foundation, make significant contributions to develop the health of Békéscsaba's citizens.

2. *Secondary building blocks*: referring to the assets located within the community but largely controlled by outsiders. The City Health Promotion Plan builds, to a large extent, upon those services which are located within the community but run by the government at national level. Such services are provided, for instance, by the district nurses who are in charge of counselling pregnant women and families with newborn babies. All pregnant women have to consult a district nurse in order to be entitled for maternity allowance by the state. Thus district nurses have direct and intense access to these population groups. Another key asset is given by the drug coordinators at schools. In Hungary all schools have to appoint a drug coordinator who is responsible for implementing drug prevention programmes. Moreover, a Drug Coordination Forum has to be set up by each local government to keep drug prevention high on the agenda. In addition, the Roma Minority Local Government, which exists in many local governments, ensures better access for the Roma population and makes notable contributions to the development programmes.
3. *Potential building blocks*: referring to resources originating outside the neighbourhood and largely controlled by outsiders. The New Hungary Development Plan and the EU Structural Funds are important catalysts in initiating development strategies at local levels and they ensure the appropriate funding for their implementation.

15.6 Conclusions

Current approaches to define development come under four headings:

- Economic growth
- Reduction of inequality
- Reduction of poverty
- Maximization of individual capability in these terms
- Investing in health is critical to economic productivity and human development
- Greater equity promotes economic growth and human development

The WHO document, Health: a precious asset makes the case that health is both an input and an outcome of development. The argument is as follows: *"If health is an asset and ill-health a liability for poor people, protecting and promoting health are central to the entire process of poverty eradication and human development. As such they should be goals of development policy shared by all sectors - economic, environmental and social" (WHO* 2000*; p 20).*

The WHO document puts forward three action proposals:

- Strengthen global policy for social development
- Integrate health dimensions into economic and social policy
- Develop health systems to meet the needs of poor and vulnerable populations

The Nobel Laureate economist Amartya Sen (1999) provided a more focused analysis. Agreeing that *"good health is an integral part of good development"*, he went on to argue that low-income countries should use "support-led" processes, focused strategically on more health care, education, and other social programs.

So there is a sound rationale to extend the conceptual framework of the assets approach in health to the key developmental investments and processes of development. We hope the example of Hungary offers some evidence for it.

References

Association for Healthier Workplaces website. http://www.emegy.hu/?base=szanyagok cited May 2009.

Baldersheim, H., Illner, M., Offerdal, A., Rose, L., Swianiewicz, P. (eds.) (1996). *Local democracy and the process of transformation in East-Central Europe*. Boulder: Westview Press.

Békés megye területi jellemzői az európai uniós csatlakozáskor. (2004). (Characteristics of the Békés county at the time of the EU accession). http://www.bekestt.hu/dokumentumok/dir3/420_5_B_k_s_Megye_ter_leti_jellemz_i.pdf cited May 2009.

ENWHP. (2004). *ENWHP Toolbox. A European collection of methods and practices for promoting health at the workplace*. Woerden: The European Network for Workplace Health Promotion

Füzesi, Z., Szőke, K., Tistyán, L. (2008). *Egészségmegőrzés a közösségekben. Kézikönyv az Egészségterv elkészítéséhez. Béres Egészség Hungaricum Program. Béres Egészség*

Hungarikum Alapítvány/Health promotion in communities. Handbook for Preparing a Health Plan. Béres Health Hungarikum Program. Béres Health Hungarikum Association.
Gergely, A. (1993). Önszervező társadalom I. – Önszervező és önépítő társadalom II. (Self-organizing society I. – Self-Organizing and Self-Building Society II.) In: Önkormányzati Szemle (Local Government Review). III. Volume, 1–2.
Government of the Republic of Hungary (2007). The New Hungary Development Plan National Strategic Reference Framework of Hungary 2007–2013 Employment and Growth http://www.nfu.hu/uj_magyarorszag_fejlesztesi_terv_2 cited May 2009.
Hankiss, E. (1982). *Diagnózisok (Diagnoses).* Magvető Könyvkiadó, Budapest-Dabas.
Healthy Settlement Association. (2006). Települési Egészségterv Program 2005–2006. Egészséges Településekért Alapítvány 2006./Settlement Health Plan Programme 2005–2006.
Healthy Settlement Association. (2008). *Partnerségi Települési Egészségterv Program 2006–2007. Egészséges Településekért Alapítvány 2008/Settlement Partnership Health Plan Programme 2006–2007.*
Kretzmann, J.P. & McKnight, J. (1993). *Building communities from the inside out: A path toward finding and mobilizing a community's assets.* Chicago: ACTA Publications.
KSH. (2007). Központi Statisztikai Hivatal (Central Statistical Office): Magyarország nemzeti számlái (National Accounts Hungary) 2004–2005. http://portal.ksh.hu/pls/ksh/docs/hun/xftp/idoszaki/monsz/monsz0405.pdf cited May 2009.
MoH. (2003). *'Johan Béla' National Programme for the Decade of Health.* Budapest: Ministry of Health. http://www.eum.hu/english/public-health-programme/national-public-health cited May 2009.
Sen, A. (1999). Health and Development. *Bulletin of the World Health Organization*, 77(8), 619–623.
Városi Egészségfejlesztési Terv, Békéscsaba. (2004). (City Health Development Plan of Békéscsaba) www.bekescsaba.hu/resource.aspx?ResourceID=I-EGESZSEGUGY-VET cited May 2009.
Weber, M. (1968). *Economy and society: An outline of Interpretive Sociology*, Guenther Roth and Claus Wittich, eds. New York: Bedminster Press.
WHO. (2000). *Health: A precious asset. (WHO/HSD/HÍD/00.1)* Geneva: World Health Organization.

Chapter 16
How Forms of Social Capital Can Be an Asset for Promoting Health Equity

Fran Baum

Keywords Health equity • Health policy • Social capital • Social determinants of health

16.1 Introduction

This chapter argues that societies that support and produce governments with a commitment to equity will be characterised by high levels of social capital including social cohesion. Commitment to action on the social determinants of health to increase equity in health status requires a proactive policy approach from governments and that governments demonstrating this proactivity will be those that have a value commitment to equity. This chapter is intended to be complementary to Chap. 9 in this volume by Kawachi that provides a review of the literature on the associations between social capital and health status. The chapter will not repeat the evidence which links social capital with health outcomes, but will pay particular attention to the notion of linking social capital and the role ascribed it by Szreter and Woolcock (2004) in giving rise to policies that are egalitarian in intention. Lomas (1998, p. 1181) has commented that: *"on the one hand, millions of dollars are committed to alleviating ill-health through individual intervention. Meanwhile we ignore what our everyday experience tells us, i.e. the way we organise our society, the extent to which we encourage interaction among the citizenry and the degree to which we trust and associate with each other in caring communities is probably the most important determinant of our health"*.

This chapter will develop Lomas' theme and extend it to examine how the ways we conceive and develop social policy has a dramatic effect upon health outcomes and the extent to which they are distributed across society. The chapter will also build on the work of Wilkinson (2005) and Wilkinson and Pickett (2009) who has argued that improvements in population health in rich countries will come from

F. Baum (✉)
Southgate Institute for Health, Society and Equity Flinders University, Adelaide, Australia
e-mail: Fran.Baum@flinders.edu.au

A. Morgan et al. (eds.), *Health Assets in a Global Context: Theory, Methods, Action*,
DOI 10.1007/978-1-4419-5921-8_16,

making them more equal. Social capital has also been seen as a means of putting the "social" back onto a policy agenda that has become increasingly dominated by neo-liberal economic considerations and to argue for a return to a focus on the community in public policy (see for example, Putnam 1996; Cox 1995; Baum 1999a). Thus it can be seen as an asset for shifting the focus of the policy agenda.

The chapter starts by examining the relationships between different types of social capital (bonding, bridging and linking), and individual and community health and well-being outcomes, including the extent of equity. It then considers why more equitable societies are higher in forms of social capital, and the extent to which the causality of the relationship is mutually re-enforcing. Finally the chapter considers the importance of government policies that create an environment in which equitable health and well-being outcomes are likely, and the roles of different forms of social capital in bringing these about. The main argument in the chapter is that despite conceptual difficulties associated with social capital, it does offer a way to insert a social aspect in to debates about public health policies. This is particularly important in the current period of rapid economic globalisation, which is stressing individualism and consumerism to such an extent that ideas of community and solidarity that give rise to egalitarian policies are significantly threatened. Social capital offers a means of highlighting the value of social factors on health and well-being at the local, regional, national and international levels for individuals and communities. The basic argument of the chapter is that equity is crucial to a healthy society, and that social capital is a means by which a constituency for health equity may be created through the promotion of solidarity both within and between societies, at the national and international level.

I acknowledge that there is a debate about the extent to which equity (measured by equity of income distribution) does indeed lead to better health outcomes. This chapter broadly accepts the argument that income equity is health promoting, as put forward by Wilkinson (2005). Lynch et al. (2004) reviewed the literature on income inequality and health and the overwhelming majority of papers showed clear relationships between income inequality and health. Another crucial part of the evidence comes from the "low income high health" countries which appear to maintain striking good health status on very low per capita income. This may, in part, be because they are very equal communities (Halstead et al. 1985; Sanders and Werner 1997).

16.2 Types of Social Capital in Relation to Health and Health Equity

There are significant theoretical debates about social capital and its meaning (Portes 1998; Macinko and Starfield 2001). The term "social capital" is used to describe very different phenomenon from a Swedish study that uses local voting levels as its sole measure of linking social capital to sociological studies that deal with it in a theoretically complex way linking social capital (Sundquist and Yang, 2007).

Muntaner (2004) points out that the term is often used to describe phenomenon that would be better described with more precise terms such as social cohesion or integration. This chapter will engage with some of these debates to make the argument that drawing on existing theories of social capital provides opportunities to determine the ways in which policies can be formed to support health equity. In order to do this it is necessary to examine the three forms of social capital that have been identified. Their potential in relation to health and equity is summarised in Table 16.1. A further analysis of different forms of social capital can be found in Kawachi's chapter, "The relationship between health assets, social capital and cohesive communities".

16.3 Bonding, Bridging and Linking Social Capital

16.3.1 Bonding

Bonding social capital is that between relatively closely-knit groups who are likely to share many characteristics in common. It may be exclusionary and may not act to produce society-wide benefits of co-operation and trust (Baum and Ziersch 2003). A number of commentators make the point that the outcomes of bonding social capital may not necessarily be beneficial (Portes 1998; Baum 1999a, b; Pearce and Davey Smith 2003). Thus a tightly bonded group might be controlling of its members and may, for example, develop racist attitudes that are rarely challenged because of the tightness of the group. In this case, the outcomes that flow from the bonded social capital infrastructure do not make a positive contribution to society and are unlikely to create the environment in which pressures in favour of health equity would flourish.

The violence that broke out in December 2005 between largely ethnically Anglo white male surfers and young men from a Lebanese background in Cronulla, New South Wales, Australia, was a classic example of the potential downside of strong bonding social capital. On both sides there are likely to be strong networks between people and a fair degree of trust, but this is operating within the groups and is not leading to bridging social capital that would help create tolerance and acceptance of diversity.

Bonding social capital is most likely to operate in local communities. It is also likely (but not always) to be highly class and ethnic specific. Working class bonding social capital is likely to be more bound by geography (Cattell 2001), while middle and upper class may be more likely to operate across space, because of the educational and professional work opportunities which form with less strong links to local communities. When upper and middle class social capital is largely of the bonding kind then acceptance of measures to reduce inequities is likely to be lower simply because people would not experience the reality of life of working class people. In addition, they would not have the chance to develop empathy with people from different economic backgrounds.

Table 16.1 Types of social capital and links to health equity

Type of social capital	Main characteristics	Ways in which it might promote health equity	Ways in which it has the potential to detract from health equity
Bonding	Vertical tight relationships between people with similar characteristics	• Provision of social support and psychological or practical assistance • There is evidence that such support can help recovery from illness • Lead to formation of groups that might take action in support of health (e.g. protection of community from threat or further strengthening support network)	• Might be threatening to outsiders and lead to exclusionary mentality therefore threatening social cohesion • Conflict within closely bonded group might become unhealthy for some members • Close bonding among more powerful may act to restrict access to material resources from other groups/classes
Bridging	Looser relationships across different or diverse groups (e.g.: ethnic groups)	• Lose bond between people from different backgrounds • Likely to help social cohesion especially when differences could be corrosive • Common in social movements many of which argue for greater equity	• Conflict within relationships might become unhealthy for some and more likely for people without emotional intelligence skills
Linking	Relationship across power barrier(often class)	• Leads to situations in which benefits flow from more powerful and influential to less powerful and influential • Potentially contributing to overcoming structural economic inequities	• Has been suggested it is means of quelling discontent with capitalist system of production and so will impede more radical change of unfair economic system

Bonding patterns will also differ by locality and level of development of a community. Bonding social capital is important in the provision of social support to people especially at times of crisis or enhanced need such as illness or childbirth. Those embedded within more middle or upper class networks might be expected to have access to networks which have the capacity to provide more support and assistance. Although it has been argued that some close knit well-functioning poor communities (for example in rural areas) can provide high degrees of social support. While upper or middle class bonding networks are likely to lead to access to resources that will assist people gain educational or employment advantage. This point has been most forcefully argued by Bourdieu (1986).

Pierre Bourdieu, the French sociologist, developed his ideas about social capital in his efforts to explain persistent inequities between groups in French society which could not be described by access to economic capital alone. He saw there were two other forms of capital, cultural and social, which determine an individual's position within the social structure. His definition of social capital was as: "*the aggregate of the actual or potential resources which are linked to possession of a durable network of more or less institutionalised relationships of mutual acquaintance and recognition*" (Bourdieu 1986, p. 248). The social capital he described was essentially concerned with a class bonded form of social capital. He shows that individuals (and collectively, a class of individuals) are able to reproduce and maintain their privilege partly because of the ways in which networks and the trust they generate lead to material benefits. A simplified way of looking at Bourdieu's theory is that he was describing the role of what is often called "an old boy's network" in which social contact established through social networks are used to gain a variety of economic benefits. His view of society is that conflict over resources is a central feature and that networks can play a key role in maintaining the existing distribution of resources. This means that they can also have the potential to bring about a re-distribution of resources if the networks of advantage can be weakened and the networks of disadvantage strengthened.

Bonding social capital can, in some circumstances, contribute to social change processes by forming the basis of social change movements. Trade unions represent such a form of social capital. An example would be the links and trust among union members in a close-knit mining town in the north of England or South Wales in the UK.

16.3.2 Bridging

Bridging ties are looser than bonding ties and operate across differences, in say, culture or ethnicity but not in terms of institutional power and influence. An example would be links made within an amateur football league between the members of different teams who also came from different ethnic groups such as English, Serbian, Italian or Greek, or social networks between people with different employment status. Bridging ties are likely to play a crucial role in creating cohesiveness within ethnically diverse societies. They may also play a role in encouraging social mobility by being a means by which the benefits that can flow from networks are extended beyond closely bonded networks. Thus they are likely to play a role in creating more equitable communities. They are also particularly important in societies undergoing rapid change especially through migration as they can play a role in creating more social cohesion.

Modern social movements that are typically focussed on one issue are an example of bridging social networks. Thus environment movements, gay or lesbian networks or broad-based professional associations provide an example. The voice of these groups is often excluded from the mainstream of society and media and the links between them can lead to strong advocacy for a more equitable society.

16.3.3 Linking

Linking social capital refers to relationships between people that operate across explicit, formal or institutionalised power or authority gradients in society (Szreter and Woolcock 2004; Szreter 2002). Szreter and Woolcock (2004, p. 655) define linking social capital as "norms of respect and networks of trusting relationships between people who are interacting across explicit, formal or institutionalised power or authority gradients in society". They used the concept to examine historical periods in which they argued that classes with power were more likely to take action to improve the conditions of those in less fortunate positions. Muntaner (2004) has pointed out that some of the examples they give may be more to do with classes conceding some ground in order to hold on to power in the face of pressure from social and trade union movements. This implies that linking social capital has to be conceived as the pressure in society towards progressive, socially just change which will involve both upward pressure and government policy commitment. Certainly Szreter's (1988) historical work that has elaborated the McKeown's (1979) thesis on the ways in which social rather than medical interventions increased life expectancy in nineteenth and twentieth century England has stressed the role played by social movements in bringing about a public health revolution. Of course linking social capital has to be understood as a process that is reflective of class, gender and other social tensions and as one that has links to the notion of solidarity. With this understanding linking social capital has the potential to be a great asset for health equity.

16.4 Social Capital and Equity

Figure 16.1 shows the ways in which health inequities are created through social and economic structures, opportunities and networks, and psychosocial and behavioural mechanisms. In the case of each of these contributors to health inequity, social capital can play a role in making the outcomes more equitable. Bonding and bridging social capital are most important to the psychosocial and behavioural mechanisms displayed in Fig. 16.1. Linking social capital will be most crucial to the structure and opportunities that flow from networks and to shaping the ideologies that drive the social structure. The idea of a society high in social capital implies one which is integrated, accepting of difference, has high social and civic participation with bonded, bridging and linking networks which produce co-operation and trust among the citizens (Kawachi et al. 1997; Kawachi et al. 1999) and a desire to provide a fair go, for all members of the community. Such a society is likely to result in more straightforward and effective ways of working together as it would minimise corruption, mistrust and the consequent problems of achieving common outcomes. High social capital society would also be low in alienation and anomie.

The growing literature on social exclusion (Hill et al. 2002) demonstrates that participation in a range of health promoting activities is structured by class, gender and ethnicity. Civic and social participation have also been shown to be linked to socio-economic factors (Baum et al. 1999). Wilkinson (2005), and Wilkinson and Pickett (2009), based upon an extensive review of the evidence, concludes that equity of income distribution in a population leads to a society with these high social capital attributes – these are displayed in Box 16.1. It is hard, however, to determine the direction of causality. One may assume that a high social capital society will result in more equitable health outcomes and that social capital is easier to generate in more equitable societies in such a way that a virtuous cycle is established in which

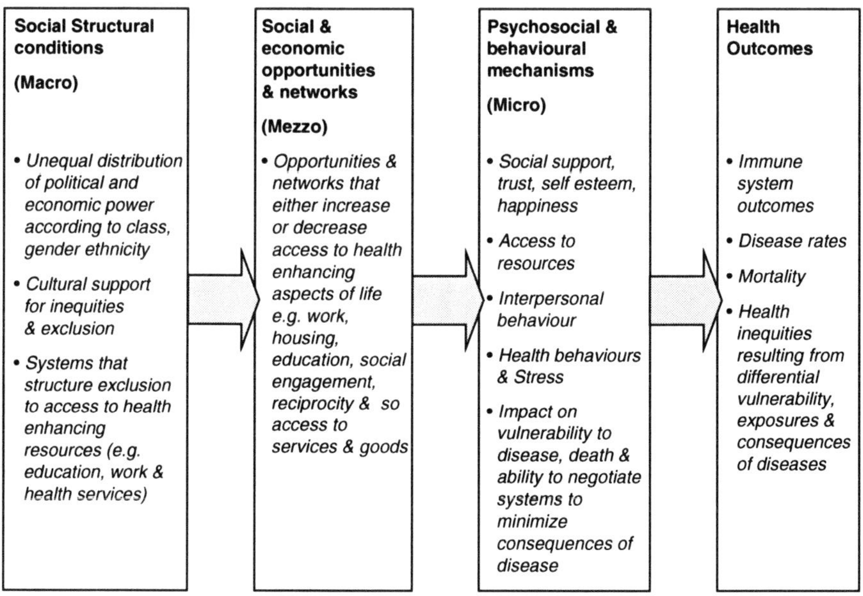

Fig. 16.1 Explanations of inequitable health outcomes (Based on Diderichsen and Hallqvist (1997) and adapted from Berkman and Glass (2000))

Box 16.1 Features associated with more equitable societies likely to promote health

Higher levels of trust
Increased political participation and engagement including higher rates of voting
Stronger and more cohesive community life
Less violent crime including homicide
Less hostility and racism
Healthier populations

Source: Wilkinson (2005) & Wilkinson and Pickett (2009).

the positive attributes are both reinforced by and help create equity. Certainly living in a more equitable society would give people a sense of fairness that is likely to make people feel inclined to behaviour in a civil manner. Veenstra (2001) notes that a society with a wide distribution of incomes is one with a pronounced status order and says *"those falling short in psycho-social comparisons with others will feel this shortcoming quite strongly, given the width of the gap, and consequently will suffer poorer health than will the "losers" of comparisons in more equal places"* (Veenstra 2001, p. 75).

That social capital has assumed such a prominent place in modern sociology dates from the attention it received from Robert Putnam, a sociologist from the United States, who brought social capital to the forefront in policy discussions. His interest in social capital was not related to understanding inequity. His original work on social capital, *Making Democracy Work*, was a longitudinal study of the reasons that accounted for the relative economic performance of regional governments in Italy (Putnam 1993). He found that the success of regional governments was significantly determined by the level of social capital in the community. In northern Italy, which has extensive voluntary associations and community groups, he concluded high social capita exists and the regional governments were more successful than those in the south where most social relationships were vertical and strictly hierarchical.

It was when Putnam applied his ideas to society in the United States that his work gained extensive coverage. His book, *Bowling Alone* (Putnam 2000), argued that there was a decline in social capital as shown by the fact less people were joining groups and voting and as a response to this less civic behaviour, crime was increasing and trust in other people declining in the US over the past half a century. This book took social capital from a scholarly idea to a popular concept that began to be used by conservative institutions such as the World Bank, politicians in many different countries and the media, including being commonly mentioned on chat shows.

In Putnam et al. 2003 he has continued the argument that social capital is in decline. His work established a focus on social capital that has essentially ignored the broader economic and political backdrop against which patterns of social capital change. Wilkinson (2005) points out that over the period Putnam saw a decline in social capital, economic inequity in the US increased significantly yet the implications of this increase are not explored in Putnam's work. In an extensive critique of Putnam's work, Arneil (2006) points out that Putnam assumes that the early periods of higher social capital was the experience of all the population. She further maintains that many groups were excluded from this, especially migrant groups and women, and that the somewhat idyllic communities of the past mourned by Putnam were less positive than he suggests. Thus she suggests that while there are changes in social capital, they should not be seen as a decline. The essence of the critique of Putnam's work was summed up in a review of one of his books.

> Putnam conceives the challenge for reforms as a matter of personal resolve – at the local level. There is nothing essentially wrong with existing political and economic arrangements. No redistribution of power or access to resources is necessary. Nor are race, ethnic and gender relations in need of fundamental reform. (Mowbray 2005, p. 461)

This pithy critique summarises the reasons why the Putnam tradition of work on social capital has little to offer the central concern of this chapter. The consideration of the ways in which the concept might assist in devising and encouraging uptake of policies designed to reduce health inequity. Critics of the use of social capital in epidemiological studies of health inequity (Muntaner 2004; Lynch et al. 2004) note that the term "social capital" is usually used in a manner that is unquestioning about the notion of a capitalist society and generally does not question the political and economic power dimensions associated with capitalism or the role of social capital within it and that the focus on social capital ignores the reality of material deprivation (Lynch et al. 2000) and is blind to class and power imbalances (Navarro 2002; Muntaner 2004). These critiques imply that social capital has little to offer the pursuit of health equity. However, much depends on the ways in which social capital is theorised and then used as a basis for policy.

The challenge is to ensure that social capital scholarship is not blind to class and power dimensions but rather explores the ways in which social and civic life act to reinforce and reproduce existing patterns of privilege and power. If this were done than social capital would be a much stronger asset in the pursuit of health equity. Social capital offers a framework with which to think through the ways in which societies have to change in order to become more equitable and which policies might assist in bringing this about. Its particular use is in offering a framework that spans local networks to policy networks influenced by linking social capital.

16.5 Policies, Forms of Social Capital and the Creation of Health Equity

Social theorists from across the right to left political spectrum have explored the policy implications of social capital. Unsurprisingly, the main division between those on the right and those on the left is the role of the state in using its power to create or influence levels of social capital. Those on the right, (for example Putnam as previously cited and Fukuyama 1996), do not see that the state has a role and see social capital as emerging from civil society action and community norms. On the left there is a much greater willingness to see the potential for government action. This was shown by the policy agenda set out by Australian social commentator Eva Cox (1995) for the way government policies could contribute to a "truly civil society" that is inclusive of previously marginalised groups. It is also shown by the policy agenda of the UK Blair Labour Government that explicitly used the language of social capital as a basis for their quest to reduce inequity (Halpern 2005). Szreter's work has also stressed the importance of state action. Some on the left (most noticeable Navarro 2002) are sceptical about the potential for social capital to change the structures that create inequity.

However, this section takes the position that governments can influence the level and distribution of social capital and uses this influence to decrease exclusion from material benefits. It is important to note that this section is written in full appreciation of the importance of material factors to understanding the existence of health inequities (for an elaboration of these see Doyal 1979; Navarro 2002). The focus here on social capital is not to suggest that the material basis of inequity is not fundamental and crucial but to explore the ways in which the concept of social capital can assist in creating a society in which a fairer distribution of material resources comes to be seen as a central expectation and goal of government. It will consider linking social capital first because it operates at the level at which policy values are formulated and is likely to set the policy agenda for initiatives that are more local and community based.

16.6 Linking Social Capital and Policy

Linking social capital implies that there is a sense of obligation from powerful institutions in society towards the less powerful. In Bourdieu's conception of social capital it is clear that the networks and reciprocities involved in exchanges most commonly work to the benefit of the already well-off and more powerful groups. They do this by giving people pathways by which they gain access to educational, cultural and employment opportunities. Policies aimed at reducing inequities should aim to ensure that the benefits that accrue to certain classes in society should be made available to other less powerful and privileged groups. Most typically this would involve action on the social determinants of health. Raphael (2003), based on his analysis of Canada, maintains that action on the social determinants is marginalized in public policy and that governments are reluctant to take this action. He sees them as acting more in the interests of capital than equity and health improvement. A society-wide concern and pressure on government to implement policies that were concerned with redistribution (for example death duties, wealth tax or more progressive taxation system) would be an example of linking social capital.

Szreter and Woolcock (2004) argue that consideration of the relationship of the state in terms of the initiation and sustaining of networks, trust and social structures is crucial. They show, with illustrations from the case study of nineteenth century England, that governments (local and central) can create and encourage the conditions in which linking social capital can operate and so make the likelihood of a progressive government committed to redistribution more likely.

We have also seen above that social capital has been interpreted differently by different theorists and that to speak of social capital alone without situating the concept in a broad set of social theories is meaningless. Social capital requires understanding within this broader theoretical landscape. Szreter and Woolcock (2004, p. 654) note that social capital is one of those concepts (like "class", "race" and "gender") that is simply too politically and ideologically important for those at any point on the political spectrum to concede to a definition of the term that they do not see as squaring with their own beliefs, assumptions and principles. One of the most important social theory debates to situate social capital within is the structure versus agency issue which involves exploring the complex interactions and interconnections between the choices individuals make and the institutional forces that shape these. This debate is central to public health and to so many strategies that are designed to improve health. So many public health strategies depend on individuals being prepared to give up some agency in favour of the greater good. Examples are laws which enforce seat belt wearing, restrict smoking, curtail food advertising, restrict gun ownership or impose safety standards on consumer products. Some countries and communities are much more prepared to accept constraints on the behaviours of individuals than others. Thus in the Nordic countries there is a far greater acceptance of the need to restrict the rights of individuals than in the United States.

A crucial question for public health is: What is it that makes this difference? Clearly in societies like those of the Nordic countries there is a greater sense of acting for the common good ("I give up my right to undertake a health damaging behaviour because it is good for me and community") while in the US the focus is on assertion of individual rights ("I have an unalienable right to own a gun regardless of the rates of gun homicides"). It is likely the notion of linking social capital, as described by Szreter and Woolcock (2004), would account for some of the willingness of society to act in the interests of the common good. Linking social capital is strongly related to solidarity – both terms imply this willingness to act in the public interest and not just to act for personal benefit. Currently many social forces act against the formation of linking social capital and solidarity. Neo-liberal economic policies places emphasis on individualism and do not value collective responses (Baum, 2008 Chapter 4 Politics and Ideology: The Invisible Hand of Public Health). Kickbusch (2006) also points out that individualism is strongly encouraged by consumer societies in which goods are marketed in terms of the benefits of lifestyle they bring to individuals and show no concern with common good, public health or equity. In fact much advertising stresses the ways in which you can be better (healthier, wealthier, wiser) following consumption of a particular product, but does this in way that also suggests it will make you superior to others thus eroding social capital. Wilkinson (2005) sees the growth of "status competition" driving consumption and maintains that this is bad for health because it contributes to unsustainable levels of economic activity and striving for status between individuals which has been shown to affect health adversely (Marmot 2004).

Thus a crucial public policy question is what are the conditions under which a society demonstrates higher degrees of linking social capital and solidarity? How can these attributes be fostered especially in an age in which economic globalisation stresses the value of individual autonomy?

Perhaps some lessons can be gleaned from periods and settings when linking social capital appeared to be prevalent. Such a period was in the UK following World War II when the welfare state, including the National Health Service (NHS), was formed. The war brought about a determination among the middle and upper classes in the UK that the post-war world would be a better one. Part of this determination sprung from the increased awareness that these people had of the health and fitness of working class people from events such as the evacuation of poor children from the cities to rural middle class England. The Fabian Society conducted a survey of the evacuation experience in 1940 and the authors comment: *"What the evacuation scheme did was to make the country-side and the comfortable classes suddenly and painfully aware in their own person of the deep and shameful poverty which existed today in the rich cities of England"* (Padley and Cole 1940, p. 73). The newspapers of the time were full of accounts of how poor the children's health was and how things had to change after the war. Thus an editorial in The Times on 1st July 1940, responding to the social and health state of city evacuees, said: *"If we speak of democracy we do not mean a democracy which maintains the right to vote but forgets the right to work and the right to live. If we speak of freedom, we do not mean a rugged individualism which excludes social organisations and economic planning. If we speak of equality we do not mean a political equality nullified by social and economic privilege"* (Marwick 1968).

A political process then ensured that such sentiments did not translate into a charity model of assistance but instead into a series of policies which were explicitly designed to be equitable in health education and housing (Marwick 1968). This political process did not evolve overnight, or even through the war, but was the culmination of many years of struggle through social and industrial movements concerned with social justice. This example suggests that familiarity with the plight of less well-off people is important to changing values but clearly it is only one aspect of the package of factors that led to the election of a post-war Labour government determined to pursue equitable social and economic policies.

A further example of the role of linking social capital comes from an analysis of the relationship between Indigenous and non-Indigenous Australians which highlights a situation of total lack of linking social capital. The history of this relationship since the European invasion of Australia has been one characterised by very low levels of linking social capital between the two groups. Indigenous Australians had their land and culture taken away and have suffered from very punitive social policies over the past two centuries that in the very recent past have included state-sanctioned removal of part-Aboriginal children – the "stolen generation" (for details see Human Rights and Equal Opportunity Commission 1997). While there have always been some non-Indigenous Australians who have shown concern for Indigenous people (see accounts in Reynolds 1998), they have remained a minority and genuine reconciliation and respect for Indigenous peoples and their culture has not been achieved. It was only in 1967 that Indigenous peoples were accorded formal citizenship rights (Chesterman and Galligan 1997). The period in which linking social capital appeared to be growing between the two groups was in the early 1990s when a favourable High Court decision laid the basis for land right claims, a Royal Commission confronted white Australia with the facts of the stolen generation and a national process of reconciliation through the Council for Aboriginal Reconciliation began. This trend stalled under the Howard Coalition Government but the formal apology made in the Federal Parliament to the stolen generations by Labor Prime Minister Rudd in February 2008 and its positive reception on the Australian community was a prime example of linking social capital. This was further enhanced by the Labor Government's formal commitment to closing the gap in life expectancy between Indigenous and non-Indigenous peoples by 2040. Yet recent indigenous policy is viewed by many of having returned to an earlier paternalism (Anderson et al. 2006; Collard et al. 2005). In response to a report on sexual abuse in Aboriginal communities in the Northern Territory (Wilde and Anderson, 2007) the Howard Government launched a draconian intervention that included compulsory child health checks, welfare reforms including compulsory income management for individuals in prescribed communities and enforcement of the measures by the army. These measures have undermined trust between many Aboriginal people and communities and the government and they been judged as leaving a negative psychological and social impact (AIDA & CHETRE, 2010). The measures have been largely continued by the Rudd Labor Government and appear to have undermined the positive impact on linking social capital of the Apology and the Close the Gap campaign. The example of the relationship between Indigenous and non-Indigenous Australia demonstrates that there has been a long term struggle for the rights of Indigenous peoples and that symbolic acts, such as the Apology, can have a powerfully positive impact on the levels of linking social capital but this impact can be eroded by other measures that are viewed as punitive and discriminatory.

These examples provide some guidance to the importance of a process of understanding and the development of empathy, but it is clear that more work needs to be done concerning the creation and maintenance of solidarity and linking social capital between groups in society. But there does seem to be sufficient evidence that linking social capital does have value in understanding the processes by which social movements come to have broad support and create a value climate in which ideas of social justice and equity can flourish. Veenstra (2001, p. 79) notes that interpersonal trust may result in more egalitarian patterns of political participation and that this will often result in *"the passage of policies which ensure the security of all its members, policies perhaps pertaining to education, transportation, pollution, child welfare and zoning laws"*. Thus he sees that the culture of social relations can have an impact on what he calls the "deep structure" of society where values, ideas and beliefs of a society are formed and have significant influence on the economy and political life of a society. It certainly seems that one of the hallmarks of neo-liberal governments that has the effect of inhibiting linking social capital, is the way that governments and media suppress information on the human consequences of their actions. Thus in Australia there has been no reporting of the experiences of people behind the razor wire in refugee detention centres or very little of the direct experience of the residents of Baghdad during the war. This has the effect of marginalizing groups of people to produce a fragmented, "them and us" society. Public sympathy relating to the importance of promoting health and well-being is reduced, and a culture is established in which sympathy and linking social capital is weakened.

A further example of linking social capital comes from the "Make Poverty History" campaign that has lobbied for reduced debt for poor countries and increased aid assistance. This campaign has been supported by large non-government organisations and has advocated at events such as the meeting of the G8. There is no doubt that this movement has increased the global linking social capital by increasing awareness of the causes of poverty and creating a constituency for change. It has also moved assistance beyond a charity model by pointing to the structural factors underpinning the gross inequities between rich and poor countries. However, the "Make History Poverty" campaign has not achieved serious institutional change that has made any inroads into the power balance between rich and poor nations. Serious redistribution and reduction in inequities is only likely to result from the establishment of global governance structures that enable the structural power differences to be challenged. Nonetheless, establishing north-south networks and creating a constituency for change will help this process happen and force governments to consider more equitable policies.

Marx, of course, noted that ruling classes in capitalist society are unlikely to give up power willingly and each of the examples provided above is of change that reflects a history of struggle, from civil society and social movements. Certainly some commentators, including Muntaner (2004), have suggested that the promotion of social capital may be a means by which the ruling classes exert control over the rest of the population. Certainly this possibility and motive needs to be considered. However, in the early twenty-first century in which international capitalism in the form of a rampant economic globalisation is ever ascendant there needs to be mechanisms by which the dominance of neo-liberal thinking and consumerism are challenged. Linking social capital seems to be one of the mechanisms by which policy windows are opened to equity.

There has been little written about linking social capital since the work by Szreter and Woolcock (2004). There needs to be more work on what might lead to a society in which those with more resources and power are willing to see some of their advantage redistributed through state endorsed mechanisms. Some policy directions that might be useful include those aimed at increasing awareness of the benefits of living in a more equitable society (see Box 16.1) through a deliberate awareness campaign and placing the topic on educational and professional training curricula. Many models of citizen engagement and involvement have been tried in a wide variety of settings. Within health promotion the importance of active (not token) participation has been widely recognised as a means of health improvement (WHO 1978, 1986). Processes of participation are often based on a desire to change patterns of inequity and involve awareness raising, planning effective action (Oakley 1989; Baum 2008). Halpern (2005) suggests the more powerful people in a society need opportunities to be aware of the situation of others (a mechanism he suggests are citizen juries). Social movements lobbying for equity should receive untied government grants to support their advocacy. It is not hard to imagine that a well-orchestrated campaign to argue for smaller wage differentials between the managers of large corporations and the average wage would attract very widespread support. Wilkinson (2005) suggests that the introduction of more industry democracy and share-holding by employees would change the social relations between managers and other workers in a way that increased trust. It would also contribute to linking social capital and provide the basis for negotiation of working conditions and salaries in a much more democratic way than is done currently and would probably lead to more equitable distribution of the profits of the company. If the system became more wide-spread and was combined with other initiatives such as co-operatives then it could lead to more sustained challenge to the current form of economic globalization based on large trans-national corporations that are divorced from, and unaccountable to, the communities in which they operate.

16.7 Bonding and Bridging Social Capital and Policy

Bonding social capital is important to health because it can result in important functions and resources flowing to people. Examples include caring in times of sickness, support with childrearing, loans of money or equipment, and help finding employment. Each of these benefits could flow from bridging ties but are more likely to be present in close knit groups. The state can help foster bonding networks through the provision of financial resources to support caring. Thus in Australia, a carer's pension is paid to a person (usually a relative) who is providing intensive home care to a sick or disabled person.

Both bonding and bridging networks will be helped by the provision of meeting places in communities. These might be community centres, neighbourhood houses or cheap, welcoming cafes. Community development workers in resource-poor communities, who have an explicit role to increase social exclusion, often help the processes of networking. Governments may also give support to inclusive sporting, hobby and cultural groups. They may also institute housing policies that encourage social mix and prevent ghettos of the poor and rich. Good public transport can help ensure that all people have access to public goods such as beaches, art galleries and other public spaces. Free, compulsory and secular education plays a major role in equipping citizens to participate effectively in community and government. Access to information (including the internet) in public libraries or through other mechanisms is also crucial for effective citizenship.[1]

Halpern (2005) suggests that policies supportive of social capital should contribute to creating "a contemporary shared 'moral' discourse" and develop processes that facilitate mutual respect. These initiatives would aim at creating "pro-social" behaviour. Explicit suggestions include the development of forums

[1]Cross government initiatives of this type are discussed extensively in Baum (2002).

appropriate to the twenty-first century for deliberating and agreeing common moral and behavioural habits (perhaps through deliberative polling or conventional citizenship education). He also suggests that television soap operas might be one way of doing this by bringing up issues that then lead to national debate contributing to greater social cohesion.

16.8 Conclusion

This chapter has argued that an important part of achieving a healthy population is ensuring equity. It asserts that forms of social capital (bonding, bridging and linking) are both contributors to greater equity and provide a benefit that follows from the social relations that typify more equitable societies. Thus each form of social capital can be an asset for health and for health equity if it is supported and encouraged by progressive government intervention aimed at increasing its extent and positive health effect. Most crucially linking social capital is a means by which progressive action on the social and economic determinants of health can be legitimised and popularised and so be more likely to be taken up by governments. This exploration of social capital has taken on board the critics of the concept who have deplored its lack of attention to broader questions of resource distribution and power and integrated consideration of these issues into the ways in which social capital operates. By giving the need for re-distribution of power and resources, serious consideration on the power of social capital as an asset for health promotion is increased significantly. It is vital that further public health work on social capital does not continue to obscure class, gender and other power relationships between groups and institutions.

There is scope for much further research on social capital and its relationship to health equity that is more strongly informed by political economy theory, especially that which is developed to understand inequity such as Bourdieu's. While social capital is just one of a range of assets that can promote understanding of the social determinants of health and health equity it is an important part of the completing the jigsaw of health equity.

Acknowledgements Thanks to Paul Laris for thoughtful comments on a draft of this chapter. Also thanks to the Australian Research Council for funding the project *Social capital and public policy: how social capital can inform public sector interventions to improve health and reduce inequalities (project ID LP0454907)* which has provided the opportunity to reflect on the role of social capital in reducing health inequities.

References

Anderson, I., Crengle, S., Leialoha Kamaka, M., Chen, T., Palafox, N., & Jackson-Pulver, L. (2006). Indigenous health in Australia, New Zealand, and the Pacific. *The Lancet*, 367, 9524: 1775–1785.

Arneil, B. (2006). *Diverse Communities: The Problem with Social Capital*. Cambridge: Cambridge University Press.

Australian Indigenous Doctors' Association and Centre for Health Equity Training, Research and Evaluation, UNSW (2010). Health Impact Assessment of the Northern Territory Emergency Response. Canberra: Australian Indigenous Doctors' Association.

Baum, F. (2008). The New Public Health, 3rd edn, Melbourne: Oxford University Press.

Baum, F. (1999a). Social capital: is it good for your health? Issues for a public health agenda. *Journal of Epidemiology and Community Health*, 53, 4: 195–196.

Baum, F. (1999b). The role of social capital in health promotion: Australian perspectives. *Health Promotion Journal of Australia*, 9, 3: 171–178.

Baum, F., Modra, C., Murray, E., Bush, R., Cox, E., Alexander, K., & Potter R. (1999). The epidemiology of participation: an Australian community study. *Journal of Epidemiology and Community Health*, 54, 6: 414–423.

Baum, F. & Ziersch, A. (2003). Social capital glossary. *Journal of Epidemiology and Community Health*, May, 57, 5: 320–323.

Berkman, L. & Glass, T. (2000). Social integration, social networks, social support and health. In Berkman L.F. & Kawachi I. (eds.), *Social Epidemiology*. Oxford: Oxford University Press.

Bourdieu, P. (1986). The forms of capital. In Richardson J.G. (eds.), *Handbook of Theory and Research in the Sociology of Education*. Greenwald Press, New York, p. 241.

Cattell, V. (2001). Poor people, poor places, and poor health: The mediating role of social networks and social capital. *Social Science and Medicine*, 52, 10: 1501–1516.

Chesterman, J. & Galligan, B. (1997). *Citizens Without Rights: Aborigines and Australian Citizenship*. Melbourne: Cambridge University Press.

Collard, K., D'Antonie, H., Eggington, D., et al. (2005). "Mutual" obligation in indigenous health: Can shared responsibility agreements be truly mutual? *The Medical Journal of Australia*, 182, 10: 502–504.

Cox, E. (1995). *A Truly Civil Society*. Sydney: Australian Broadcasting Corporation.

Doyal, L. (1979). *The Political Economy of Health*. London: Pluto.

Fukuyama, F. (1996). *Trust: The Social Virtues and the Creation of Prosperity*. New York: The Free Press.

Halpern, D. (2005). *Social Capital*. Cambridge: Polity Press.

Halstead, S.B., Walsh, J., & Warren, K.S. (eds.) (1985). *Good Health at Low Cost*. New York: Rockefeller Foundation.

Hill, J., Le Grand, J., & Piachaud, D. (eds.) (2002). *Understanding Social Exclusion*. Oxford: Oxford University Press.

Human Rights and Equal Opportunity Commission. (1997). *Bring them Home: Findings of the National Inquiry into the Separation of Aboriginal and Torres Strait Islander Children from Their Families*. Sydney: Human Rights and Equal Opportunities Commission.

Kawachi, I., Kennedy, B.P., Lochner, K., et al. (1997). Social capital, income inequality, and mortality. *American Journal of Public Health*, 87, 9: 1491–1498.

Kawachi, I., Kennedy, B., & Glass, B. (1999). Social capital and self-rated health: a contextual analysis. *American Journal of Public Health*, 89, 8: 1187–1193.

Kickbusch, I. (2006). Mapping the future of public health: action on global health. *Canadian Journal of Public Health*, Jan/Feb, 97, 1: 6–8.

Lomas, J. (1998). Social capital and health: implications for public health and Epidemiology. *Social Science and Medicine*, 47, 9: 1181–1188.

Lynch, J., Davey Smith, G., & Kaplan, G., & House, J.S. (2000). Income inequality and mortality. *British Medical Journal*, 320: 1200–1204.

Lynch, J.G., Davey Smith, S., Harper, M., Hillemeier, M., Ross, N., Kaplan, G.A., et al. (2004). Is income inequality a determinants of population health? Part 1. A systematic review. *Millbank Quarterly*, 82, 1: 5–99.

Macinko, J. & Starfield, B. (2001). The utility of social capital in research on health determinants. *Milbank Quarterly*, 79, 3: 387–427.

Marmot, M. (2004). *The Status Syndrome. How Social Standing Effects Our Health and Longevity*. New York: New York Times Books.

Marwick, A. (1968). *Britain in the Century of Total War, Peace and Social Change, 1900-1967.* London: Bodley Head.
McKeown, T. (1979). *The Role of Medicine: Dream, Mirage or Nemesis?* Oxford: Basil Blackwell.
Mowbray, M. (2005). How to make social capital: Bowling alone's sequel, better together, *Community Development Journal*, 40, 4: 459–465.
Muntaner, C. (2004). Commentary: Social capital, social class, and the slow progress of psycho-social epidemiology. *International Journal of Epidemiology*, 33: 1–7.
Navarro, V. (2002). A critique of social capital. *International Journal of Health Services*, 32, 3: 423–432.
Oakley, P. (1989). *Community Involvement in Health Development: an Examination of the Critical Issues*. Geneva: World Health Organization.
Padley, R. & Cole, M. (eds.) (1940). *Evacuation Survey: A Report to the Fabian Society*. London: Routledge.
Pearce, N. & Davey Smith, G. (2003). Is social capital the key to inequalities in health? *American Journal of Public Health*, 93, 1: 122–129.
Portes, A. (1998). Social capital: Its origins and applications in modern sociology. *Annual Review of Sociology*, 24: 1–24.
Putnam, R.D. (1993). *Making Democracy Work: Civic Traditions in Modern Italy*. Princeton: Princeton University Press.
Putnam, R.D. (1996). The strange disappearance of civic America. *Policy*. Autumn, 3–15.
Putnam R.D. (2000). *Bowling Alone: The Collapse and Revival of American Community.* NewYork: Simon & Schuster Ltd.
Putnam, R.D., Feldstein, L.M., & Cohen, D. (2003). *Better Together: Restoring the American Community*. New York: Simon and Schuster.
Raphael D. (2003). Barriers to addressing the societal determinants of health: public health units and poverty in Ontario, Canada. *Health Promotion International*, 18, 4: 397–405.
Reynolds, H. (1998). *This Whispering in our Hearts*. St. Leonards: Allen and Unwin.
Sanders, D. & Werner, D. (1997). *Questioning the Solution. The Politics of Primary Health Care and Child Survival.* Palo Alto: Health Wrights.
Sundquist, K. & Yang, M. (2007). Linking social capital and self-rated health: a multilevel analysis of 11,175 men and woman in Sweden, Health & PLace, 13, 2: 324–331.
Szreter, S. (1988). The importance of social intervention in Britain's mortality decline c.1850–1914: A reinterpretation of the role of public health. *The Society for the Social History of Medicine*, 1, 1: 1–37.
Szreter, S. (2002).The state of social capital: bringing power politics and history back. *Theory and Society*, 31: 573–621.
Szreter, S. & Woolcock, M. (2004). Health by association? Social capital, social theory, and the political economy of public health. *International Journal of Epidemiology*, 33: 650–667.
Wild, R. & Anderson, P. (2007). Ampe Akelyernemane Meke Mekarle. "Little Children are Sacred": Report of the Northern Territory Board of Inquiry into the Protection of Aboriginal Children from Sexual Abuse. Darwin: Northern Territory Government.
Wilkinson. R. (2005). *The Impact of Inequality. How to Make Sick Societies Healthier*. New York: The New Press.
WHO. (1978). *Primary Health Care. Report of the International Conference on primary Health Care, Alma –Ata, USSR, 6–12 September 1978*. Geneva: World Health Organization.
WHO. (1986). *Ottawa Charter for Health Promotion. The Move Toward A New Public Health, Ottawa, 17–21 November 1986*. Geneva: World Health Organization.
Veenstra, G. (2001). Social capital and health. *ISUMA – Canadian Journal of Policy Research*, Spring, 2, 1: 72–81.

Chapter 17
Internal and External Assets and Romanian Adolescents' Health: An Evidence-Based Approach to Health Promoting Schools Policy

Adriana Baban and Catrinel Craciun

Keywords Adolescents • Health behaviour of school-aged children • HIV/AIDS • Romania • School community • Sense of coherence

17.1 Introduction

Adolescence has gained recognition as a crucial developmental period to be targeted by health promotion interventions (Williams et al. 2002). There are several factors that have led to this state of affairs. Firstly, adolescence represents a period when health behaviours such as physical exercise or eating a healthy diet are strengthened and when risk behaviours (i.e. smoking, alcohol consumption, unprotected sex) emerge. Moreover, stress protective factors such as social competences that contribute to establishing and maintaining supportive social relations also develop during adolescence and need to be addressed in this age group (Wilkinson et al. 1998). Secondly, mortality for teenagers results predominantly from unintentional injury following accidents (National Centre of Health Statistics 1993), while morbidity is determined mostly by substance abuse and dependence, sexually transmitted infection or mental health problems (Holden and Nitz 1995). These factors differ from those causing death and illness in adults and thus require specific health promotion intervention for teenagers. Furthermore, it has been argued that due to the particular developmental characteristics of young people, intervention efforts designed for adults are not effective with adolescent populations (Williams et al. 2002). Consequently, it is the task of health promoters to develop programmes that are tailored to the needs and age characteristics of teenagers.

A. Baban (✉)
Babes-Bolyai University, Cluj, Romania
e-mail: adrianababan@psychology.ro

A. Morgan et al. (eds.), *Health Assets in a Global Context: Theory, Methods, Action*,
DOI 10.1007/978-1-4419-5921-8_17,

The health of adolescents is influenced both by individual factors such as health beliefs (Marcell and Halpern-Felsher 2005), self-efficacy (Schwarzer and Luszczynska 2006) or sense of coherence (SOC) (Torshein et al. 2001), but also by social factors like social capital (Smylie et al. 2006) or parental support and monitoring (Li et al. 2000). As young people spend significant time at school next to family and friends this plays an important role in the development of their mental and physical health. Previous research has shown that a cohesive school environment is protective of emotional well being and fosters health behaviour as opposed to risk factors such as unsafe sexual practices, substance abuse or violence (Rowe et al. 2007). Moreover, a sense of belonging and connectedness inside the school community is not only protective of health but also contributes to improved academic achievement and engagement (Croniger and Lee 2001). Therefore, the school environment provides great opportunities for intervention to promote health behaviour and mental health among teenagers.

Health promotion for adolescents can be addressed at individual, organizational or community level. Restricting access to cigarettes, alcohol or illicit drugs while improving access to health care, prohibiting smoking in public areas and providing health education are all regulated by health policy. All these actions have an impact on teenagers' emotional health and behavioural choice (Weisz et al. 2005). Effective health promotion needs to be regulated by policy that aims to increase personal health skills and create health supportive environments in accordance with a proactive health promotion approach that enables teenagers to increase control over the determinants of their own health (Nutbeam 1997). Earlier public health policies have been largely based on a deficit model and as a result have focused on the failure of individuals and communities to avoid illness rather than on factors that contribute to health fostering and maintenance. In order to compensate for this drawback, current trends in health policy support the adoption of an asset approach that sustains the creation of health rather than disease prevention (Morgan and Ziglio 2007).

17.2 Mapping Internal and External Assets in Romanian Adolescents

Romania is one of the new European Union (EU) member states, located in South-Eastern Europe. It has a population of 22 million, out of which 24% is below 19 years of age and 12.6% fall within the 10–19 age subgroup. The majority of young people live with their families, however, there are currently 20,000 youths reported to be living in state care. Theoretically, all children in Romania are integrated in the school system, but there is concern regarding the increased school abandonment rate, especially among the Roma ethnic group and the poor residents of rural areas. Most affected are vocational schools, with an abandonment rate of 5.5%, followed by high schools (2.3%), secondary (2.0%) and primary schools (1.3%).

The mortality rate for young people is estimated at 0.3/1,000 inhabitants for the 10–14 age group and at 0.6/1,000 for adolescents between 15 and 19 years old. Gender differences emerge within mortality statistics, boys being at a disadvantage in comparison to girls. On the other hand, there are specific problems that mainly affect the mental and physical health of the female population such as the abortion rate, estimated to be 0.84 for the 15–19 age group (Ministry of Health 2005). HIV/AIDS affects a large number of Romanian teenagers, as 60% of Romanians living with HIV/AIDS can be integrated in the 15–19 years old age group (Ministry of Health 2004). According to UNICEF (2006) between 1986 and 1991 more than 10,000 Romanian children were infected with HIV, making it the largest group with this condition in Europe. Transmission within the 0–14 age category is mainly nosocomial (transmitted accidentally during hospital care), while after the age of 15, HIV/AIDS is mostly sexually transmitted. Unfortunately, in terms of the mental health of the young population, the national evidence base on youth suicide, depression, anxiety, eating disorders and other mental illness is sparse and needs further development. Work in this area is being progressed and the Ministry of Public Health has developed a document, already signed by the Prime Minister, which defines the mental health of children and adolescents as a policy priority.

Health assets have been defined in Chap. 1 as any factor or resource that enhances the ability of individuals, groups, communities or institutions to sustain health and well-being and reduce health inequalities. They have been categorised as individual (i.e. social competence, self-efficacy), community (i.e. supportive social networks) and organizational (i.e. health system in a community). In this context, school as an organization can play a major role as an active health promotion agent and contribute to the development of both internal and external assets in young people, empowering them to achieve and maintain health and well-being. However, the process of developing health-promoting schools requires generating evidence-based policy in the realm of young people's health. In line with this, this chapter sets out to present research data on how internal and external assets relate to mental health and health behaviour of Romanian adolescents. Also, we will discuss the existence of a "gender gap" in relation to the internal and external assets of boys and girls in relation to their health behaviour and mental well-being. We then proceed to describe the current Romanian policy concerning health promoting schools and make recommendations for its further development based on existing evidence.

The first step in applying the asset model framework to adolescent health promotion is represented by asset mapping in a particular community or describing the existing evidence base for health policy development, as outlined in Chap. 1. We choose to explore the internal and external assets which are available to Romanian adolescents, and that play a role in their mental well-being and health behaviour adoption.

Internal assets can be described as personal resources that individuals rely on in order to guide their behavioural choices and foster their well being. In this chapter, we examine self-efficacy, self-esteem and sense of coherence as previous research has shown them to be relevant internal factors that affect health of young people (Schwarzer and Luszczynska 2006; Torshein et al. 2001).

Self-efficacy has been defined as a sense of personal control over one's own behaviour or environment (Bandura 1997). Numerous studies have shown self-efficacy to be an important predictor of health behaviour initiation and maintenance as well as for mental health. In terms of adolescent health, self-efficacy has been studied in connection to risk and health behaviour and proved to be a predictor of contraceptive use (Wang et al. 2003), quitting smoking (Aung et al. 2003), physical activity (Nahas et al. 2003; Wu et al. 2003), and healthy nutrition (Wilson et al. 2002).

Self-esteem relates to the extent to which an individual values them self, and is considered to be another relevant internal determinant of health (WHO 1997). It is seen as important in relation to building social networks and acting as a protective factor against experiencing negative emotions (Wilkinson 1999). Studies have shown adolescent self-esteem to be a predictor for adult well-being and behaviour. For instance, teenagers with low self-esteem have been found to have poorer physical and mental health, worse economic circumstances and engage in more criminal behaviour when they reach adulthood (Trzesniewsky et al. 2006).

One of the most studied personal concepts in relation to mental health is the SOC theory. It is defined as a global orientation, or belief about the world, to view life situations as comprehensible, manageable and meaningful (Antonovsky 1987). Comprehensibility refers to the level of cognitive control people feel they can exercise over their environment, manageability relates to the extent to which individuals believe they have coping resources available and meaningfulness is the motivational ingredient that makes life situations worth committing to (Feldt et al. 2003). SOC is thought to influence stress by several paths: stressors appraisal, coping mechanisms choice and the level of experienced stress related tension that leads to health consequences (Antonovsky 1993). The original theoretical approach viewed SOC as a developmental construct that becomes crystallized around the age of 30. This definition led to there being few studies on the relation between SOC and young peoples' health. However, more recent findings show that SOC plays an important role in stress and coping in young people as well as in adults. For example, in relation to the school environment of children and adolescents, SOC represents a salutogenic factor that helps coping with school stress (Torshein et al. 2001).

The recent interest in the role of social capital in school health has led to our decision to explore *school social capital* (SSC) as an external asset for health promotion among Romanian adolescents. Social capital reflects the quality and quantity of social interactions within a community (Drukker et al. 2005). It is defined as "features of social organization-such as networks of secondary associations, high levels of interpersonal trust and norms of mutual aid and reciprocity-which act as resources for individuals and facilitate collective action" (Kawachi et al. 1997). The components of social capital in most models include structural (i.e. number of friends, family members, number of organizations available) and cognitive dimensions (i.e. trust, shared identity, shared values and aspirations, engagement). The school as an organization offers the possibility to explore both structural and cognitive components of the social capital concept. Previous studies have shown that SSC represents an important factor for positive health in the school environment (Sampson et al. 1999) and for academic achievement (Coleman 1988). A combination of supportive school climates (caring and supportive relationships) and school bonding (trust and sense of school community) foster positive health in young people (Sun and Stewart 2007a). SSC came out as a protective factor in the school environment, enabling adolescents to resist teenage pregnancy, substance abuse, delinquency, academic failure or maltreatment (Coleman and Hoffer 1987; Frustenberg and Hughes 1995; Putnam 2000; Teachman et al. 1996). In order to operationalise and measure SSC we have adapted the conceptualisation of social capital used by Morrow (1999) and applied it to the school context. The following components emerged:

- Social networks (the quality of school social networks, relations with peers)
- Engagement (the extent to which students can influence decisions at school)
- School identity (the extent to which students feel they belong to the school, and feel safe at school)
- Teacher support

17.3 Research Methods

The Health Behaviour of School-Aged Children (HBSC) study represents a World Health Organization (WHO) Collaborative Cross National project. A self-report questionnaire-based survey was designed to monitor well-being and health of European and North American children (Currie et al. 2004). The Romanian survey was conducted in (Aung et al. 2003) on a national representative sample of 11, 13 and 15 year olds. In this chapter we discuss data collected in schools from a 1,562 sample of 15 year olds, out of which 591 were boys (38%) and 971 girls (62%).

Internal and external assets, as well as mental health and behaviours, were measured using several scales from the HBSC questionnaire. Self-efficacy was measured using the General Self-efficacy scale (Schwarzer and Jerusalem 1995), comprising ten items (Cronbach's alpha:[1] 0.82). Social self-esteem was assessed with a five item subscale from the self-perception profile for adolescents (Harter 1988) (Cronbach's alpha: 0.71). Antonovsky's SOC scale was used in order to measure the three components of SOC: comprehensibility, manageability and meaningfulness (Cronbach's alpha: 0.81).

In order to assess external assets we computed a SSC index that included four components mentioned above: social networks, engagement in school decisions and activities, school identity and teacher support. *Social networks* comprise three

[1]Cronbach's alpha measures how well a set of items (or variables) measures a single unidimensional latent construct. When data have a multidimensional structure, Cronbach's alpha will usually be low. Technically speaking, Cronbach's alpha is not a statistical test – it is a coefficient of reliability (or consistency). A reliability coefficient of 0.70 or higher is considered "acceptable" in most social science research situations (UCLA website: http://www.ats.ucla.edu/stat/Spss/faq/alpha.html).

items that refer to the quality of student relations inside the classroom ("The students in my class enjoy being together"), characteristics of classmates that can have a positive influence on communication ("Most of the students in my class are kind and helpful") and the feeling of belonging to the social network inside the class ("Students accept me"). The *engagement* component includes two items that measure the level of participation in developing school rules ("In our school the students take part in making the rules") and involvement in organization of school events ("Students get involved in organizing school events"). Possessing a *school identity* was assessed by five items describing the school climate ("the students are treated too severely in this school"; "the rules in this school are fair"; "our school is a nice place to be"); the feeling of belonging to the school ("I feel I belong to this school") and feeling of security inside the school ("I feel safe at this school"). The level of *teacher support* was measured with four items describing getting emotional support ("I am encouraged to express my own views in my class"; "My teachers are interested in me as a person"); instrumental support ("When I need extra help I can get it") and fair treatment ("Our teachers treat us fairly").

17.4 Results

The descriptive data show that more than half of the Romanian teenagers included in the HBSC survey have above average self-efficacy and self-esteem. Also, the majority consider themselves to have cognitive control over their environment. However, most adolescents in the sample are believed to be low on the instrumental SOC dimension and fewer than half of the sample score high on the motivational SOC component. In what concerns SSC, almost 60% of the sample considered themselves to be involved with deciding upon school rules or organizing events at school. Moreover, more than half of the teenagers said they have a friendly peer group at school and thought they receive support from their teachers. Nevertheless, only around 47% declared they have a school identity comprising feelings of belonging to their school and feeling safe at school (Table 17.1).

Table 17.1 Descriptives for internal and external assets (median, SD)

Assets	M (SD)	>M	<M
Self-efficacy	32.86; 4.93	59.6%	40.4%
Self-esteem	15.47; 3.00	53.4%	46.6%
SOC manageability	12.71; 3.27	40%	60%
SOC meaningfulness	13.84; 2.51	39%	61%
SOC comprehensibility	15.16; 3.88	57.8%	42.2%
School engagement	8.00; 2.00	59.4%	40.6%
School identity	9.53; 3.03	46.9%	53.1%
Student network	6.70; 2.11	50.2%	49.8%
Teacher support	8.59; 1.88	51.2%	48.8%

Table 17.2 Gender differences in internal and external assets (median, SD)

Assets	Boys M (SD)	Girls M (SD)	Mean difference
Self-efficacy	33 (5.55)	32.77 (4.52)	$F=6.54$, $p<0.01$
Self-esteem	15.48 (3.16)	15.47 (2.90)	$F=1.35$, $p=0.24$
SOC manageability	13 (3.32)	12.59 (3.22)	$F=0.90$, $p=0.75$
SOC meaningfulness	13.66 (2.63)	13.94 (2.44)	$F=2.69$, $p=0.10$
SOC comprehensibility	15.82 (4.05)	14.77 (3.72)	$F=5.81$, $p<0.05$
School engagement	8.20 (2.26)	7.91 (1.93)	$F=18.15$, $p<0.01$
School identity	9.76 (3.31)	9.39 (2.84)	$F=9.12$, $p<0.01$
Student network	6.60 (2.11)	6.76 (2.11)	$F=0.10$, $p=0.90$
Teacher support	8.54 (1.99)	8.62 (1.82)	$F=4.80$, $p<0.05$
School social capital index	33.12 (7.10)	32.73 (6.18)	$F=10.06$, $p<0.01$

A "gender gap" in internal and external assets was identified among the adolescents who participated in the study, suggesting the need for specific intervention to develop strengths. Significantly, more boys than girls were shown to have above average self-efficacy and a sense of cognitive control over their environment. Boys also emerged as having higher SSC. They consider themselves to be more involved in developing school rules and organizing events and feel they have a school identity more than girls do. On the other hand, girls said they receive more social support from teachers in comparison to boys (Table 17.2).

17.5 Internal and External Assets and Adolescent Mental Health

Mental health of adolescents was measured by using several scales from the HBSC survey: the mental health index (Cronbach's alpha: 0.70), the life satisfaction scale, the perceived health scale and one item measuring perceived school stress level.

The *mental health* index is a non-clinical list of ten items with five point answer categories which aims to measure children's and adolescents' mental health status (Ravens-Sieberer et al. 2005). Several dimensions of psychological well-being are included: affective (i.e. "Have you felt sad?"), cognitive (i.e. "Have you been able to pay attention?"), physiologic (i.e. "Have you felt full of energy?") and social (i.e. "Have you got on well at school?").

We also chose to use more general evaluators of mental health and measure general well being in teenagers with the life satisfaction scale (Cantril 1965). This scale requires adolescents to rate their global satisfaction with life, from 1 (worst) to 10 (best). As yet another general indicator of mental health, we included in our analysis the self-reported health item ("How healthy do you think you are?") as it was proven by previous studies to be effective in epidemiological studies (Idler and Benyamini 1997). The item has four point answer categories with options ranging from very healthy to not very healthy.

School stress represents an important influence on adolescent mental health and well-being, and it is the result of an existing imbalance between school requirements and student coping resources (Karvonen et al. 2005). The item measures how stressed teenagers perceive themselves to be due to school requirements and has four point answer categories from very much to not at all.

Previous research has shown *body image* to play an important role in self-evaluation and mental well-being of teenagers (Mendelson et al. 2000; Williams and Currie 2000). On the other hand, high dissatisfaction with one's bodily appearance emerged as a predictor of depression, eating disorders and psychosomatic complaints (Siegel 2002; Thompson and Chad 2002). Body image was measured with a six item Body Investment Scale from the HBSC survey referring to feelings of satisfaction, comfort and liking ones looks and body (Orbach and Mikulincer 1998).

More than half of the Romanian 15 year olds included in the HBSC study proved to have above average mental health and almost two thirds declared they were very satisfied with their lives. Perceived health was also considered good or excellent by the majority of the questioned adolescents (79.4%), while 20.6% declared their health to be fair or poor. However, almost half of the sample considered themselves to be stressed by school in different degrees: of these, 44.2% said school stresses them a little, 34.5% reported medium school stress and 9.9% said they are very stressed by school. Only 10.7% of the questioned adolescents said they are not at all stressed by school. In relation to body image the majority of the teenagers feel their looks are average (46.7%), many believe their looks to be very good or quite good and only 10.2% say they don't like their looks. When looking at the results for body image index, 41.4% of the sample find themselves below the mean when it comes to being satisfied with their body (Table 17.3).

The mental health index correlates well with self-efficacy and self-esteem, as well as with the three components of SOC (manageability, meaningfulness, comprehensibility). There are also significant correlations between all internal assets and life satisfaction, showing that the more teenagers possess self-efficacy, self-esteem and find life situations meaningful the more they are satisfied with their life. Adolescents with high self-efficacy, self-esteem, and manageability consider themselves as being healthy. As expected, youths that have high self-efficacy, self-esteem, meaningfulness and manageability also have a more positive body image. Having a high self-efficacy also means that the teenagers feel themselves less pressured by school work.

Table 17.3 Descriptives for mental health (median, SD)

Mental health	M (SD)	>M	<M
Mental health index	34.01 (6.61)	54.1%	45.9%
Life satisfaction	7.18 (1.89)	75.8%	24.2%
Perceived health	1.99 (0.70)	79.4%	20.6%
Perceived school stress	2.44 (0.81)	45%	55%
Body image index	23.80 (4.67)	58.6%	41.4%

In terms of *external assets*, the higher the SSC, the better the scores for mental health, life satisfaction, perceived health, and positive body image. Teenagers that possess high social capital tend to perceive less stress at school.

Regression analysis results show that both internal and external assets predict mental health. Internal assets explain 30% of mental health variance with self-efficacy, self-esteem and SOC components (comprehension, manageability, meaningfulness) all being significant predictors. SSC explains only 9% of teenagers' mental health variance with school identity and peer social networks and perceived teacher support as significant predictors.

Internal and external resources play an important role in predicting mental health of Romanian adolescents and therefore would constitute a good basis for formulating targeted intervention and evaluation criteria for fostering mental and emotional well being in schools. Increasing self-efficacy, self-esteem and SOC dimensions could be included in the school health education curriculum both as content and as teaching methods that encourage building up of these resources in young people. Although they emerged as playing a smaller role in mental health, external resources have to be considered when designing health policy for Romanian schools. Asset enhancement goals could focus on increasing support provided by teachers, fostering the creation of peer social networks by structural interventions such as group study centres and provision of social extra-curricular activities and building a school identity favourable to adolescent well being.

17.6 Internal and External Assets and Health Behaviour

Health behaviours were shown to be predicted by both internal resources like self-efficacy (Schwarzer and Luszczynska 2006) and external ones such as social capital (Smylie et al. 2006). Therefore, it is important to explore the role of internal and external assets in determining health behaviour and use this information to develop comprehensive health education policy.

The following *health behaviours* were measured using items from the HBSC questionnaire: physical exercise, eating fruit and vegetable and not smoking. In order to find out how much *physical exercise* is done by adolescents we asked them about the level of sustained physical activity (meaning activity that makes one sweat or loose breath, like bicycle riding or swimming) performed during the last 7 days for at least 60 min. *Fruit and vegetable consumption* were measured with two items were teenagers could choose on a seven scale how many fruit and vegetable they eat during 1 week. A score of one meant they never eat any fruit or vegetables while a score of seven means they eat the recommended portions daily. *Smoking* behaviour was assessed by asking adolescents whether they have smoked before or not.

Less than half (36.1%) of the teenage sample said they eat fruit once or more than once every day. Vegetables are even less liked since only 24% said they eat these on a daily basis. About 10% of the adolescents in our study said they practice sports for at least 60 min every day, most (25.5%) declaring they have intense physical activity for 2 days per week. In relation to smoking, there are almost an equal number of smokers (48.2%) and non-smokers (50.6%) among the questioned teenagers.

There is a significant relation between self-esteem and smoking with teenagers who have high self-esteem tending to smoke less. Also, having higher self-efficacy relates to eating more fruit and vegetables and practicing more sport. The small correlations suggest that although these internal factors are significant, there might be other external determinants that influence healthy eating like availability in the environment or peer group norms. SSC correlates significantly with all health behaviours. The higher the social capital of teenagers, the less likely they are to smoke and the greater the probability that they practice physical activity.

Both internal and external assets predict the adoption of health behaviour. In so far as internal resources are concerned, self-esteem is a good predictor for not taking up smoking, together with SOC meaningfulness component. Self-efficacy significantly predicts eating fruit, vegetables and practicing physical activity. From the external assets peer support predicts the adoption of physical activity. Having a school identity predicts not taking up smoking together with the feeling of being engaged with making school rules and organizing events at school.

As shown by previous research, both internal assets like self-efficacy (Schwarzer and Luszczynska 2006) and external ones such as social capital (Smylie et al. 2006) play an important role in the adoption of teenage health behaviour. Present data validate the role of self-efficacy in eating fruit and vegetable as well as practicing physical activity. Taking up smoking is more influenced by self-esteem and the motivational component of SOC, as self-efficacy probably becomes more important in quitting smoking or withstanding peer pressure to smoke. Therefore, the enhancement of internal assets should also represent a target for school health promotion in order to influence the adoption and maintenance of health behaviour. From the SSC dimensions, peer social networks, school identity and school engagement emerged as predictors of health behaviour. These could also be increased by asset promoting policy that focuses on structural dimensions such as providing spaces at school for practicing sports and offering healthy menus at the school canteen to be shared with ones' peer group. In terms of school health policy an important aspect could be making teenagers more involved with organizing health promoting events at school and having a say in deciding school rules related to health behaviour such as smoking policy.

17.7 The "Asset Promoting School": Providing a Framework for Policy Development

Asset mapping represents the first step in developing effective evidence-based health policy and needs to be followed by concrete action strategies as well as designing rigorous evaluation criteria and methodology. The role played by school in fostering young peoples' health has received global recognition through the *health promoting school (HPS) approach* (Anderson 2004) and was further developed by ideas about increasing resilience (Knight 2007) and social capital (Sun and Stewart 2007b). The HPS model is based on the belief that school health can be enhanced by establishing health promotion actions at organizational level and stipulates change in three domains:

1. Curriculum, teaching and learning
2. School organization, ethos and environment
3. Partnerships and services

The HPS approach has been shown to be successful in promoting health in the school setting (Clift and Bruun Jensen 2006) and has been effectively implemented in Europe (Parsons et al. 1996), USA (Allensworth and Kolbe 1987), Australia (St Leger 1999) and the Asia-Pacific region (Rowling and Richie 1996/1997). Based on this evidence we employed the HPS model to analyse the Romanian school health education policy, present its strengths, discuss existing challenges and make recommendations based on the assets evidence base.

In Romania, following WHO recommendations, the Ministry of Public Health decided to prioritise mental health prevention interventions on its working agenda. This resulted in the development of several laws and associated strategies that targeted the improvement of child and adolescent health. The *"Health education in Romanian schools"* policy stands as a successful example of intersectorial collaboration between ministries (Ministry of Education and Research, the Ministry of Public Health, local authorities, non government groups (NGOs) universities and schools), that led to the implementation of a health promotion programme aimed at increasing health in young people. The programme was developed in 2003 by the joint efforts of the Ministry of Education and Research, and Ministry of Public Health and had as its main objective the introduction of health education as an extracurricular activity to develop responsible attitudes towards one's own health and the health of others.

In terms of *curriculum, teaching and learning,* there is a balance of themes dealing with mental health (i.e. building a positive self-image, developing stress management skills, preventing negative attitudes towards self, others and life) and health behaviour promotion (i.e. developing a healthy lifestyle, preventing accidents and reducing risk behaviour). However, the curriculum, teaching and health component of the HPS model is concerned not only with content but also with participatory teaching methods and student-centred learning activities which enhance the students' role in decision making at school (Bruun Jensen and Jensen 2006). A successful illustration of the inclusion of these interactive teaching methods in Romanian curricula is represented by the recent publishing of two manuals for teachers and educators, aimed at training them on how to develop social and emotional competences in pre-schoolers (Stefan and Kallay 2007). However, the Romanian health education curricula still have to improve on applying the student-centred learning approach. This will result in higher engagement from the students and help develop their internal assets like self-efficacy and self-esteem. Student participation has been shown to help build the strengths of young people (Rowe et al. 2007), and cooperation among students leads to higher social capital (Barker et al. 1997). Teaching and learning activities that have been proven to build social capital include small group work, class discussions, cooperative learning activities, shared tasks and peer tutoring. Cooperative learning strategies that involve small, heterogeneous groups of students of different abilities and backgrounds working together as learning partners enhance social relations and school identity (Rowe et al. 2007). Experiential learning has also been proposed by several authors as an effective means of building SSC (Barker et al. 1997). The Romanian health education curriculum for high schools also includes clear recommendations on the use of interactive teaching methods (Ministry of Education and Research 2003), but needs to be augmented with student involvement strategies and an effective evaluation system to measure the internal and external assets that are targeted to be developed in adolescents. Moreover, extra-curricular activities dealing with health education such as peer tutoring programs could be introduced. These kinds of activities have been shown to enhance SSC (Korinek et al. 1999) as students can learn from each other how to deal with peer pressure towards adopting risk behaviour or model how to deal with school stress.

The school *organization, ethos and environment* of the HPS framework refers to the use of formal and informal school structures (i.e. school organisation, rules, physical environment) to promote health. The term *ethos* describes the psychosocial environment within the school (WHO 1995) and includes the underlying values of school structures and procedures (i.e. codes of discipline) that regulate relations between staff, students and parents (Parsons et al. 1996) mostly at an informal level. Schools that value positive personal relations and are oriented towards a shared set of values and goals have been shown to have a strong sense of community and connectedness (Barker et al. 1997). Involving students in school organisational structures like school council committees (Babiuk 1999) and student run organizations has been shown to promote SSC. In Romania, students take part in school decisions through student council representatives. However, as reflected by the HBSC data, few Romanian adolescents feel they take part in developing school rules or help organize school events. Consequently, there is need for strategies at the organizational level to make teenagers feel more involved in shaping the school environment. For example, students could take part in making decisions about health education curricula in order that the topics chosen will meet their interests and needs. Also, adolescents can participate in deciding and implementing internal school policy such as rules about smoking on school premises or violence and bullying prevention.

The environmental component of HPS refers to the psychological as well as physical environment. In terms of psychosocial aspects it proposes that teachers act as role models within the school environment by developing caring and accepting rapport with students. Experiencing positive and caring interactions with teachers, helps students feel supported and valued and contributes to their developing internal assets (Baker et al. 2003). Previous research has shown that professional development of teachers in relation to improving their positive relation skills and applying them in communication with students contributes to building up SSC (Thomas and Smith 2004). In this context, the health education in Romanian schools project provides a good example of intersectorial collaboration between the ministries, universities and schools. For example, the psychology department from Babes-Bolyai University, Cluj-Napoca offers the "MAGISTER" training program for teachers, focusing on themes like socioemotional development, communication skills improvement, stress management, risk behaviour prevention and positive health promotion. Several county school inspectorates are involved as partners in the implementation of the project. The programme was accredited by the Ministry of Education and Research in June 2003 and since then, 6,000 teachers from all regions of Romania have been trained. "MAGISTER" is being financed by the Ministry and funds are being administered through the County school inspectorates. However, this training programme needs to be further improved by development and implementation of process and outcome evaluation, informing on the effectiveness of the intervention.

The other environmental feature refers to physical aspects that facilitate building social capital. The playground layout, the building and classroom design and appearance including lighting or use of colour (Hebert 1998; WHO 1996) all constitute areas of structural intervention to develop SSC and influence adolescent well being. The Romanian health education school programme still has to integrate recommendations referring to structural interventions to change the physical environment of schools in order to foster social capital growth, health behaviour adoption and the mental health of teenagers. One example of an intervention would be making school cafeterias friendly places for socialising and offering healthy menus (i.e. including the necessary portions of fruit and vegetables) that adolescents could try out and enjoy with their peer groups. Another important aspect for encouraging physical activity would be making sure there are enough spaces for practicing sports at school. In order to help build social capital and promote student collaboration, special places where teenagers can study together should be created. These could be built inside the school library or as pleasant group study centres on school premises. Designing school health centres can also contribute to making health information and counselling on mental and physical health issues more available and accessible to students.

The *partnership and services* component has been presented as the most essential dimension of the HPS (WHO 1996) due to its potential to build SSC by linking the school to the larger community (Coleman and Hoffer 1987). Health services and community agencies need to develop partnerships with schools for the mutual goal of promoting youth health. Relationships between these institutions have to be characterised by equal partnerships and provision of resources and expertise (St Leger 1999; WHO 1996). The Romanian health education program offers a fine illustration of existing intersectorial collaboration between NGOs and schools. Several international and national NGOs (i.e. United Nations Children's Fund (UNICEF), United Nations Development Programme (UNDP), United States Agency for International Development (USAID), Open Society Institute and Soros Foundation, Youth for Youth, and Romanian Association of Health Psychology) have provided human and financial resources to facilitate the process of implementing the health education programme in Romanian schools. This collaboration needs to be continued and further improved by involving international as well as national NGOs and Universities. Elaborating and disseminating reports of the health education activity and effectiveness within school premises will encourage new investments, both national and international and partnerships to raise necessary funds and not rely completely on the state financing.

17.8 Conclusions

Social changes in family structures and parenting patterns as well as the availability of temptations in the environment (i.e. fast food, cigarettes, alcohol and drugs) have made the role played by school in the health education of teenagers more important (Knight 2007). School health education should be regulated by an asset approach, as discussed in Chap. 1, rather than a deficit model. The approach should focus on building internal and external resources in young people and making them active agents in the promotion of their own mental well being and health behaviour. Evidence base from the HBSC study shows that internal and external assets play an important role in fostering mental health and health behaviour adoption in Romanian adolescents. Also, gender differences emerged, boys having more internal and external resources than girls.

These data can form the base for the improvement of the health education program in Romanian schools. Curricula can be developed by including student-centred methods that help increase self-efficacy and self-esteem and take gender differences into account when developing these resources in teenagers. In order to develop SSC, structural interventions should be designed. Providing spaces where students can study together or practice sports help with building social capital that influences well being and adoption of health behaviour. Moreover, involving teenagers in forming school policy relating to health behaviour like smoking or fast food eating and giving them the opportunity to organise health promoting events can help them become more active in the health education process. Last but not least, further developing the intersectoral collaboration between ministries, school inspectorates, universities, NGOs and schools will help to provide the necessary human and financial resources to sustain the improvement and implementation of school health education policy.

References

Allensworth, D., & Kolbe, L. (1987). The comprehensive school health program: exploring an expanded concept. *Journal of School Health*, vol. 57, 409–412.

Anderson, A. (2004). Health promoting school: a community effort. *Physical and Health Education Journal*, vol. 70, no. 2, 4–9.

Antonovsky, A. (1987). *Unraveling the mystery of health. How people manage stress and stay well*. San Francisco, CA: Jossey-Bass.
Antonovsky, A. (1993). The structure and properties of the sense of coherence scale. *Social Science and Medicine*, 36, 725–733.
Aung, A. T., Hickman, N. J. 3rd & Moolchan, E. T. (2003). Health and performance, reasons for wanting to quit: gender differences among teen smokers. *Substance Use and Misuse*, 38, 1095–1107.
Babiuk, G, (1999). Making holistic changes to the school structure. *Education Canada*, vol. 39, no. 1, 20–21.
Baker, J. A., Dilly, L. J., Aupperlee, J. L., & Patil, S. A. (2003). The developmental context of school satisfaction: schools as psychologically healthy environments. *School Psychology Quarterly*, vol. 18, no. 2, 206–221.
Bandura, A. (1997). *Self-efficacy: the exercise of control*. New York: Freeman.
Barker, J. A., Terry, T., Bridger., R., & Winsor, A. (1997). Schools as caring communities: a relational approach to school reform. *School Psychology Review*, vol. 26, no. 4, 586–603.
Bruun Jensen, B., & Jensen, B. (2006). Inequality, health and action for health: do children and young people in Denmark have an option? In Clift, S., & Bruun Jensen, B. (Eds.). *The health promoting school-international advances in theory, evaluation and practice*. Copenhagen: Danish University of Education Press.
Cantril, H. (1965). *The pattern of human concern*. Rutgers University Press. Adapted for HBSC survey 2001/02.
Clift, S., & Bruun Jensen, B. (2006). *The health promoting school-international advances in theory, evaluation and practice*. Copenhagen: Danish University of Education Press.
Coleman, J. S., & Hoffer, T. B. (1987). *Public and private schools: the impact of communities*. New York: Basic Books.
Coleman, J. (1988). Social capital in the creation of human capital. *American Journal of Sociology*, 94(Suppl), S95–S120.
Croniger, R. G., & Lee, V. E. (2001). Social capital and dropping out of high schools: benefits to at risk students of teachers support and guidance. *Teachers College Record*, vol. 103, no. 4, 548–581.
Currie, C. E., Roberts, C., Morgan, A., Smith, R., Settertobulte, W., & Samdal, O., et al. (2004). *Young people's health in context*. Copenhagen: WHO Regional office for Europe.
Drukker, M., Buka, S., Kaplan, C., McKenzie, K., & Van Os, J. (2005). Social capital and young adolescents' perceived health in different socio-cultural settings. *Social Science and Medicine*, 61, 185–198.
Feldt, T., Leskinen, E., Kinnunen, U., & Ruoppila, I. (2003). The stability of sense of coherence: comparing two age groups in a 5-year follow up study. *Personality and Individual Differences*, 35, 1151–1165.
Frustenberg, F. F., & Hughes, M.E. (1995). Social capital and succesful development among at risk youth. *Journal of Marriage and Family*, 57, 580–592.
Harter, S. (1988). *Subscales for the self-perception profile for adolescents*. Denver: University of Denver.
Hebert, E. (1998). Design matters: how school environment affects children (realising a positive school climate. *Educational Leadership*, vol. 56, no. 1, 69–71.
Holden, E. W., & Nitz, K. (1995). Epidemiology of adolescent health disorders. In Wallander J. L., & Siegel L. J. (Eds.). *Adolescent health problems: behavioural perspectives*, (pp. 7–21). New York: Guilford Press.
Idler, E. L., & Benyamini, Y. (1997). Self-rated health and mortality: a review of twenty-seven community studies. *Journal of Health and Social Behaviour*, 38, 21–37.
Karvonen, S., Vikat, A., & Rimpela, M. K. (2005). The role of school context in the increase in young people's health complaints in Finland. *Journal of Adolescence*, 28(1), 1–16.
Kawachi, I., Kennedy, B. P., Lochner, K., & Prothrow-Stith, D. (1997). Social capital, income inequality, and mortality. *American Journal of Public Health*, 87(9), 1491–1498.

Knight, C. (2007). A resilience framework: perspectives for educators, *Health Education*, vol. 107, no. 6, 543–555.

Korinek, L., Walter-Thomas, C., Mclaughlin V., & Williams, B. (1999). Creating classroom communities and networks for student support. *Intervention in School and Clinic*, vol. 35, no. 1, 3–9.

Li, X., Stanton, B., & Feigelman, S. (2000). Impact of perceived parental monitoring on adolescent risk behaviour over 4 years. *Journal of Adolescent Health*, 27(1), 49–56.

Marcell, A., & Halpern-Felsher, B. L. (2005). Adolescents' health beliefs are critical in their intentions to seek physician care. *Preventive Medicine*, 41, 118–125.

Mendelson, M. J., Mendelson, B. K., Andrews, J. (2000). Self-esteem, body esteem, and body-mass in late adolescence: is a competence x importance model needed? *Journal of Applied Developmental Psychology*, 21: 249–266.

Morgan, A., & Ziglio, E. (2007). Revitalizing the evidence base for public health: an assets model. *Promotion and Education Supplement*, 2: 17–20.

Ministry of Education and Research. (2003). *Health Education Curriculum.* Available http://www.didactic.ro/files/16/edsan112.pdf cited March 2008.

Ministry of Health. (2004). *HIV/AIDS in Romania, 1985-2003.* Prof.Dr.Matei Bals, Infectious Diseases Institute, HIV/AIDS Monitoring and Evaluating Department. Available http://www.stopsida.ro/informatii_hiv_sida_cifre.php cited March 2008.

Ministry of Health. (2005). *Reproductive Health Survey Romania.* Available http://siteresources.worldbank.org/INTROMANIA/Resources/study.pdf cited March 2008.

Morrow, G. (1999). Conceptualising social capital in relation to the well-being of children and young people: a critical review. *The Sociological Review*, 44, 744–765.

Nahas, M. V., Goldfine, B., & Collins, M. A. (2003). Determinants of physical activity and young adults: the basis for high school and college physical education to promote active lifestyles. *Physical Educator*, 60, 42–56.

National Centre of Health Statistics. (1993). *Losing generations: adolescents in high risk settings.* Washington DC: National Academy Press.

Nutbeam, D. (1997). Promoting health and preventing disease: an international perspective on youth health promotion. *Journal of Adolescent Health*, 20, 396–402.

Orbach, I., & Mikulincer, M. (1998). Body investment scale: construction and validation of a body experience scale. *Psychological Assessment*, 10(4), 415–425.

Parsons, C., Stears, D., & Thomas, C. (1996). The health promoting school in Europe: conceptualizing and evaluating change. *Health Education Journal*, 55, 311–321.

Putnam, R. D. (2000). *Bowling alone: the collapse and revival of American community.* New York: Simon & Schuster.

Ravens-Sieberer, U., et al. (2005). KIDSCREEN-52 quality-of-life measure for children and adolescents. *Expert Review of Pharmacoeconomics and Outcomes Research*, 5(3), 353–364.

Rowe, F., Stewart, D., & Patterson, C. (2007). Promoting school connectedness through whole school approaches. *Health Education*, vol. 107, no. 6, 524–542.

Rowling, L., & Richie, J. (1996/1997). Health promoting schools: issues and future directions for Australia and the Asia-Pacific region. *Asia Pacific Journal of Public Health*, 9, 33–37.

Sampson, R. J., Morenoff, J. D. & Earls, F. (1999). Beyond social capital: spatial dynamics of collective efficacy for children. *American Sociological Review*, 64, 5, 633–660.

Schwarzer, R., & Jerusalem, M. (1995). Generalized self-efficacy scale. In Weinman, J., Wright, S., & Johnston, M. *Measures in health psychology: a user's portfolio. Causal and control beliefs*, (pp. 35–37). Windsor: NFER-NELSON.

Schwarzer, R., & Luszczynska, A. (2006). Self-efficacy, adolescents' risk-taking behaviours, and health. In Pajares, F., & Urdan, T., (Eds.). *Self-efficacy beliefs of adolescents*, (pp. 139–159). Greenwich: Information Age Publishing.

Siegel, J. M. (2002) Body image change and adolescent depressive symptoms. *Journal of Adolescent Research*, 17, 27–41.

Smylie, L., Medaglia, S., & Matika-Tyndale, E. (2006). The effect of social capital and sociodemographics on adolescent risk and sexual health behaviours. *The Canadian Journal of Human Sexuality*, 15(2), 95–109.

St Leger, L. (1999). The opportunities and effectiveness of the health promoting primary school in improving child health- a review of the claims and evidence, *Health Education Research*, vol.14, no.1, 51–69.

Stefan, C. A., & Kallay, E. (2007). *Dezvoltarea competentelor emotionale si sociale la prescolari – ghid pentru parinti*. Editura ASCR, Cluj-Napoca.

Sun, J., & Stewart, D. (2007). How effective is the health promoting school approach in building social capital in primary schools? *Health Education*, vol. 107, no. 6, 556–574.

Sun, J., & Stewart, D. (2007). Development of population based resilience measures in the primary school setting. *Health Education*, vol. 107, no. 6, 575–599.

Teachman, J. D., Paasch, K., & Carver, K. (1996). Social capital and dropping out of school early. *Journal of Marriage and Family*, 58, 773–783.

Thomas, S. P., & Smith, H. (2004). School connectedness, anger behaviors, and relationships of violent and non-violent American youth. *Perspectives in Psychiatric Care*, vol. 40, no. 4, 135–148.

Thompson, A. M., & Chad, K. E. (2002). The relationship of social physique anxiety to risk for developing an eating disorder in young females. *Journal of Adolescent Health*, 31, 183–189.

Torshein, T., Aaore, L. E., & Wold, B. (2001). Sense of coherence and school related stress as predictors of subjective health complaints in early adolescence: interactive, indirect or direct relationships? *Social Science and Medicine*, 53, 603–614.

Trzesniewsky, K. H., Donnellan, M. B., Moffitt, T. E., Robins, R. W., Poulton, R., & Caspi, A. (2006). Low self-esteem during adolescence predicts poor health, criminal behaviour, and limited economic prospects during adulthood, *Developmental Psychology*, vol. 42, no. 2, 381–390.

UNICEF. (2006). *Children on the brink, a focused situation analysis of vulnerable, excluded and discriminated children in Romania*. United Nations Children's Fund, Bucharest, Romania. Available http://www.unicef.org/romania/sitan_engleza.pdf cited September 2009.

Wang, R. H., Wang, H. H., & Tsu, M. T. (2003). Factors associated with adolescent pregnancy: a sample of Taiwanese female adolescents. *Public Health Nursing*, 20, 33–41.

Weisz, J. R., Sandler, I., Durlak, J., & Anton, B. (2005), Promoting and protecting youth mental health through evidence-based prevention and treatment. *American Psychologist*, 6, 628–648.

WHO. (1995). *School health promotion-series 1: report of the workshop on school health promotion sydney*. Manila: World Health Organization.

WHO. (1996). *The status of school health*. Geneva: World Health Organization.

WHO. (1997). *Life Skills Education for children and adolescents in schools*. Geneva: World Health Organization (rif. WHO/MNH/PSF/93.7A.Rev.2).

Wilkinson, R. G., Kawachi, I., & Kennedy, B. (1998). Mortality, the social environment, crime and violence. In Bartely, M., Blane, D., & Davey-Smith, G., (Eds.). *The sociology of health inequalities*, (pp. 19–38). Oxford: Oxford Sociology of Health and Illness Monograph.

Wilkinson, R. G. (1999). *Putting the picture together: prosperity, redistribution, health, and the welfare state*. In Marmot, M., & Wilkinson, R. G., (Eds.). *Social determinants of health*. New York: Oxford University Press.

Williams, J. M., & Currie, C. (2000). Self-esteem and physical development in early adolescence: pubertal timing and body image. *Journal of Early Adolescence*, 20:129–149.

Williams, P. G., Holmbeck, G., & Greenley, N. (2002). Adolescent health psychology. *Journal of Consulting and Clinical Psychology*, vol. 70, no. 3, 828–842.

Wilson, D. K., Friend, R., Teaseley, N., Green, S., Reaves, I. L. & Sica, D. A. (2002). Motivational versus social cognitive interventions for promoting fruit and vegetable intake and physical activity in African American adolescents. *Annals of Behavioral Medicine*, 24, 310–319.

Wu, S. Y., Pender, N., & Noureddine, S. (2003). Gender differences in the psychosocial cognitive correlates of physical activity among Taiwanese adolescents: a structural equation modelling approach. International Journal of Behavioral Medicine, 10, 93–105.

Chapter 18
Bringing It All Together: The Salutogenic Response to Some of the Most Pertinent Public Health Dilemmas

Monica Eriksson and Bengt Lindström

Keywords Ottawa charter • Salutogenic theory • Sense of coherence • Empowerment • Antonovsky • Resource adjusted life year

18.1 Introduction

The 19th International Union for Health Promotion and Education (IUHPE) World Conference of Health Promotion and Education was held in Canada in June 2007. Before the conference, the key actors involved in the development of the Ottawa Charter in 1986 (WHO 1986b) were asked to comment on the development of health promotion over the past 20 years. Two of the key actors were Morgan and Ziglio, who, in a 2007 paper titled "*Revitalizing the evidence base for public health: an assets model*", emphasized the need to move in the direction of promoting health instead of only preventing diseases (Morgan and Ziglio 2007). They encouraged people to focus on the resources of health, abilities and assets rather than risks of diseases, obstacles and inabilities. This chapter is a direct response to the paper by Morgan and Ziglio, which is also reproduced as the first chapter of this book.

Epidemiology is the study of the distribution and determinants of health states or events in specified populations, and the application of this study to the control of health problems (Nutbeam 1998). Nutbeam points out epidemiological information drives the core activity of public health and its focus on physical environmental risks (ibid p. 7). This approach is representative of biomedical or pathogenic approach where health is generated through the elimination of risks for diseases. This approach is still the dominating paradigm. Is it possible to integrate and manage the impact of the challenges of the global world on everyday life without becoming over-stimulated or stressed? The salutogenic approach, focusing on assets for health and health promoting processes, could give some indications of

M. Eriksson (✉)
Folkhälsan Research Centre, Helsinki, Finland
e-mail: monica.eriksson@folkhalsan.fi

A. Morgan et al. (eds.), *Health Assets in a Global Context: Theory, Methods, Action*, DOI 10.1007/978-1-4419-5921-8_18,

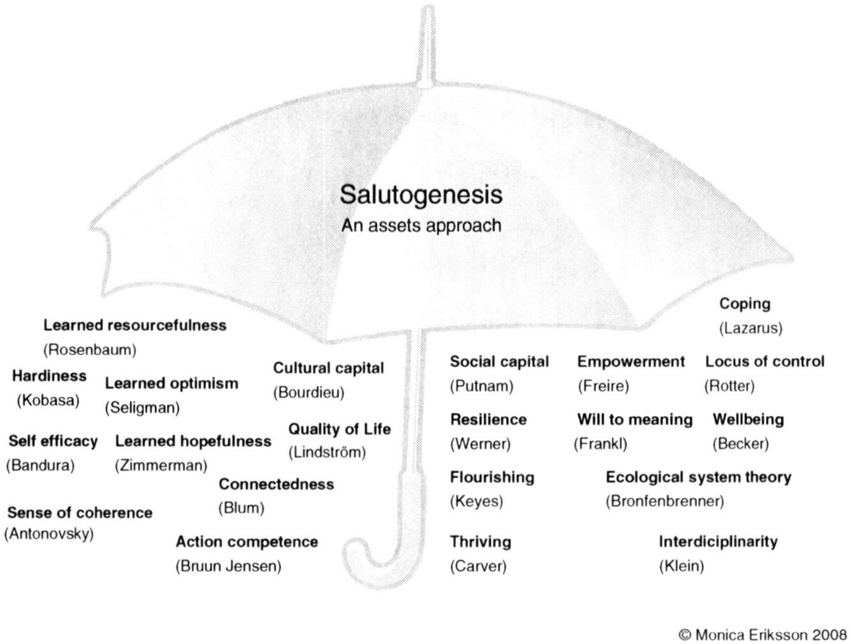

Fig. 18.1 The salutogenic umbrella – some convergent concepts and theories contributing to the explanation of health and quality of life

future direction. Morgan and Ziglio proposed an asset model for public health, consisting of three parts: (1) the salutogenesis as the theoretical foundation and evidence base; (2) the asset mapping for actions, and (3) the evaluation and asset indicators (see Fig. 1.1). In the following text we first comment on the parts of the asset model for public health and health promotion.

18.2 The Theory of Salutogenesis

Salutogenesis is a life-orientation theory with a strong evidence base, as described in Chap. 2. The theory orignated from the "Sense of Coherence" (SOC) scale, a valid and reliable instrument constructed from interviews with Holocaust survivors. The present evidence base brings forward detailed proof on the effectiveness of the salutogenic model and demonstrates its potential as a positive and health-promoting construct both for research and practice (Eriksson and Lindström 2005, 2006, 2007; Lindström and Eriksson 2006; Eriksson 2007). Overall, this corresponds closely with the key concepts, intentions, principles and values of the WHO's Ottawa Charter (Eriksson and Lindström 2008). Furthermore, the salutogenic model is valuable and useful in the making of healthy public policy, that is to implement health in all policies (Lindström and Eriksson 2009). However, there is more to the salutogenesis than only the measurement of SOC through the SOC questionnaire. Salutogenesis, i.e. the emphasis on resources (or assets), is a much broader framework than simply the measurement via the SOC. One of the most important challenges now is to implement the salutogenic approach on all societal levels in all policies, i.e. building healthy public policy the salutogenic way.

18.3 Asset Mapping

In his second book Antonovsky discussed similarities with some other concepts for the explanation of health (Antonovsky 1987; Chap. 2). He mentioned the concepts of hardiness (Kobasa), sense of permanence (Boyce), domains of social climate (Moos), resilience (Werner and Smith), and the family construction of reality (Reiss), Furthermore, the concept of self-efficacy, learned resourcefulness/helplessness, will to meaning and locus of control.

Part 2 of this publication deals with the concept of resilience. Research on resilience, the ability to survive despite adversities and risk factors for a negative health development, has a long tradition in health research (Werner and Smith 1982, 2001). From resilience research we have learned much about protective factors and how to survive in spite of adversity. This has formed a good basis leading to the next step, focusing on factors that promote health or considers salutogenic factors. Again, salutogenesis is more than measuring SOC. Figure 18.1 shows some other convergent concepts and theories for explaining health and quality of life which all bear some resemblance to the salutogenic theory. There are similarities and differences between the salutogenic theory and the theories behind the concepts in the figure. However, salutogenic dimensions and elements are included. Some of the concepts are examined more in detail in this chapter. To review all of them is beyond the scope of this publication.

The concept of resilience is complex (Werner and Smith 1982, 2001; Luthar 2003; McCubbin 1999; Lindström and Spencer 1995; Glantz and Johnsson 1999). There is no generally accepted definition nor is there a common specific theory. Resilience is further defined in different ways depending on what specific disciplinary framework is used. The core theoretical foundation has emerged from a convergence of psychological, psychoanalytical and social cognitive theories of child development. Garmetzy and his colleagues were among the first to emphasize the importance of examining protective factors in high-risk populations. Their research created the basis for the resilient approach (Luthar 2003). Some view the concept as a personality trait (Werner and Smith 1982, 2001), some describe resilience as the adjustment and recovery from adversities as a process in a continuum at an individual, group or societal level (McCubbin et al. 1999; Lindström and Spencer 1995; Glantz and Johnsson 1999; Carver 1998). In the late 1980s Michael Rutter centred on four main processes in resilience: reduction of risk impact, reduction of negative chain reactions, establishment and maintenance of self-esteem and self-efficacy, and opening up of opportunities (Rutter 1987). There is a common agreement that resilience emerges when individuals faced with negative life events or strains, have the capacity to mobilize protective factors or internal and external resources and stay well. Antonovsky (1987) saw the connections between the resilience construct and the salutogenic concept. He personally met the scientist behind the Hawaiian longitudinal study on children on the Kauai Island (Werner and Smith 1982, 2001). Both Werner and Antonovsky asked the same question: why some people, regardless of severe hardships, stay healthy and others do not? Antonovsky referred to stress whilst Werner referred to risk and adversities. A comparison of resilience and salutogenesis brings forward both differences and similarities. Firstly, both concepts emphasize resources: the salutogenic framework uses "General Resistance Resources" (GRR), and resilience uses protective factors. Secondly, they both consider the maintenance and development of health as a process in a continuum. Thirdly, both the SOC and resilience are applicable at an individual, group (i.e. families) and societal level. The two frameworks differ when it comes to the adjustment process. Resilience is always connected with risk factors. Rutter concludes: *"The phenomenon of resilience is due in part to vulnerability and protection processes by which there is a catalytic modification of a person's response to the risk situation."* (Rutter 1987; p. 329) If Rutter's conceptualisation of resilience was seen through salutogenic eyes the development of a strong SOC would serve as such a catalytic converter in buffering the stress exposure of young people through the life span. Lindström describes this transition from childhood to adulthood through several social arenas, the family, the social and geographical context, cultural and historical context, learning systems, peer systems and workplaces. The better these arenas are interconnected regarding structure and function the easier it is for the adolescent to make life coherent (Lindström 2001; p. 10).

Next to review is the concept of the health proneness construct of *hardiness* (Kobasa 1982). Both Antonovsky and Kobasa asked the salutogenic question: why some people exposed to stressful situations stayed well and others did not. The hardiness concept, derived from the existential theory of personality, use different terms but relates to the same dimensions, i.e. control (Antonovsky manageability), commitment (meaningfulness) and challenge (comprehensibility and meaningfulness). Antonovsky was aware of the potential overlap with the concept of hardiness and discussed this in his second book (Antonovsky 1987; p. 35–38). He considered the hardiness and the SOC to be two separate theories. Later, some other authors have tried to investigate the relationship between the hardiness and the SOC concept. In a study on patients with coronary heart disease, Kravetz used five health proneness and three negative affect measures (Kravetz et al. 1993). The results of the correlations between these measures and confirmatory factor analysis indicated that although the measures of health proneness were negatively related to measures of negative effect, these two sets of measures and the constructs could be differentiated from each other. The SOC was less independent of negative affect than was hardiness. Support for an overlapping construct between hardiness and SOC were found among American students (Smith and

Meyers 1997). Here the SOC was related to other personality measures such as learned helplessness, self-efficacy, hardiness and locus of control. The results showed that SOC was predicted by greater general self-efficacy, less perceived stress, greater hardiness, a more internal locus of control and also being female, i.e. in the same direction as Antonovsky assumed. SOC and hardiness and self-efficacy seemed to be measuring very similar constructs. Finally, a difference between the SOC and the hardiness is the measurement of the two concepts. Hardiness is measured by different kinds of measures (Kravetz et al. 1993; Smith and Meyers 1997; Newton 1999). The SOC is measured by one measure, the Orientation to Life Questionnaire, however, either by using the original scales (29-item or 13-item) or the modified versions with differing scoring alternatives but the same questions (Eriksson 2007).

Self-efficacy, stemming from social learning theory, is a generative capability of organized cognitive, social, emotional and behavioural skills. It is not about the number of skills, but the belief in what to do with the skills under a variety of conditions (Bandura 1997). Antonovsky discussed the similarities and differences between the SOC and self-efficacy, concluding that it was a far-fetched explanation to consider the self-efficacy to be analogous with the SOC construct (Antonovsky 1987, p. 59). Similar to the salutogenic theory and its core concept, sense of coherence, the concept of self-efficacy is a multi-dimensional construct applicable at an individual and a group level (Bandura 1997; Antonovsky 1993a, Antonovsky, 1991). Only a few studies in the research synthesis have used both self-efficacy and SOC simultaneously. The reported correlations with the SOC concept range between 0.10 and 0.66 among students, (Smith and Meyers 1997; Newton 1999; Bandura 1997; Antonovsky 1991, 1993b; Amirkhan and Greaves 2003) and retired subjects (Wells and Kendig 1999). None of them have employed discriminant analysis for the two concepts. There is consequently a need for further research to discriminate between self-efficacy and SOC. Furthermore, an additional concept with possible overlap with the SOC is the *locus of control* construct (Rotter 1966). Amirkhan and Greaves explored the underlying mechanism behind the SOC among undergraduates ($n = 116$) aiming to discriminate between coherence and controllability measured by The Generalized Self-efficacy Scale and The Spheres of Control Battery (locus of control) (Amirkhan and Greaves 2003). Three possible mechanisms were examined: perceptual, attributional and behavioural. The findings demonstrated distinctiveness of the two concepts, coherence and control. Coherence was not identical to control. The SOC seemed here to operate via a perceptual influence. Persons with a strong SOC perceived a majority of life events to be coherent. There was also evidence of a behavioural mechanism. Individuals with a strong SOC tended to have a more adaptive coping.

The concept of *empowerment* has raised considerable interest and involved researchers from many different fields such as social psychology, community psychology, social science, education and public health and health promotion (Eklund 1999). The Brazilian educationalist, Paulo Freire, is the person that symbolizes the shift of education practice towards empowerment in the sense of making learning available to all and especially to the oppressed. Freire used empowerment as a way of learning, focusing on populations who have difficulty acquiring learning in ordinary institutions. His aim was to reduce inequity through this learning process thus mobilizing the uneducated. The core was on the creation of a respectful dialogue thereby enhancing a sense of social community, i.e. building social capital (Freire 1996). Empowerment is about giving people control and mastery over their lives similar to the enabling process in health promotion. It is about the development of abilities and coping skills and endowing people with the ability to work for active critical conscious-raising. It is also a democratic concept looking at the structure of power and a process of professional activity and a relinquishment of the professionals' power. Health promotion again focuses on the positive, dynamic and empowering aspects of health (WHO 1986a). According to the essential principle document of health promotion, i.e. the Ottawa Charter, the key objective was the process of enabling individuals and communities in order to empower them and thereby increase their control over the determinants of health. Furthermore, health promotion research was not seen just as research but as research and development, stressing action and encouraging multi disciplinary approaches promoting core values such as equity, participation and empowerment. These basic values can also be derived from the salutogenic concepts and its perspective on health.

The concept of empowerment is still largely seen as a principle or an idea rather than a solid theory. It still lacks a theoretical underpinning and therefore becomes difficult to make the concept operational and measurable (Koelen and Lindström 2005; Rissel 1994). There are also many interpretations of the concept. However, empowerment has more and more been given the meaning of a multilevel construct coming from within an individual, group, organisation or society rather than from a top-down hierarchy. According to the World Health Organization (WHO), empowerment for health is defined in health promotion *"as the process through which people gain greater control over decisions and actions affecting their health"* (Nutbeam 1998). There is a consensus, independent of the level of implementation (individual, group or society), that the empowerment is an ongoing process (Koelen and Lindström 2005; Rissel 1994; Rappaport 1987). The main objective of this process is to alter the level of awareness, identify areas necessary to change, strategic planning, action for change and finally evaluation of the actions and the activities. This process should lead to an increased level of awareness and more effective strategies for the next step. The enabling process continues.

At the end of the 1980s an interesting article was published by Rappaport, discussing the ecological nature of the concept of empowerment, definitions, conditions and distinctions related to prevention (Rappaport 1987). He considers the concept not to be only an individual psychological construct, but also to be of organizational, political, sociological, economic and spiritual character (ibid p. 130). He points out the importance of developing a sound theoretical base and asking questions for research. Koelen and Lindström define individual empowerment based on elements of salutogenic thinking, the only definition so far, *"as a process by which people gain mastery (control) over their lives, by which they learn to see a closer correspondence between their goals and a sense of how to achieve these goals, and by which people learn to see a relationship between their efforts and the outcomes thereof*" (Koelen and Lindström 2005). The focus is on resources, both internal as external, on the learning process in order to create a SOC. According to Antonovsky, life experiences (consistency, load balance, participation in shaping outcomes, emotional closeness) shape the SOC whilst the GRR provide the individual with sets of meaningful and coherent life experiences (Antonovsky 1987). Participation in shaping outcomes, i.e. empowerment, seemed to be the most relevant childhood experience related to the adult SOC (Sagy and Antonovsky 2000).

The concept of *habitus* and *cultural capital* stems from sociology and represents an expression of a "common consciousness". Bourdieu (1993) developed the theory of the cultural field trying to describe how works of art are situated in the social conditions of their production, circulation and consumption. Habitus is about the creation of coherence of systems. He dissects the relationship between systems of thought, social institutions and different forms of material and symbolic power. Furthermore, the theory is dispositional, which means that it takes into account possibilities of the individuals and the societal structures. The key concepts are habitus, field and cultural capital. Habitus, embodied in individuals, is derived from a set of dispositions which generate practices and perceptions. This is the subjective habitus. The collective habitus on the other hand, is connected to a social group or class. It creates a common view of society as coherent. The next key concept is the field. This is the social room where individuals, or to use Bourdieu's expression "agents" are active in multiple fields of activities. Cultural capital, the third key concept and the most important of what Bourdieu called symbolic capital. According to Bordieu the different forms of capital together with habitus and field are analytical tools by which the motivation, actions and ways of thinking of both individuals and groups can be described. There are some interesting similarities between Bourdieu's way of thinking and the salutogenesis. Both have the ambition to create coherence between structures and systems. Therefore the focus on the creation of SOC would be a good synthesis of both frameworks. This could be taken one step further to answer the question on how to create coherence thus addressing the learning process itself. There is a model within general education theory called the "Action Competence Approach", exemplified in environmental education which could be developed (Bruun Jensen and Schnack 1997; Bruun Jensen 2000) This concept comprises of two components: first, an analysis of the nature of environmental problems and second, an idea of education as something more than academic schooling or behaviour modification. The fundamental assumption is that environmental problems are structurally anchored in society and our ways of living. It is necessary to find solutions to the problems through changes at both the societal and the individual level. Citizens have to be capable to act on both levels. The structure and the content of the education have to be adjusted to demands of solving environmental problems and demands from the citizens.

To conclude, all the above mentioned theories and concepts could be interpreted to have a salutogenic approach. The challenge now is to use this new knowledge in a systematic way. Western countries have excellent statistical profiles, but people's assets, abilities and internal and external resources are not systematically measured. Longitudinal population studies are rare due to the cost; therefore evidence is often based on occasional cross-sectional studies asking people about their perceived health. We strongly emphasize the need for building up vital statistics on health resources and assets for understanding health and quality of life as a whole.

18.4 Asset Indicators

The work for developing a set of mental health indicators for a comprehensive health monitoring system has for several years been run within the European Commission and the Health Monitoring Programme (HMP) and the European Union consortium on Health Promotion Indicators Development (Bauer et al. 2003; Korkeila et al. 2003). In a review, Korkeila and colleagues list a set of indicators of mental health: sociodemographic (sex, age, marital status, ethnicity, socioeconomic status), social networks (social support, social isolation), stressful events (life events), positive mental health (subjective well-being, personal resources/resilience), subjective experience of the individual (self-perceived health, quality of life), services/ supply/ use and demand (beds in hospitals, number of staff, use of services and others), morbidity/generic (psychological distress), morbidity/disease specific (measures on specific disorders, major depression, anxiety disorders), disability (cut down in activity level) and mortality (cause of death) (Korkeila et al. 2003). Independent on the fact that Antonovsky's SOC concept is not mentioned as a separate health indicator in the above list, the authors discuss and consider the SOC to be an indicator of positive mental health. With the evidence base of the salutogenic research on hand, an integration of the SOC as an indicator should strengthen the health indicator system. Using SOC as a health indicator systematically on a population level has not been done before. We propose it is time to do that as soon as possible.

Based on the assumption that it causes a decreased level of functioning, disability has been seen as a negative indicator of mental health. The concept of Disability Adjusted Life Years (DALY) is a well known and frequently used concept in vital statistics. The DALY is a health gap measure that extends the concept of potential years of life lost due to premature death to include equivalent years of 'healthy' life lost by virtue of being in states of poor health or disability (Murray et al. 2002). In accordance to what we earlier have described and discussed we want to make a salutogenic interpretation introducing a new concept RALY meaning Resource Adjusted Life Year as a measure to include in vital statistics of societies. The authors are aware of the revised version of the International Classification of Functioning (ICF), where some sections of abilities and competences are involved (WHO 2001). However, to our opinion the ICF still is in the main extent focused on diseases and loss of function. The new concept, RALY, should be systematically applied on the general population including disabled people. Let us start a discussion about how to systematically measure abilities and assets of general populations. Our suggestion of the new concept, RALY, could serve as the starting point.

The use of the SOC as an indicator of health in populations is part of a deeper integration of the salutogenic perspective on healthy public policy or health in all policies, one of the main action strategies in the Ottawa Charter for health promotion (Murray et al. 2002; Eriksson and Lindström 2008; WHO 1986b). This principle can be applied on both the individual and system level. The key elements of the health promotion process are firstly, the determinants for health (that can be identified within the individual, in the social context and on the socioeconomic and societal level). Secondly, people have to be able to not only gain control over these health determinants but also be able to use them for the best of their health, in other words, one has to identify the mechanisms that makes this possible. Finally, the overall objective of this process is to give people the possibility to live the life they want to live or enjoy a good quality of life. In public health policy there is a further ethical/value requirement or prerequisite due to the importance of the issue of equity and equal distribution of health in society. This means that people should not attain health and quality of life at the cost of other people or by damaging or harming the ecological systems. At the heart of it all is the recognition of human rights where people are seen as active participating subjects in charge of their own lives. The main strategy to conceptualize this is the making of a healthy public policy. A paper, recently accepted for publication in Promotion & Education (from 2009 Global Health Promotion), outlines how the salutogenic framework is applied to the making of healthy public policy and is illustrated by a case study (Lindström and Eriksson 2009).

Mainstream public health policy research and development is still focused on the development of health policy within the health sector. It seems health policy experts do not easily conceive the term healthy public policy. Another problem regarding the more theoretical approach to health policy is that the ideas and models are largely taken out of organizational theory and management theory because this is the tradition within policy research. One problem in policy making on macro level is to keep the framework together and comprehensive, since it is hard to maintain the policy coherent when it is applied on a country level across regions, sectors, disciplines and organizations. There are only a few instruments and models that encompass this capacity. Appropriate health promotion theory needs to be applied to this sector. One of the most promising theoretical approaches is the salutogenic model, which explores the origin of health (Antonovsky 1996). The model emphasizes the importance of developing the determinants of health focusing on how health is created instead of disease. Its operative concept SOC appeals to policy making, as the broad policies have to become one coordinated, coherent movement in every sector of society to be effective. This has never been described before.

The salutogenic model has been used in health outcome studies both on the individual, group and population level (Eriksson and Lindström 2005). It has also been used as a tool for the learning process making it operational in problem solving, education and communication (Nilsson and Lindström 1998; Nilsson 2004). We know from research that people (and organizations) who have developed skills to use the available resources and focus on problem solving and positive outcomes tend to have: better perceived health; adjustment to chronic disease; positive health behaviours; a longer life span; better general well-being; mental health; quality of life and a stronger SOC (Eriksson, 2007). Transferring the salutogenic framework to policy making, the main question raised is, what has to be considered in order to make a salutogenic process out of making a healthy public policy? What salutogenic questions have to be addressed and how can healthy policy be made comprehensive, manageable and meaningful to all involved. There are several logical steps in the process of creating a healthy public policy the salutogenic way. It is of course essential, on the one hand, to identify what the health problems are and what causes them. At the same time it is just as important to identify the salutogenic factors i.e. what health resources are available and identify what mechanisms can support a positive development and on the basis of this, form them into a comprehensive vision. In policy making the available resources and mechanisms are often not made explicit, thus the salutogenic question is not raised.

After the situation analysis, where the health problems are identified through an overall presentation of the present situation and the processes involved, it is necessary to consider what could serve as GRR. From this, the mechanisms that can improve the SOC can be formulated from the individual to the structural-organizational and societal level. In a comprehensive salutogenic approach it is necessary to consider the overall situation - what would be the coherent movement which would make most sense out of the situation (coherence). In salutogenic terms it is an empowerment process where it is necessary that the population becomes aware of what factors serve as strong motivators for themselves and their context (motivation/meaning). It is important that people become involved and understand (comprehensibility); furthermore that good arguments are formulated and that it is clear what would be the most sensible chain of activities for the population. For the professionals, it is necessary to use the right language and have good communication skills. Besides the involvement and knowledge of the population concerned, the process requires considerable historical, socioeconomical, anthropological and cultural competence of all actors. Furthermore, it is necessary to find the best direction, and the best strategic choices to manage the development that will induce the right processes and behaviours to empower the people (manageability). Antonovsky said *"Think salutogenically and act salutogenically!"* (Antonovsky 1993a). In policy making this means one automatically is directed towards positive outcomes and solutions to problems.

The salutogenic framework has so far been discussed in terms of mental health indicators and building healthy public policy. To demonstrate the usefulness of the salutogenic framework for public health and health promotion research we'd like to introduce a coherent process-oriented health promotion research model. The structure of the model consists of an individual level (micro), a group (meso), social environment (exo) and a global (macro) level. The model combines research on risks and protective factors (resilience) with salutogenic or promotional factors (Lindström and Eriksson 2009).

The theories behind this model are Bronfenbrenner's health ecological system theory (Bronfenbrenner 1979), Bourdieu's concept of habitus (Bourdieu 1993), Antonovsky's salutogenic theory (Antonovsky 1996), the concept of resilience as developed and applied by Sun and Stewart (2007) and the concept of connectedness by Blum et al. (2002). This theoretical model could be useful in research and practice for building Healthy Public Policy (WHO 1988)/Health in All Policies (Ministry of Social Affairs and Health 2006). This model creates a synergy between research on risk factors for vulnerability and adversities, protective factors for survival and a good health outcome with salutary factors promoting health and quality of life, i.e. creates a balance between the risk approach and the salutogenic approach of health research. In addition, the model integrates a solid ethical foundation and adopts the core values and principles of the Ottawa Charter (Lindström 2001; Koelen and Lindström 2005; Poland 2007). Up to now, most of the research on the salutogenic model has focused on the level of the individual. However, many of the serious stressors in life are collective stressors and must be viewed in terms of the social context in which they occur. The important question of how the salutogenic model contributes to the understanding of the role of a network orientation (family, community, workplace) in promoting health. Finally, the model corresponds well to the Lindström model of quality of life integrating the personal, interpersonal, external and global resources for the enhancement of an active and productive life (Lindström 1994). In addition, the model is coherent to the spirit and ethics of The Declaration of Human Rights (UN 1948), the Convention on the Rights of the Child (UNICEF 1990) and the Ottawa Charter (WHO 1986b). The need for an ethical agenda for health promotion has recently been revitalized (Mittelmark 2008).

References

Amirkhan, J. H., & Greaves, H. (2003). Sense of coherence and stress: The mechanics of a healthy disposition. *Psychol Health,* 18(1):31–62.

Antonovsky, A. (1987). *Unraveling the Mystery of Health. How People Manage Stress and Stay Well.* San Francisco: Jossey-Bass.

Antonovsky, A. (1991). The salutogenic approach to family system health: promise and danger. In. European congress on "Mental Health in European Families", 1991, p. 9. http.// www.angelfire.com/ok/soc/agolem.html cited May 2009.

Antonovsky, A. (1993a). Some salutogenic words of wisdom to the conferees. In; The Nordic School of Public Health in Gothenburg, Sweden;1993; p.3. http://www.angelfire.com/ok/soc/ agoteborg.html cited May 2009.

Antonovsky, A. (1993b). The structure and properties of the sense of coherence scale. *Soc Sci Med,* 36(6):725–733.

Antonovsky, A. (1996). The salutogenic model as a theory to guide health promotion. *Health Promot Int,*11(1):11–18.

Bauer, G., Davies, J. K., Pelikan, J., Noack, H., Broesskamp, U., Hill, C., et al. (2003). Advancing a theoretical model for public health and health promotion indicator development. Proposal from the EUHPID consortium. *Eur J Publ Health,* 13(Suppl 3):107–113.

Bandura, A. (1997). *Self-efficacy. The Exercise of Control.* New York: W.H. Freeman and Company.

Blum, R. W., McNeely, C., & Nonnemaker, J. (2002). Vulnerability, risk, and protection. *J Adolescent Health,* 31S:28–39.

Bourdieu, P. (1993). *The Field of Cultural Production. Essays on Art and Literature.* Cambridge: Polity Press.

Bronfenbrenner, U. (1979). *The Ecology of Human Development – Experiments by Nature and Human Design.* Cambridge Massachusetts: Harvard University Press.

Bruun Jensen, B. (2000). Health knowledge and health education in the democratic health-promoting school. *Health Educ*, 100(4):146–153.
Bruun Jensen, B., & Schnack, K. (1997). The action competence approach in environmental education. *Environ Educ Res*, 3(2):163–178.
Carver, C. S. (1998). Resilience and thriving: Issues, models, and linkages. *J Soc Issues*, 54(2):245–266.
Eklund, L. (1999). From citizen participation towards community empowerment. An analysis on health promotion from citizen perspective. Tampere: Faculty of Medicine, University of Tampere. (Doctoral thesis).
Eriksson, M. (2007). Unravelling the mystery of salutogenesis. The evidence base of the salutogenic research as measured by Antonovsky's Sense of Coherence Scale. (Doctoral thesis). Åbo Akademi University Vasa, Fakulty of Social and Caring Science, Department of Social Policy. Folkhälsan Research Centre, Health Promotion Research Programme, Research Report 2007:1. Turku: Folkhälsan.
Eriksson, M., & Lindström, B. (2005). Validity of Antonovsky's Sense of Coherence Scale – a systematic review. *J Epidemiol Community Health*, 59(6):460–466.
Eriksson, M., & Lindström, B. (2006). Antonovsky's Sense of Coherence Scale and the relation with health – a systematic review. *J Epidemiol Community Health*, 60:376–381.
Eriksson, M., & Lindström, B. (2007). Antonovsky's Sense of Coherence Scale and It's relation with quality of life: A systematic review. *J Epidemiol Community Health*, 61:938–944.
Eriksson, M., & Lindström, B. (2008). A salutogenic interpretation of the Ottawa Charter. *Health Promot Int*, 23(2):190–199.
Freire, P. (1996). *Pedagogy of the Oppressed.* Harmondsworth: Penguin.
Glantz, M. D., & Johnsson, J. L, editors. (1999). *Resilience and Development. Positive Life Adaptations*. New York: Kluwer Academic/Plenum.
Kobasa, S. (1982). The hardy personality: toward a social psychology of stress and health. In: Sanders, G., & Suls, J. editors. *Social Psychology of Health and Illness*. Lawrence Erlbaum Associates: New Jersey.
Koelen, M. A., & Lindström, B. (2005). Making healthy choices easy choices: The role of empowerment. *Eur J Clin Nutr*, 59(Suppl 1):10–16.
Korkeila, J., Lehtinen, V., Bijl, R., Dalgard, O-S., Kovess, V., Morgan A., et al. (2003). Establishing a set of mental health indicators for Europe. *Scand J Public Health*, 31(6):451–459.
Kravetz, S., Drory, Y., & Florian, V. (1993). Hardiness and sense of coherence and their relation to negative affect. *Eur J Personality*, 7(4):233–244.
Lindström, B. (1994). The essence of existence. On the quality of life of children in the Nordic countries – theory and practice in public health. (Doctoral thesis.). Göteborg: Nordic School of Public Health.
Lindström, B. (2001).The meaning of resilience. *Int J Adolesc Med Health*, 13(1):7–12.
Lindström, B., & Eriksson, M. (2006). Contextualising salutogenesis and Antonovsky in public health. *Health Promot Int*, 21(3):238–244.
Lindström, B., & Eriksson, M. (2009). The salutogenic approach to the making of HiAP/Healthy Public Policy: illustrated by a case study. *Global Health Promotion*, 16(1): 17–28.
Lindström, B., & Spencer, N, editors. (1995). *Social Pediatrics*. Oxford: Oxford University Press.
Luthar, S. S., (ed). (2003). *Resilience and Vulnerability. Adaptation in the Context of Childhood Adversities*. Cambridge: Cambridge University Press.
McCubbin HI, Thompson EA, Thompson AI, Futrell JA (1999). (Eds.) *The dynamics of resilient families*. Thousand Oaks: Sage Publications.
Ministry of Social Affairs and Health. (2006). *Health in All Policies: Prospects and Potentials*. Finland, Helsinki: Ministry of Social Affairs and Health.
Mittelmark, M. B. (2008). Setting an ethical agenda for health promotion. *Health Promot Int*, 23(1):78–85.
Morgan, A., & Ziglio, E. (2007). Revitalising the evidence base for public health: an assets model. IUHPE – *Promotion & Education*, 2(Suppl):17–22.

Murray, C., Salomon, J., Mathers, C., Lopez, A., editors. (2002). *Summary Measures of Population Health: Concepts, Ethics, Measurement and Applications*. Geneva: World Health Organization.

Nilsson, L. A. (2004). Health promotion as school development. *Scand J Nutr,* 48(2):70–76.

Nilsson, L., & Lindström, B. (1998). Learning as a health promoting process – the salutogenic interpretation of the Swedish curricula in state education. *Int J Health Promot*, 14.

Newton, S. E. (1999). Relationship of hardiness and sense of coherence to post-liver transplant return to work. *Holist Nurs Pract,* 13(3):71–79.

Nutbeam, D. (1998). *Health Promotion Glossary.* Geneva: World Health Organization.

Poland, B. (2007). Health promotion in Canada: Perspectives & future prospects. *Brazilian J Health Promot*, 20(1):3–11.

Rappaport, J. (1987). Terms of empowerment/exemplars of prevention: Toward a theory for community psychology. *Am J Community Psychol*, 15:121–148.

Rissel, C. (1994). Empowerment: the holy grail of health promotion? *Health Promot Int,* 9(1):39–47.

Rotter, J. (1966). Generalized expectancies for internal versus external control of reinforcements. *Psychological Monographs*, 80, Whole No. 609.

Rutter, M. (1987). Psychosocial resilience and protective mechanisms. *Am J Orthopsychiatry,* 57(3):316–331.

Sagy, S., & Antonovsky, H. (2000). The development of the sense of coherence: A retrospective study of early life experiences in the family. *J Aging Hum Dev,* 51(2):155–166.

Smith, T. L., & Meyers, L. S. (1997). The sense of coherence: Its relationship to personality, stress, and health measures. *J Soc Behav Pers*, 12(2):513–527.

Sun, J., & Stewart, D. (2007). Development of population-based resilience measures in the primary school setting. *Health Education*, 107(6):575–599.

UN. (1948). *Universal Declaration of Human Rights*. Paris: General Assembly of the United Nations.

UNICEF. (1990). *Convention on the Rights of the Child.* New York: United Nations Children's Fund.

Wells,Y. D., & Kendig, H. L. (1999). Psychological resources and successful retirement. *Aust Psychol,* 34(2):111–115.

Werner, E., & Smith, R. (1982). *Vulnerable but Invincible. A Longitudinal Study of Resilient Children and Youth*. New York: McGraw Hill.

Werner, E, & Smith, R. (2001). *Journeys from Childhood to Midlife. Risk, Resilience, and Recovery.* Ithaca: Cornell University Press.

WHO. (1986a) A discussion document on the concepts and principles of health promotion. *Health Promot Int,* 1:73–76.

WHO. (1986b). Ottawa charter for health promotion: an *International Conference on Health Promotion, the Move Towards a New Public Health, November 17–21 1986*. Geneva: World Health Organization.

WHO. (1988). Adelaide Recommendations on Healthy Public Policy. *Second International Conference on Health Promotion, Adelaide, South Australia, April 5–9 1988.*

WHO. (2001). *International Classification of Functioning, Disability and Health.* (Endorsed at the Fifty-fourth World Health Assembly on May 22 2001) http://www.who.int/classifications/icf cited August 19th 2008.

Conclusions

Antony Morgan, Maggie Davies, and Erio Ziglio

The Asset Model described in Chap. 1 aims to revitalise how policy makers, researchers and practitioners think and act to promote a more resourceful approach to tackling health inequities. The model outlines a systematic approach to asset based public health which can provide scientific evidence and best practice on how to maximise the stock of key assets necessary for promoting health.

Taken together the 18 chapters serve to illustrate how the model can be advanced towards its ultimate goal of producing a credible evidence base that can stand side by side the more well developed pathogenic approach to public health, helping to provide answers on how best to sustain health and minimise health inequities in different country contexts.

Of course, there is some way to go before we reach this goal. However the challenge lies not only in creating new data and evidence but harnessing what we already know using an asset frame of reference. Specifically knowledge needs to be organised to:

1. Illustrate how health assets operate in different communities and to quantify the value of assets to population health compared to other more, well established determinants of health.
2. Identify policies and programmes that enhance the stock of health assets available in individuals, communities and organisations.
3. Secure the best ways of measuring the health assets known to be protective of health.

The generation of this knowledge must then be accompanied by support at the international level with a range of tools and practical guides to assist countries to develop contextualised health and development programmes that combine need-reduction and asset-maximisation considerations.

This edited volume has hopefully sparked an interest in all those interested to promote health, whether they are researchers, policy makers or practitioners, to work towards a set of theories, methods and action that focus on the positive rather than the negative, capabilities rather than need and health and wellbeing rather than disease. The test of course is whether the asset model in the future can provide answers to how best to develop cost effective public health strategies which achieve equitable and sustainable rises in the general level of population health and well-being across the globe. Hopefully revised editions of this book will include such success stories and those assets known to be protective of health are brought to the fore and applied appropriately for all.

Index

Lightning Source UK Ltd.
Milton Keynes UK
16 November 2010

162902UK00008B/51/P

9 781441 959201